AF658180

PHYSICAL PHARMACEUTICS

PHYSICAL PHARMACEUTICS

Dr. R. Manavalan
M.Pharm. Ph.D.
Professor and Head
Institute of Pharmaceutical Technology
Annamalai University
Chidambaram – 608 002
Tamil Nadu

and

Dr. C. Ramasamy
M.Pharm. Ph.D.
(Formerly Professor of Pharmacy, Madras Medical College)
Professor and HOD
Department of Pharmacy Practice
S.R.M. College of Pharmacy
S.R.M University
Kattankulathur,
Kanchipuram (Dist), Tamil Nadu

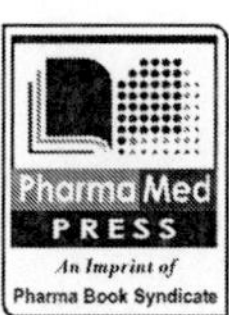

PharmaMed Press
An imprint of Pharma Book Syndicate
A Unit of BSP Books Pvt. Ltd.
4-4-309/316, Giriraj Lane,
Sultan Bazar, Hyderabad - 500 095.

Physical Pharmaceutics by *Manavalan and Ramasamy*

Published by

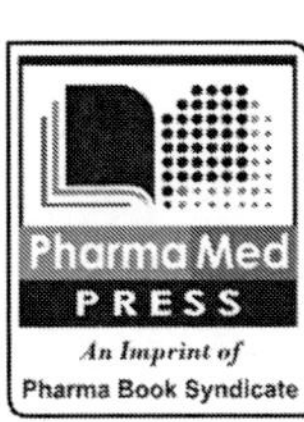

PharmaMed Press

An imprint of Pharma Book Syndicate

A unit of BSP Books Pvt. Ltd.

4-4-309/316, Giriraj Lane, Sultan Bazar, Hyderabad - 500 095.
Phone: 040-23445605, 23445688; Fax: 91+40-23445611
e-mail: info@pharmamedpress.com

ISBN: 978-93-5230-078-5 (HB)

PREFACE

It has been a long standing desire to bring out a book on PHYSICAL PHARMACEUTICS which will suit the student community in India. Our aim has been to present the book with schematic representations in such a way that it chalks out the basic principles involved in a methodical manner and at the same time comprehensible. In the preparation of this book more importance has been given to clarity than to brevity. We believe the students may be able to learn the contents of the book by themselves with added explanation of pharmacy teachers.

In keeping with above aims, the first edition of the book was brought out in the year 1995. The contents of the book was expanded and revised in the second edition 2001. The second edition has now been revised with some additions.

The study of the principles discussed in the book forms basis for carrying ou preformulation study of drugs to develop suitable and acceptable. dosage form as well as the route of administration. For example, the solubility data allow selection of most appropriate salt for development. Stability studies in solution indicate the feasibility of parenteral or other liqUid dosage forms and can identify the methods of stabilization. Solid state study by DSC, TLC and HPLC will predict drug excipient interaction and subsequent selection of suitable excipients for solid dosage forms such as tablets and capsules to avoid interactions with the drug.

At the end of each chapter, suggestions for practicals, though not a complete treatise, have been included to enable the teachers plan their experiments to see the theory in practice.

It is hoped that this revised edition will also be readily accepted by the students and any suggestion for the improvement of this book from the teachers as well as from the students will be thankfully acknowledged.

- C. Ramasamy **- R. Manavalan**

CONTENTS

INTRODUCTION

Physical pharmaceutics deals with the physico-chemical principles involved in the practice of pharmacy. By proper application of the principles, one is sure to get a better, efficacious, and reasonably stable dosage form. It will be helpful to improve an already existing dosage form or to formulate a new dosage form and it is of immense help in advanced study.

1. Dimensions and units

It is worthwhile to refresh the knowledge about dimensions and units involved in the study of physical pharmaceutics.

Matter is something that occupies space and has mass. The properties of matter are expressed by three chosen base quantities- length, mass and time. Each of these quantities has been assigned a definite unit and a reference standard.

We are mainly concerned with Metric and SI system. In the Metric system, the units are the centimeter (cm), the gram (g) and the second (s) and hence it is called cgs system. The *International Union of Pure and Applied Chemistry* (IUPAC) has introduced "Systeme International" or SI units in view of establishing an internationally uniform set of units. The basic SI units are the meter, the kilogram and the second and hence **mks** system.

Base quantities and the corresponding base units for both the metric system and the 'Systeme International' are shown in the following table:

Quantity	Length (L)	Mass (M)	Time (T)
Cgs unit	Centimeter (cm)	Gram (g)	Second (s)
SI unit	Meter (m)	Kilogram (kg)	Second (s)
Reference standard	Meter	Kilogram	Mean solar day

Base quantities used in SI System

Quantity	Unit	Symbol
Length	meter	m
Mass	kilogram	kg
Time	second	s
Electric current	ampere	A
Thermodynamic temperature	kelvin	°K
Luminous intensity	candela	cd.

Other quantities such as area, density, pressure, energy etc are derived from the three fundamental quantities- length, mass and time. Hence they are termed as derived quantities.

Density and specific gravity

Density is mass per unit volume at a fixed temperature and pressure. It is expressed in cgs system as g/cc or g/cm^3 or gcm^{-3}

Density is a derived quantity while specific gravity is a pure number

$$\text{specific gravity} = \frac{\text{density of a substance}}{\text{density of water}}$$

and for practical purpose, specific gravity

$$= \frac{\text{mass of a substance}}{\text{mass of an equal volume of water}}$$

Force

The **cgs** unit of force is **dyne.** It is the force that is imparted to a mass of 1 g with an acceleration of 1 cm/sec^2

Weight of a body is the gravitational pull (attraction) on it by the earth.

Expressing the weight in force units,

$$W = m \times g$$

where g is the gravitational attraction.

Weight of a body of 1 g mass is

$$W = 1g \times 980.7 \ cm/sec^2$$

$$\equiv 980.7 \ g \ cm/sec^2 \text{ or } 980.7 \text{ dynes.}$$

The weight of 1 *g* mass is actually 980.7 dynes. However, it is common practice to express weight directly in mass units since weight is directly proportional to mass as the gravitational attraction is almost constant.

Pressure

Pressure is force per unit area. The unit of pressure is $dyne/cm^2$. Pressure is also given in atmospheres.

Mean pressure at sea level is taken as one atmosphere and is equal to 760 mm or 76 cm of Hg (mercury) i.e., it supports a column of mercury of 760 mm or 76 cm in height in a tube of 1 cm^2 cross sectional area in a barometer. This barometric pressure may be converted into fundamental pressure units $dyne/cm^2$ as follows

Weight of 76 cm column of Hg is obtained by multiplying the volume (which is height × cross sectional area) and the density of Hg.

$$76cm \times 1cm^2 \times 13.595 g/cm^3 \text{ at } 0°C$$

The force exerted is obtained by multiplying this by acceleration due to gravity (980.7 cm/sec^2)

$$76cm \times 1cm^2 \times 13.595 g/cm^3 \times 980.7 cm/sec^2$$

$$= 1.0133 \times 10^6 \text{ dynes}$$

$$\left(\text{i.e. } cm \times cm^2 \times \frac{g}{cm^3} \times \frac{cm}{sec^2} = gcm/sec^2 = \text{dyne}\right)$$

Pressure is force per unit area and hence the result obtained is divided by cm^2 to get the pressure in atmosphere

That is, 1.0133×10^6 $dynes/cm^2$ = 1 atmosphere.

The **SI** unit of force is **Newton**. The pressure is expressed as Newton per square meter (N/m^2) This unit is too small and hence a unit known as 'bar' is often used (1 bar = 10^5 N/m^2 = 1 atm.)

Energy, work and Heat

Energy is the capacity for doing work. Energy may be kinetic energy or potential energy. The kinetic energy of a body is the energy possessed by virtue of its motion while the potential energy of a body is the energy possessed by virtue of its position.

Work is the mechanical equivalent of energy and heat is the thermal equivalent of energy.

Work performed on a body is equal to the force multiplied by its displacement when a constant force is applied to the body in the direction of its movement.

$$W = f \times l \quad (l = \text{distance of displacement})$$

The cgs unit of work is the **erg** and it is the work performed when a force of 1 dyne acts through a distance of 1 centimeter.

1 erg = 1 dyne × 1 cm

The SI unit of work is 'joule'. One joule of work is said to be done when a force of 1 Newton acting on a body moves it through a distance of 1 meter in the direction of the force

$$1 \text{ joule} = 1 \times 10^7 \text{ ergs}$$

Heat and work are equivalent forms of energy. The thermal unit of energy is gram calorie (small calorie). The kilogram calorie (large calorie) is equal to 1000 gram calories.

1 g. calorie = 4.184 joules.

Temperature

The base SI unit of temperature is the Kelvin (K). The practical unit, degree celsius (°C) is also retained and is often used to express temperatures. The degree celsius and the Kelvin are identical but are separated by a temperature interval of 273.16°K.

i.e. 0°C = 273.16°K

10°C = 273.16°K + 10°C = 283.16°K

In general T°K = t°C + 273.16°K

2. Exponent, Power, and Root

Consider the expression,

$$2^5 = 32$$

In this, 32 is called the *power* of the *base* 2, and 5 is the *exponent* of the power

The following laws should be remembered

1. $2^5 \times 2^4 = 2^{5+4} = 2^9$
2. $2^{10} \div 2^2 = 2^{10-2} = 2^8$
3. $(2^3)^4 = 2^{3\times4} = 2^{12}$
4. $(2 \times 4 \times 6)^2 = 2^2 \times 4^2 \times 6^2$
5. $\left(\frac{4}{5}\right)^2 = \frac{4^2}{5^2}$
6. Any number other than 0 with exponent 0 equals 1; eg $2^0 = 1$ or $10^0 = 1$
7. $2^{-4} = \frac{1}{2^4}$
8. The root of a power is obtained by dividing the exponent of the power by index of the root

$$\sqrt[2]{2^8} = 2^{8/2} = 2^4$$

In general, $\sqrt[3]{a^2} = (a^2)^{1/3} = a^{2/3}$

Logarithms

Logarithms offer a means of expressing very large or very small numbers in a very simple fashion. Lengthy problems can be performed rapidly and easily with the aid of logarithms (or simply logs)

The log of a number is the exponent of the power to which a given base must be raised in order to equal that number. For example, $a^b = x$ can be expressed in logarithmic notation as

$$\log_a x = b \qquad \text{... (1)}$$

The exponent 'b' to which the base 'a' is raised to give x is referred to as the logarithm of x.

Thus, the equity

$$2^3 = 8$$

is expressed in logarithmic notation as

$$\log_2 8 = 3$$

The exponent 3 to which the base 2 is raised to give the value 8 is therefore the logarithm of 8. i.e. logarithm of 8 is 3.

John Napier of Scotland discovered logs over three hundred years ago and he used the Natural log number, 2.7/828....., as the base. Henry Briggs, a few years later introduced 10 as the base which is the most convenient for practical purposes. Napier's system is called natural logs (or simply ln) and Brigg's system is called common logs.

Natural logarithms

Equation 1 in natural logarithm is written as

$$\log_{2.71828....} x = b$$

or simply $\log_e x = b$

The above equation may be written without the use of the base 'e' as

$$\ln x = b \qquad \text{... (2)}$$

It indicates $e^b = x$

Thus, $\ln 100 = 4.605$ means $e^{4.605} = 100$ and it actually means $(2.71828.....)^{4.605} = 100$

Since $e^0 = 1$, $\ln 1 = 0$

Common logarithms (or Briggsian logarithms)

It uses 10 as the base. Then the equation can be written in common logarithms as

$$\log_{10} x = b$$

The above equation is generally written as

$$\log x = b \qquad \text{... (3)}$$

Thus $\log_{10} 100 = 2$

or simply $\log 100 = 2$ (It indicates $10^2 = 100$)

Since $10^0 = 1$, $\log 1 = 0$

Conversion of natural logarithms into common logarithms and vice versa

The relationship of common logarithm to natural logarithms is given as

$$\log x = \frac{\ln x}{2.303}$$

$$\text{or } \ln x = 2.303 \log x$$

Thus, to convert common logarithms into natural logarithms, multiply common logarithm by 2.303 and to convert natural logarithms into common logarithms divide natural logarithm by 2.303

Important rules of logarithms

Common logs	Natural logs
$\log (a)(b) = \log a + \log b$	$\ln (a)(b) = \ln a + \ln (b)$
$\log (a/b) = \log a - \log b$	$\ln (a/b) = \ln a - \ln b$
$\log 1/a = -\log a$	$\ln (1/a) = -\ln a$
$\log a^b = b \log a$	$\ln a^b = b \ln a$
$\log a^{1/b} = \frac{1}{b} \log a$	$\ln a^{1/b} = \frac{1}{b} \ln a$
$\log a^{-b} = -b \log a$ $= b \log (1/a)$	$\ln a^{-b} = -b \ln a$ $= b \ln (1/a)$
$\log (a \times b) = \log (a + b)$	$\ln (a \times b) = \ln (a + b)$
$\log (a \div b) = \log (a - b)$	$\ln (a \div b) = \ln (a - b)$
$\log 10 = 1$	$\ln e = 1$
$\log 10^a = a$	$\ln e^a = a$
$\log 10^{-a} = -a$	$\ln e^{-a} = -a$
$\log \sqrt{a} = \log a^{1/2}$ $= \frac{1}{2} \log a$	

Examples

1. Find the log of 0.08001

The number 0.08001 is first written as 8.001×10^{-2}. The characteristic of a number may be either positive or negative; the mantissa of a log always must be positive. The characteristic is this case is -2 and the mantissa is .9031

Therefore $\log 0.0800 = -2 + 0.9031$
$= -1.0969$

2. Find the antilog of − 2.6990

The number -2.6990 can be separated as $-2 + (-0.6990)$

(a) Add -1 to the characteristic, so that it becomes -3 (i.e. $-2 + (-1)$)

(b) Add $+1$ to the mantissa. This yields 0.301 (i.e. $+1 - 0.6990 = 0.301$). This step is to make the mantissa positive

It results in

$$\log x = \bar{3} \cdot 301$$

From the log table the antilog of 0.301 is found to be 2.

Then, the antilog of $\bar{3} \cdot 301$ is 2×10^{-3}

Thus if $\log x = -2.6990$, then the $x = 2.0 \times 10^{-3}$

Graphic Methods

It is usual to represent experimental data graphically. It helps to observe the relationship between variables more clearly. It is also possible to obtain an empiric equation from the plot of the data.

Usually the independent variable is measured on the horizontal line called x-axis and the dependent variable along the vertical line called the y-axis. The x-value is known as the x co-ordinate or the abscissa and the y-value as the y co-ordinate or the ordinate. Where the x and y meet is referred to as the origin. (Fig. 1)

The simplest relationship between two variables may be given by a first degree equation in which the value of the exponent of the variables is equal to

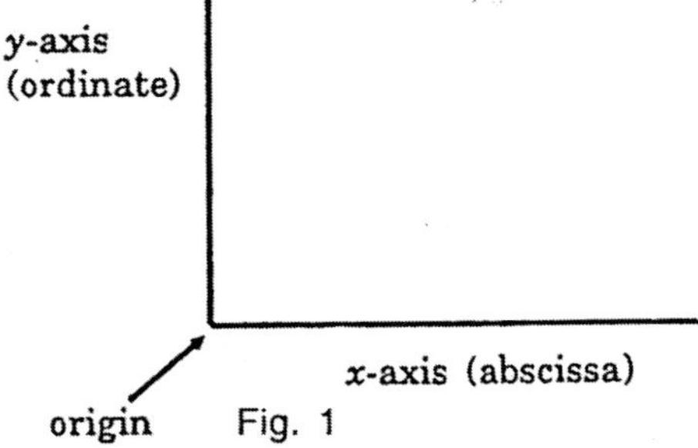

Fig. 1

one. This equation, on plotting on a rectangular graph paper yields a straight line. The equation is given as

$$y = b + mx \quad \text{... (4)}$$

where

y = the dependent variable,

b = the y intercept,

m = the slope of the straight line, and

x = the independent variable

The y–intercept: It indicates the point at which the straight line intersects the y-axis. y intercept gives the value of y when $x = 0$. When the value of y intercept is zero, the straight line passes through the origin. In that case, the equation becomes

$$y = 0 + mx$$

$$\text{or } y = mx \quad \text{... (5)}$$

The slope: It is represented by the letter 'm' in the equation of the straight line. The slope gives the change in the value of y, as a result of change in the value of x. Mathematically, it is given by

$$m = \frac{\Delta y}{\Delta x} \text{ or } \frac{y_2 - y_1}{x_2 - x_1} \quad \text{... (6)}$$

Negative slope indicates a decrease in the value of 'y' on increasing the value of x. In this case, the line slants downward to the right.

Positive slope indicates an increase in the value of 'y' on decreasing the value of x. In this case, the line slants upward to the right.

A steeper slope indicates a large value for m and a less-steeper slope indicates a small value for m.

When the value of slope is unity (or one), it indicates the change in the value of 'y' equals the change in the value of 'x'.

Plotting the graph

A rectangular graph paper (two-dimensional) is used to plot a graph using dependent and independent variables. In general, the independent variable is represented on the x axis and the dependent variable on the y axis. For example, if we want to plot degradation of drug as a function of time, the time is then, the independent variable and the amount of drug degraded is the dependent variable. When plotting a graph, it is advisable to use the entire length of each axis.

Suppose some experimental data, when plotted, produce a straight line with a negative slope as shown in Fig. 2. the equation of the line ($y = b + mx$) may then be given as

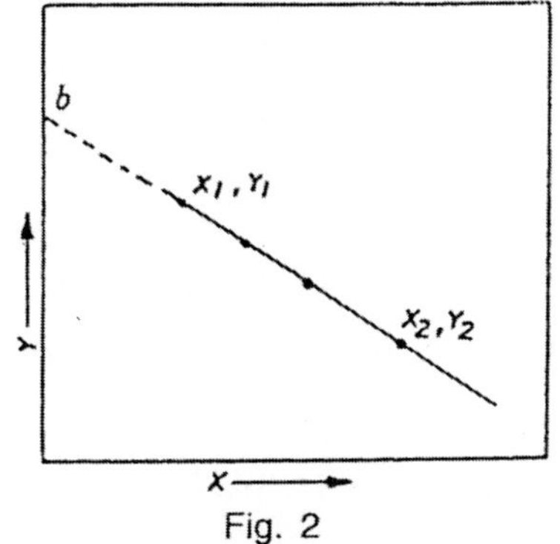

Fig. 2

$$y - y_1 = \frac{y_2 - y_1}{x_2 - x_1}(x - x_1) \text{ or,}$$

$$y = \frac{y_2 - y_1}{x_2 - x_1}(x - x_1) + y_1. \quad \text{... (7)}$$

The values of the two widely separated points are substituted into the two point equation to obtain the value of 'b'. It may also be obtained simply by extrapolating the line upwards to intersect the y-axis. The point at which it intersects the 'y' axis gives the value of 'b' (the value 'y' intercept). The slope of the straight line 'm' may be obtained from the equation

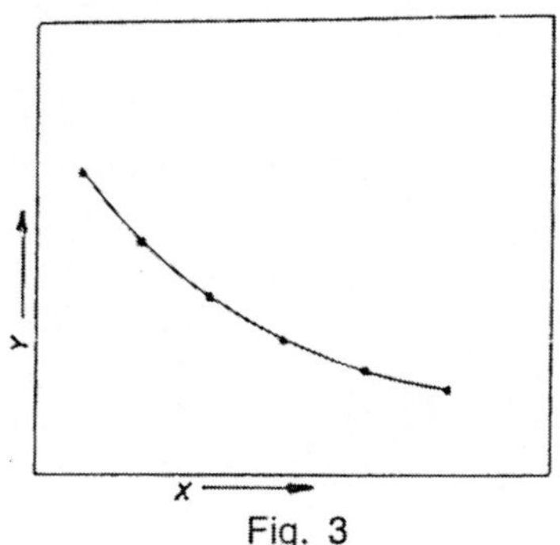

Fig. 3

The derived quantities from length, mass and time are shown below.

Quantity	Area (A)	Volume (V)	Density (ρ)	Velocity (v)	Acceleration (a)	Force (f)	Pressure (p)	Energy
	(Square of length)	(cube of length)	$\left(\frac{\text{mass}}{\text{volume}}\right)$	$\left(\frac{\text{length}}{\text{time}}\right)$	$\left(\frac{\text{length}}{\text{time}^2}\right)$	(mass × acceleration)	$\left(\frac{\text{force}}{\text{area}}\right)$	force × length
Dimension	L^2	L^3	ML^{-3}	LT^{-1}	LT^{-2}	MLT^{-2}	$ML^{-1}T^2$	ML^2T^2
cgs unit	cm^2	cm^3	g/cm^3 or $g.cm^{-3}$	cm/sec or $cm.sec^{-1}$	cm/sec^2 or $cm.sec^{-2}$	g cm/sec^2 or dyne	$dyne/cm^2$ or $dyne.cm^{-2}$	ggm^2/sec^2 = erg
SI unit	m^2	m^3	kgm^{-3}	ms^{-1}	ms^{-2}	$kgms^{-2} = Jm^{-1} = N$	$kgm^{-1}S^{-2} = Nm^{-3} = Pa$	$kgm^2S^{-2} = Nm = J$

where J = Joule ; N = Newton ; P = Pascal

$$\frac{y_2 - y_1}{x_2 - x_1} = \frac{\Delta y}{\Delta x} = m \quad \ldots (8)$$

Assume the data x and y values obtained from a certain experiment when plotted yield a curve shown in Fig. 3.

Then with such a curve, it is dif**ficult to draw** a smooth line through the **points or to** extrapolate the curve to **meet the y axis**. However, a straight line can be obtained if logarithms of y values are plotted against x values (Fig. 4). This indicates that it follows a logarithmic or exponential relationship. The slope and the y intercept are then obtained from the graph. But in this method, it is essential to obtain the logarithms of y values for the construction of the curve and then to obtain antilogarithm of the ordinate. Such an inconvenience of converting to logarithms and then to antilogarithms may be avoided by the use of *semilogarithm graph paper*.

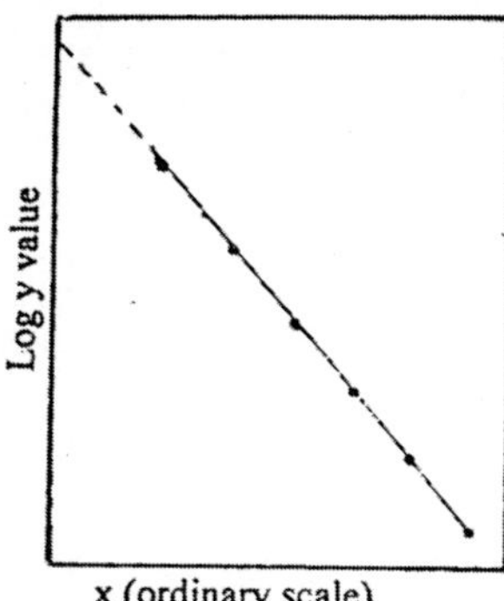

Fig. 4

In this the x and y values are plotted directly on the semilogarithm graph paper. The **semilogarithm paper may be used for natural logarithm (ln) or for log plots.**

Semi-logarithmic graph paper

Semi-logarithmic graph paper is one half logarithmic and one half non-logarithmic i.e. one of the two axes (x or y) of this graph paper is in the logarithmic scale and the other half is in the non-logarithmic scale (ordinary scale)

The plotting of data on a semi-logarithmic paper is different from plotting the data on a rectangular co-ordinate graph paper in several respects. The following points should be noted while plotting the data on a semi-logarithmic graph paper.

1. In this one of the two axes is in logarithmic scale, and the other axis is in regular co-ordinate scale.
2. Negative numbers cannot be plotted on the logarithmic scale.
3. The logarithmic scale of a semi logarithmic paper (usually y-axis) is divided into 9 main divisions. Each main division is subdivided into 5, 10, or 20 sub-divisions. These main divisions are subdivided in a logarithmic fashion. The nine main divisions on the logarithmic scale constitute one cycle of semi-logarithmic graph paper.
4. There is no zero on the y-axis of logarithmic scale, as there is no logarithm of zero. The lowest point must have a numerical value equal to 1×10^n. When n can be any positive or negative whole number.
5. A semi-logarithmic paper with 4 main divisions on its entire y axis is termed one-cycle logarithmic graph paper. The highest point on the one cycle graph paper has a numerical value that is equal to 10 times the numerical value of the lowest point. For example, if the lowest point has the value 1×10^n, then the highest point has the value $1 \times 10^{n+1}$. If the highest value is expected to be more than 10 times the value of the lowest value, then one should use a two-cycle or, more than two cycle graph paper depending upon the values to be plotted.
6. In a two-cycle semi-logarithmic graph paper, one cycle is placed on the other cycle and both the cycles occupy the same space as is occupied by a single logarithmic

cycle on one cycle semi-logarithmic graph paper.

7. If the first cycle starts with 1 and ends with 10, the next cycle starts with 10 and ends with 100. If it is a three cycle logarithmic cycle graph paper, the third cycle starts with 100 and ends at 1000. Simply saying if the first cycle starts with (i.e. the lowest point) 1×10^0, the next cycle starts in 1×10^1, the third 1×10^2, the fourth 10^3 and so on. Similarly if the numerical value of the lowest point (i.e. where the y axis and x axis meet) is 0.01, the highest point in the first cycle will be 0.1 (i.e. $0.01 \times 10 = 0.1$), the highest point in the second cycle will be 1 (i.e. $0.1 \times 10 = 1$), and in the third cycle it will be 10 (i.e. $1 \times 10 = 10$) and so on. In other words, the numerical value of second cycle will be 10 times the numerical values of the first cycle and the numerical values of the third cycle will be 10 times the numerical values of the second cycle and so on.

8. Be it a one cycle, two cycle or three cycle logarithmic graph paper, it will occupy the same space as occupied by the one-cycle graph logarithmic paper. Because of the above fact, the accuracy of plotting the data decreases as the number of cycles increases. Hence, we should be careful in choosing the right type of the semi-logarithmic graph paper. For example, the highest value of the data collected is equal to 10 times or below 10 times the lowest value, it is wise to select a one-cycle logarithmic graph paper. When the highest value of the data collected is more than 10 times and is equal to 100 times or less than 100 times the lowest value of the data, we can choose a two-cycle logarithmic paper for plotting the data.

9. It is worthwhile to mention at this juncture that we should take logarithms of the points on the y axis to calculate the slope of the straight line (i.e. to reflect the change in y with x)

Some useful expressions relating the variables with suggested methods of plotting to yield straight lines are

1. $y = mx + b$	Plot y vs x on rectangular co-ordinate graph paper. The slope gives the value of m and the intercept on y axis at $x = 0$ gives the value of b.
2. $y = ax^n$ ($\log y = \log a + n \log x$)	Plot y vs x on logarithmic co-ordinate. The slope gives the value of n and the intercept on the 'y' axis at $x = 1$, gives the value of a
3. $y = a^{bx}$	Plot y vs x on semi-logarithmic co-ordinate. The slope is equal to $\frac{b}{2.303}$ and the intercept on the y axis at $x = 0$, gives the value of a
4. $y = a + cx^n$	Plot y vs x, the intercept gives the value of 'a'. Then plot $(y - a)$ vs x on logarithmic co-ordinate to get the slope.
5. $y = a + \frac{b}{x}$	Plot y vs $\frac{1}{x}$ on a rectangular plot. The values of a and b are obtained from the intercept and the slope respectively.

Method of Least Squares

This method is used to fit the best straight line to a set of data.

Consider the equation $y = mx + b$

First, the values of m and b are formed to N pairs of x and y values. The values of x and y being experimental, it is unlikely that any pair of values (x, y) will satisfy the best fit line exactly.

The values of m and b are obtained using the following equation.

$$m = \frac{N\sum xy - \sum x \sum y}{N\sum x^2 - (\sum x)^2} \quad \text{... (9)}$$

$$b = \frac{\sum x^2 y - \sum xy \sum x}{N\sum x^2 - (\sum x)^2} \quad \text{... (10)}$$

All sums must be taken over all experimental points.

The best way to use the above formula is to construct a table with four columns headed x, y, x^2, xy and complete the table for the experimental data. The sums of the columns will give all the values required.

Example

Let the relation between x and y be represented by the equation of the form

$$y = ax^n$$

If the values of x and y are as given below

x	4530	5010	5780	9600	12600	15600
y	0.0097	0.0095	0.0092	0.0081	0.0075	0.0071

we can obtain the best values of a and n.

Writing the above formula in logarithmic terms, we get

$\log y = n \log x + \log a$

(i.e. $y = mx + b$ form)

where $y = \log y$; $x = \log x$; $b = \log a$

For the data presented above, the following table is evaluated.

$\log x$	$\log y$	$\log x^2$	$\log x \cdot \log y$
3.656	−2.103	13.366	−7.360
3.700	−2.022	13.690	−7.481
3.762	−2.036	14.153	−7.659
3.982	−2.092	15.856	−8.330
4.100	−2.125	16.810	−8.213
4.193	−2.149	17.581	−9.011
$\Sigma x =$ 23.393	$\Sigma y =$ 12.437	$\Sigma x^2 =$ 91.456	$\Sigma xy =$ −48.554

The best fit values of n and a are

$$n = \frac{6(-48.554) - (23.393)(-12.437)}{6(91.456) - (23.393)^2}$$

$$= -0.256$$

$$a = \frac{(91.456)(-12.437) - (-48.554)(23.393)}{6(91.456) - (23.393)^2}$$

$$= -1.074$$

Thus the relationship between y and x becomes ($\log y = -0.256 \log x - 1.074$)

$$y = (0.084\, x)^{-0.256}$$

3. Statistics

Statistics may be defined as a logic that utilises mathematics in the science of collecting, analysing and interpreting data for the purpose of making decisions. Logic and reasoning play a major part in arriving at decisions.

Statistics is gaining importance as an useful tool in the design, analysis and interpretation of experiments. Statistical methods and appropriate statistical analysis are routinely applied in the pharmaceutical field in sampling, in quality control testing, in stability testing and in process validation. Moreover, the statistical techniques are gaining more importance in pharmaceutical research also.

The practice of statistical methods may comprise (1) design of the experiment, (2) collection of data, (3) analysis of data, and (4) interpretation of the analysis.

After proper design of the experiment, the collection of data starts. In the collection of data, possible errors that may be introduced because of various factors involved should be minimized.

First of all, it is necessary to know about the two types of errors — determinate and indeterminate errors, so that one may be able to locate and eliminate them as far as possible. Such errors will affect accuracy and precision and hence they must be avoided to an extent of possibility.

Determinate errors

These are errors which can be determined and possibly eliminated. These errors may be introduced by defective instruments, unskilled operators, and faulty experiments.

For example, an error due to instrument may occur when a 20 ml. pipette which actually measures 20.1 ml is used. It may arise even from the environmental factors. For example, a pipette which measures 10 ml at 25°C may not measure the same volume at some other temperatures. Errors due to instruments may be eliminated to a greater extent by calibrating the instruments periodically and also by the use of appropriate blanks.

Errors may be introduced by operators themselves, in reading a meniscus, in pouring and measuring, in weighing, in doing calculations and in matching colours. These errors may creep in due to carelessness, fatigue or inadequate instructions received. The errors due to operators may also be called as *biased personal errors* and are usually introduced because of variation of personal judgement. Biased personal errors may be avoided by checking calculations and results with others involved in the same practice.

Errors may also be introduced by defective experimental methods. They may include the use of an improper procedure and the use of an improper indicator (For example using methyl orange in the place of phenolphthalein in volumetric analysis). These errors may be eliminated only by understanding the theoretical background of the experiment properly and are usually difficult to detect.

Indeterminate errors

These errors are also called accidental or random errors. For example, one may measure the boiling point of a liquid successively and report the values as 99.8°C, 100.1°C, 100.2°C and 100°C. Here there is an obvious error in his measurements. Such an error is called indeterminate error which cannot be predicted or determined accurately and they follow a random distribution. Indeterminate errors cannot be controlled by the experimentalist and it cannot be pinpointed. For example, when pipetting out a liquid, the speed of draining, the angle of holding the pipette, the position at which the pipette is held at the time of draining etc., could introduce indeterminate error in the volume of liquid pipetted out.

Precision and Accuracy

Precision is defined as the agreement among the numerical values in a group of data. Precision is affected by indeterminate errors.

Accuracy is the closeness between the data and the true value. It is affected by determinate errors.

Accuracy refers to closeness to a true or expected value whereas precision shows how closely the measurements agree with each other.

The term accuracy is denoted in terms of absolute error and mean error. The absolute error, E, is the difference between the observed value X_i and the expected or true value X_t.

$$E = | X_i - X_t | \qquad \text{... (11)}$$

(the vertical lines on either side indicate that the algebraic sign of the deviation (+ or −) should be disregarded)

The value E depends on the reliability of X_i and X_t.

The difference between sample arithmetic mean and true value is termed as mean error and this also gives a measure of the accuracy of an operation.

Sometimes, the term relative error is used to express the uncertainties in the data. The relative error is the percentage of error compared to the expected or true value. It is given as

$$\frac{| X_i - X_t |}{X_t} \times 100 \qquad \text{... (12)}$$

Precision is expressed in terms of mean deviation and standard deviation.

Analysis of Data

Scientific data are subjected to certain mathematical and statistical tests before accepting and reporting the results.

Analysis of the data collected consists of graphing, applying statistical formulaes and drawing inferences.

It is useful to plot the data before beginning the statistical analysis. A graph is obtained by plotting one variable x (independent variable) against another variable y (dependent variable). Such a graph is called rectangular coordinate. The most common type of curve often obtained by plotting x against y is the normal frequency distribution curve or bell shaped curve (Fig. 5). It is also called normal probability curve. Many statistical formulaes and interpretations are based on the assumption of a normal frequency distribution curve of data.

When such a normal distribution curve is obtained for the data collected, the arithmetic mean is taken as the central value of the distribution. A bell shaped curve obtained by plotting particle size against frequency is shown in Fig. 5.

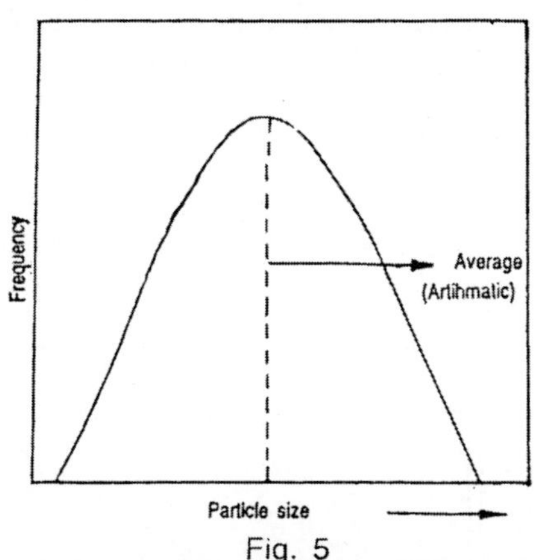

Fig. 5

The arithmetic mean $(\overline{X})$ is usually obtained by dividing the sum of various measurements (X_i) by the number of measurements N. It is expressed mathematically as follows.

$$X = \frac{\Sigma (X_i)}{N} \qquad \dots (13)$$

X_i = individual measurement

N = number of values.

This arithmetic mean is also called as mean value or average.

Measures of variation

As mentioned before, these are variations that exist in nature and they may also be man-made. Hence, it is necessary to express variation or scatter about the central value (arithmetic mean) to estimate the variation among the results.

The simplest measure of variation is the range. It is the difference between the largest and smallest value in a series of observations (or measurements). The range is valuable when N (number of observations or values) is less than 10.

When $N = 2$, the range is as efficient as the standard deviation in expressing the measure of variation. When N is greater than 10, standard deviation gives a better estimate of the variation.

The other measure of variation is the mean deviation 'd'. It is the ratio of the difference between each individual value X_i and the arithmetic mean $\overline{X}$ without considering the algebraic signs and the number of values N.

$$d = \frac{\Sigma \mid X_i - \overline{X} \mid}{N} \qquad \dots (14)$$

The use of mean deviation is discouraged and it is considered to give a biased estimate and therefore, the standard deviation is much commonly used especially in research work. The standard deviation 'σ' is the square root of the mean of the square of the difference between the individual measured values X_i and the mean of the number of measurements (μ).

$$\sigma = \sqrt{\frac{\Sigma (X_i - \mu)^2}{N}} \qquad \dots (15)$$

N = number of values measured.

This equation is applicable only for a set of measurements. The value σ is known as *population standard deviation.*

If a random sample is taken from a population (the sample is the subset of the population), then, the standard deviation for the population is known as the *sample standard deviation* and is given as

$$S = \Sigma\sqrt{\frac{(X_i - \overline{X})^2}{N-1}} \quad \text{... (16)}$$

where $\overline{X}$ is the mean of the sample values. The symbol '*S*' instead of σ is used here to indicate that the standard deviation obtained is only an approximation of the true value.

The standard deviation of the sample is called standard error and this is denoted by *s*, where

$$s = \frac{S}{\sqrt{N}} \quad \text{... (17)}$$

Another term used to denote precision is the coefficient of variation (c.v). This is given as

$$\text{C.V} = \frac{\text{standard deviation}}{\text{mean}} \times 100$$

$$= \frac{S}{d} \times 100.$$

Population is the whole of what is under consideration whereas the sample is that portion of the population used in the analysis.

The operation becomes more and more precise when the standard deviation estimate gets smaller and smaller and therefore, the mean deviation and standard deviation are used as measures of precision of a method.

It is possible for a result to be precise without being accurate.

Significant figures

Data have to be reported with care, keeping in mind the reliability about the number of figures used. Every measured value has some uncertainty associated with it. For example, a number may have as many as six decimal numbers when one uses a calculator. It is meaningless to report all these six numbers because there may be uncertainty about the first decimal itself. Therefore, experimental data should be rounded off so that they contain only the digits known with certainty plus the uncertain one. Thus, if the refractive index of a liquid is known with certainty only upto two decimals, the value can be reported upto three decimals. This practice is called *significant figure practice.*

Significant figures are used to indicate the precision of a result. For example, the number 37.56 is more precise than the number 37.5

Linear Regression Analysis

An effective way of predicting a trend or relationship is, as mentioned before, by plotting two variables *x* and *y* one against the other.

For example, for the following *x* and *y* values, the trend is shown in Fig. 6 as linear relationship between the values of *x* and *y*

x	1	2	3	4	5	6
y	10.0	20.5	29.9	40.0	50.9	60.1

Frequently such good linear relationship may not be obtained (may be because of poor techniques) or may not exist. In such cases, the points may deviate from the best fit for the given or collected data i.e. there would be scatter of points about a line and we will not obtain a straight line with any degree of confidence. Then, we must

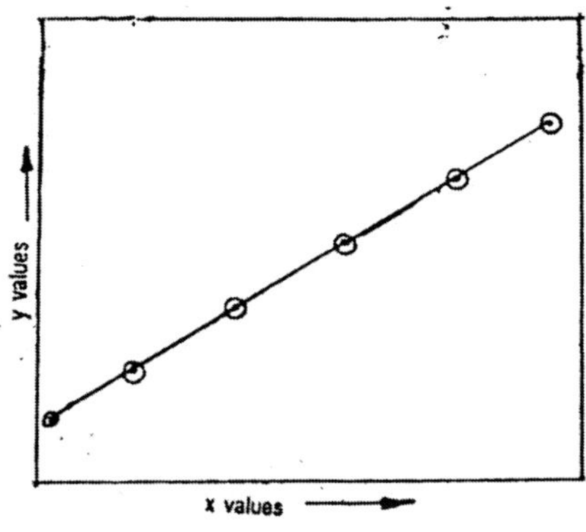

Fig. 6

employ a better means of analysing the available data and for that we can make use of statistics to calculate whether the data fit a straight line. For this purpose, we employ linear regression analysis.

We must, as a first step, calculate the correlation co-efficient 'r' which helps to examine the appropriateness of the linear relationship between x and y

**The 'r' is given by

$$r = \frac{\Sigma (x - \bar{x})(y - \bar{y})}{[\Sigma (x - \bar{x})^2 \cdot \Sigma (y - \bar{y})^2]^{1/2}} \quad \text{... (18)}$$

$\bar{y}$ = mean of y values

When the value of 'r' is 1 it would mean a perfect linear relationship. If the 'r' value is more than 0.75, the linearity may be considered excellent.

When both x and y increase or decrease simultaneously the correlation coefficient (r) is positive and it is negative when one increases as the other decreases. A value of 0 (zero) for 'r' indicates no relationship between x and y. It is not worthwhile to proceed with the analysis if the 'r' value falls below 0.25. That is, if the value of 'r' indicates lack of correlation, the data do not fit a straight line

When there is significant correlation between x and y, the slope (m) and intercept (b) of the line can be calculated by using the equation,

$$m = \frac{\Sigma (x - \bar{x})(y - \bar{y})}{\Sigma (x - \bar{x})^2} \quad \text{... (19)}$$

where m is regression coefficient or slope

The intercept (b) is given by

$$b = \bar{y} - m\bar{x}$$

The equation of straight line is, then, given by $y = b + mx$ and this can also be obtained from the equation,

$$y = \bar{y} + \frac{\Sigma (x - \bar{x})(y - \bar{y})}{\Sigma (x - \bar{x})^2}(x - \bar{x}) \quad \text{... (20)}$$

4. Forces between molecules, ions and atoms

Molecules, ions and atoms have both attractive and repulsive forces. Liquid and solid states exist because of coherence between molecules. This coherence is due to attractive forces that exist between molecules (ions and atoms). However in the absence of repulsive forces, attractive forces may cause mutual destruction of molecules. Therefore, both attractive and repulsive forces operate between molecules, ions and atoms and within them.

Repulsive forces

A general type of repulsive forces exists when two atoms are brought close together due to overlapping of electron clouds. This type of repulsive forces decreases with distance of separation between atoms.

A second type of repulsion is columbic repulsion that exists between similarly charged ions. However this repulsive force will be less if the ions are in a dielectric medium.

* **Dipole Moment**: When a covalent bond is formed between two unlike atoms (A and B), the atom (say A) which is more electronegative has a tendency to attract the shared pair of electrons and the molecule becomes $A^{\partial -} \cdot B^{\partial +}$. Now the dipole moment (μ) of the molecule is defined as the vector equal in magnitude to the product of electric charge (expressed in electrostatic units, *esu* and the distance of separation of the charges joining the positive and negative charges (expressed in angstrom units Å). Thus an electron separated from a unit positive charge by a distance of 1Å (i.e. 10^{-8}cm) is given by

$$\mu = 4.8 \times 10^{-10}\ esu \times 10^{-8}\ \text{cm}$$

$$= 4.8 \times 10^{-18}\ esu \text{ per cm or} = 4.8 \text{ Debyes (Debye is the unit for } \mu)$$

For polyatomic molecule containing the net dipole moment is the resultant addition of in dividual charge moments multiplied by the distance of separation between the changes. In a linear molecule, the individual bond moments exactly cancel each other or vector addition and the dipole moment is zero and hence the molecule is said to be non-polar.

Attractive forces

First type of attractive forces arises between the oppositely charged ions. Ions result from the transfer of electrons from one atom to another. The bond formed between oppositely charged ions is termed electrovalent bond (eq. NaCl)

Second type of attractive forces exists in covalent bonds. This bond arises due to sharing of electrons. Equal sharing of electrons will form a non-polar covalent bond and precisely equal sharing of electrons will occur in molecules of same element (eg. H_2,Cl_2 etc). These molecules have a dipole moment of zero.

In the case of molecules containing atoms of different elements, the electron affinity may not be exactly the same. When a covalent bond between them is formed, the shared electron pair will always be nearer to the more electronegative atoms. Then, the positive and negative centers do not coincide resulting in separation of charges. This separation of charges is permanent and it gives rise to a permanent dipole moment* associated with the bond. The dipole moment will possess a value and will act in a particular direction. Several bonds within a molecule may give rise to various bond moments and these bond moments contribute to an overall value for the dipole moment* of the molecule. If a molecule has a permanent dipole moment greater than zero, it is said to be polar.

A molecule with a dipole moment of zero is said to be non-polar. If an ion (carrying charge) is brought close to a non-polar molecule, the shared electron pair may get displaced towards one or other of the atoms in the non-polar molecule and this gives rise to an induced dipole moment in the bond of the non-polar molecule. If the ion is withdrawn, this effect also disappears. In the same way, a molecule with a permanent dipole moment may also induce a dipole moment in a non-polar molecule.

The three types of components - ions, permanent dipole and induced dipole give rise to six types of attractions.

1. Ion-ion attraction
2. Ion-permanent dipole attraction
3. Ion-induced dipole attraction
4. Permanent dipole - permanent dipole attraction (*Keesom forces*)
5. Permanent dipole - induced dipole attraction (*Debye interaction*)
6. Induced dipole - induced dipole attraction (*London forces*)

The last three types of attractions are in general known as *Van der Waals* forces.

The attractive forces between non-polar molecules (i.e. induced dipole - induced dipole attraction) are known as London or dispersion forces. This type of attraction arises in non-polar molecules because of vibrations of electrons that produce induction of dipoles within the molecules.

One more type of attraction between molecules is hydrogen bonding. This bond arises when hydrogen atom is covalently bonded to a highly electronegative atom such as O, N or F. In the molecule HF (H:F), the shared electron pair is strongly held close to fluorine which is more electronegative resulting in a strong dipole in the molecule.

$$\overset{\delta+}{H} : \overset{\delta-}{F}$$

The hydrogen atom which is nearly stripped of its surrounding electron exerts a strong electrostatic attraction on the lone pair of electron in another F in HF nearby

$$\overset{\delta+}{H} - \overset{\delta-}{F}: + \overset{\delta+}{H} - \overset{\delta-}{F}: \longrightarrow$$

$$\overset{\delta+}{H} - \overset{\delta-}{F} \ldots\ldots \overset{\delta+}{H} - \overset{\delta-}{F}$$

↑ hydrogen bond

Hydrogen bond is indicated by a dashed or dotted line.

Thus, the hydrogen bond or hydrogen bonding is the electrostatic attraction between 'H' atoms covalently linked to an electronegative atom 'X' (such as O, F and N) and a lone pair of electron on X in another molecule.

The energy of hydrogen bond is about $\frac{1}{10}$ th of a covalent bond. The hydrogen bond may be intermolecular if it occurs when electronegative atoms are contained in different molecules (i.e. between two separate HF or H_2O molecules) or intramolecular if the electronegative atoms are in the same molecule as in 2-nitrophenol and salicylic acid.

Intra Type Inter type

Salicylic acid showing intra and inter hydrogen bonding

In general, attractive forces between like molecules are termed as ***cohesive forces*** and the attractive forces between unlike molecules are termed as ***adhesive forces***. For example attractive forces between (H_2O) water molecules are cohesive forces and the attractive forces between H_2O molecules and C_2H_5OH (ethyl alcohol) molecules are adhesive forces.

Based on the forces of interaction occuring in solvent molecules, solvents can be broadly classified as follows

Polar solvents: These are solvents made up of strong dipolar molecules which form hydrogen bonding (e.g. water, hydrogen peroxide)

Semipolar solvents: These are solvents made up of strong dipolar molecules which do not form hydrogen bonding (e.g. acetone, pentyl alcohol)

Nonpolar solvents: These are solvents made up of molecules with a small or no dipolar character (e.g. benzene, vegetable oils)

Dielectric constant

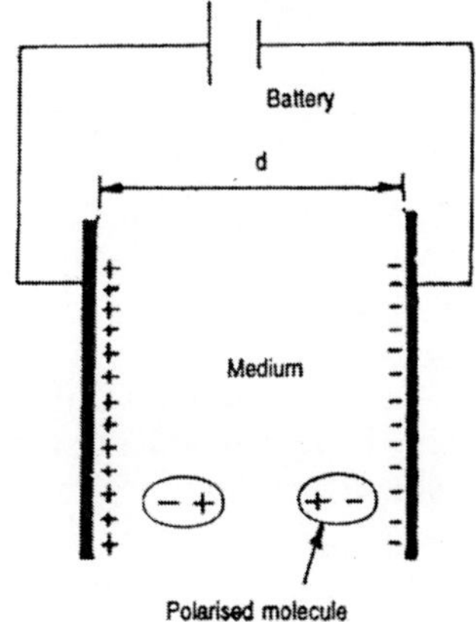

Fig. 7

Consider two parallel electricity conducting plates (parallel plate condensers) separated by some medium across a distance of d and connected to a battery as shown in the Fig. 7.

Electricity will flow from the left plate to the right plate until the potential difference of the plates is equal to that of the battery supplying the initial potential difference.

The capacitance of the condenser (c) in *farads* is then equal to the quantity of electric charge q (in *coulombs*) stored on the plates divided by the potential difference V between the plates.

$$c = \frac{q}{V} \qquad \text{... (21)}$$

When vacuum fills the space between the plates, the capacitance C_o is

$$C_o = \frac{q_o}{V_o} \quad \text{... (22)}$$

If water fills the space, the capacitance C_x is given by

$$C_x = \frac{q_x}{V_x} \quad \text{... (23)}$$

When water fills the space, the capacitance is increased. The ratio between these two capacitances i.e. the capacitance when water or any other liquid fills the space and the capacitance when vacuum fills the space gives the dielectric constant (ε) of water or for any other liquid.

$$\varepsilon = \frac{C_x}{C_o} \quad \text{... (24)}$$

Water is an unique solvent and has a high dielectric constant (i.e. 78.5). The dielectric constant indicates the effectiveness of a substance it has, when it acts as a medium, on the ease in separating two oppositely charged ions in a molecule.

Coulomb's law for the force of attraction between two oppositely charged ions is given as

$$F = \frac{Z_1 Z_2}{\epsilon r^2} \quad \text{... (25)}$$

where Z_1 and Z_2 = charges on the ions

r= distance separating the oppositely charged ions.

ϵ = dielectric constant of the medium

Thus, the interactive force between sodium and chloride ions in water at a distance r would be 78.5 times less than that when it is in vacuum separated by the same distance. That is, it is 78.5 times easier to separate the sodium and chloride ions in sodium chloride molecule in water than in vacuum

The ease of solution of salts in solvents like water and glycerin can be explained based on the high dielectric constants. In general, the more polar is the solvent, the greater is the dielectric constant

There exists a close relationship between dielectric constants and the two types of interactions i.e. dipole-dipole interaction (*Keesom* forces) and the induced dipole-induced dipole interaction (London forces). The dielectric constant is related to these two forces by the equation

$$P = \frac{\varepsilon - 1}{\varepsilon + 2} \frac{M}{D} \quad \text{... (26)}$$

where P = total molar polarisation indicating the measure of relative ease with which a charge separation may be made within a molecule.

ε = dielectric constant of the substance (i.e. solvent)

M = molecular weight of the substance (i.e. solvent)

D = density of the solvent

Solvents with large dipole moments will have large dielectric constants. It is also to be noted that as temperature increases, the dielectric constant of dipolar solvents will tend to decrease.

Dielectric constants of some liquids at 25°C are

N-methyl formamide	182.00
Hydrogen cyanide	114.00
Formamide	110.00
Water	78.50
Glycerol	42.50
Methanol	32.60
Isopropanol	18.30
Chloroform	4.80
Benzene	2.27
Carbon tetrachloride	2.23

I. STATES OF MATTER

Matter normally exists in one of the three states-solid, liquid, or gas. The two common factors which usually determine the three states of matter are the intensity of intermolecular forces and the temperature. Solids have the strongest forces and the gases have the weakest forces.

The molecules, atoms, or ions (in general called particles) in the solid are strongly held in close proximity by intermolecular, interatomic or ionic forces respectively. The particles of a solid can oscillate only about fixed positions. As the temperature of a solid substance is raised, the particles acquire sufficient energy to disrupt the ordered arrangement (intermolecular forces are weakened and intermolecular distances are increased) and pass into the liquid state. On further increasing the temperature, the molecules pass into the gaseous state. In gaseous state, the intermolecular distances are greatly increased and the intermolecular forces are reduced almost to nil.

As solid goes into a liquid state and then to gaseous state, heat is absorbed and the enthalpy (heat content) increases and the entropy (degree of molecular randomness) also increases.

During a change of state, the temperature remains constant but heat is absorbed and that absorbed heat is called **latent heat.** Thus ice turns to water at 0°C. During this change, the quantity of heat absorbed is termed as the latent heat of fusion. Likewise the latent heat of vapourisation is the quantity of heat absorbed when a change of state from liquid to vapour is involved at its boiling point.

When a change of state occurs directly from solid state to the gaseous state, it is termed **sublimation.**

Gaseous state

The physical behaviour of gases is independent of chemical nature of the molecules. Therefore, almost all gases respond in an identical way to the variations in pressure, temperature and volume.

Two important characteristics of gases are pressure and volume with respect to temperature. Gases exert pressure on the containers in which they are contained. Gases tend to occupy completely any available space (volume)

The general behaviour of gases with variations of pressure, volume and temperature can be given by the *ideal gas equation.* (Ideal gas molecules exhibit no intermolecular forces of attraction)

$PV = RT$ for 1 mole of ideal gas ... (27)

$PV = nRT$ for 'n' moles of ideal gas. ... (28)

where P = pressure,

V = volume of 1 mole of gas at the given temperature and pressure

n = number of moles of gas,

R = gas constant and

T = absolute temperature

The ideal gas law expresses three facts

(i) volume of a gas is directly proportional to the number of moles.

*In general, vapour of a liquid above its critical temperature is considered as gas.

(ii) volume of a gas is directly proportional to the absolute temperature, and

(iii) volume of a gas is inversely proportional to the pressure.

Although the ideal gas law does not precisely apply to any actual gas, where the intermolecular attraction and the volume of the molecules themselves are not negligible, a great majority of gases and vapours* at ordinary temperatures and pressures obey the law sufficiently accurately.

The value of R (gas constant) can be given in different terms.

(i) when P and V are given in atmospheres and liters respectively, the value of R is 0.821 lit. atm. $mole^{-1}$ deg^{-1}.

(ii) When P and V are given in $dynes/cm^2$ and cm^3 respectively the value of R is 8.314×10^7 ergs $mole^{-1}$ deg^{-1}.

Since 1 joule is 1×10^7 ergs, R is 8.314 joules $mole^{-1}$ deg^{-1}

R is also 1.987 cal $mole^{-1}$ deg^{-1} since 4.184 joules is 1 calorie.

The deviation of a gas from ideal behaviour depends on the nature of the gas, its temperature and pressure.

Real or actual gas deviates from ideal behaviour as the molecules tend to attract one another. The deviation from ideal behaviour becomes significant when the pressure becomes very high and the temperature very low because the molecules are in close proximity to attract each other.

The modified equation for real gases is given by *Van der Waals* and for 1 mole of gas

$$(P + \frac{a}{V^2})(V - b) = RT \qquad \ldots (29)$$

where $\frac{a}{V^2}$ accounts for intermolecular forces of attraction when the molecules are very close to each other under high pressure and low temperature or simply the internal pressure per mole (the internal pressure is also used for describing the cohesive forces in liquids) and b accounts for the incompressibility of the gas molecules i.e. excluded volume.

Pharmaceutical gases: They include the anaesthetic gases such as nitrous oxide and halothane. Compressed gases include nitrogen, carbon-di-oxide and oxygen (for therapy). liquefiable gases used in pharmaceutical field are used as propellants (a propellant is one that causes the liquid/solid in the container to move upward and out of the container) in aerosol products. They include certain halohydrocarbons and hydrocarbons. Volatile liquids such as ether, halothane and methoxy fluorane are used as inhalation anaesthetics. Amyl nitrite is a volatile liquid which can be inhaled for its vasodialating effect in the treatment of acute angina.

Liquid State

The liquid state may be considered as an intermediate state as matter goes from solid state to gaseous state. Liquids can be considered as highly compressed gases or slightly released solids.

Regarding the concept of molecular motion, there must be space in liquids. Liquids may have holes and this concept explains the expansion of volume when materials undergo fusion, or diffusion in liquids, and the decrease in viscosity and density as the temperature is raised. The liquids may be considered as solution of holes in material and that gases as solutions of matter in free space.

The molecules of a gas are in a state of constant motion owing to their kinetic energy which is proportional to the absolute temperature of the gas. When the gas is cooled, its kinetic energy is gradually reduced. As the temperature is being reduced, a stage is reached where the molecules almost loose their kinetic energy and are not able to overcome the forces of attraction. As a result, the gas molecules come closer and ultimately the gas gets into the liquid state. At this juncture, it is worthwhile to know about critical point. It refers to a certain value of temperature or pressure. Above or below this critical point changes in phase will not take place. Thus, the critical point can be defined as the temperature above which a gas can not be liquified whatever be the amount of pressure applied. That is, pressure can be effective in liquefying the gas only below this critical temperature. The critical temperature is, then, defined as the temperature below which a gas can be liquified. The critical temperature is different for different gases or vapours. The critical pressure is the pressure required to liquify a gas at its critical temperature. At critical temperature, the gas and its liquid become indistinguishable and hence the entropy of vapourisation as well as the enthlpy of vapourisation is zero. The critical temperature of water is 374°C or 647°K and its critical pressure is 218 atmospheres.

Gases can be liquefied by the following methods.

(a) By subjecting the gases to intense cold by the use of freezing mixtures

(b) By the use of **adiabatic expansion** (for ideal gases)

(c) By the use of **Joule Thomson effect** (for real gases).

The intermolecular forces of attraction (van de waals forces) in liquids impose some ordering or regular arrangement among the molecules. Hydrogen bonds also promote cohesion of molecules in liquids. However these forces in liquids are much weaker than covalent or ionic forces, and hence they tend to display short range rather than long range order. The properties of liquids such as surface and interfacial tensions and rheology are discussed under the respective chapter.

Vapour pressure

When a liquid is in contact with its vapour, two opposing processes are in operation. One is the process of vaporisation which tends to change the liquid to the gaseous state. The other one is the process of condensation that tends to change the vapours back into the liquid. These two opposing processes continue till the pressure of the vapour ultimately reaches a value at which the rate of vapourisation equals the rate of condensation and hence an equilibrium is established. The pressure exerted by the vapour at equilibrium conditions is termed as the *vapour pressure* or *equilibrium vapour pressure* of the gas.

Equilibrium vapour pressure depends on temperature and the effect of temperature on the vapour pressure of a liquid is given by the ***Classius-Clapeyron*** equation. (See under *Thermodynamics*)

Vapour pressure of a mixture of liquids

In the case of ***miscible liquids*** (solution of a liquid in liquid), the partial vapour pressure exerted by each component is proportional to its molar concentration in the mixture solution. The total vapour pressure *P* is given by

$$P = P_A + P_B = P_A^o X_A + P_B^o X_B \quad \ldots (30)$$

where X_A and X_B are mole fractions of components A and B respectively.

P_A^o and P_B^o are the vapour pressures exerted by the pure components A and B respectively.

P_A and P_B are the partial vapour pressures exerted by A and B respectively in the liquid mixture.

In the case of a mixture containing two ***immiscible liquids*** each liquid exerts its own vapour pressure independently of the other. The total vapour pressure *P* is then given by

$$P = P_A^o + P_B^o \quad \ldots (31)$$

Other properties of liquids such as surface tension and viscosity are discussed under *interfacial phenomena* and *rheology* respectively.

Solids

The most significant property of solid state is the high degree of order in which solid substances exist. Solids like liquids are practically incompressible.

Solids exist in different crystalline forms. They may be *cubic* (sodium chloride) *tetragonal* (urea) *hexagonal* (iodoform) *rhombic* (iodine) *monoclinic* (sucrose), *triclinic* (boric acid), etc.

There are different types of bonds that hold solids together. The bond types are metallic (metals), ionic (salts), valence (diamond), and molecular (organic compounds). In some solids, the atoms or molecules or ions are arranged in a regularly repeating pattern and those solids may be termed as crystalline solids. In some other solids, there is no such characteristic regularity and hence they are termed as non-crystalline or amorphous substances.

The distinguishing attributes for the crystalline and amorphous substances may be given as follows.

Crystalline solids

1. They have fixed molecular order (i.e the molecules occupy set positions in a specific array in the solid)
2. They have sharp melting points.
3. They exhibit anisotropicity with the exception of cubic crystals. Anisotropicity refers to their properties which are not the same in all directions.

Amorphous solids

1. In these, the molecules are randomly arranged.
2. They do not have a sharp melting points.
3. They exhibit isotropicity (i.e their properties are the same in all directions)

The melting point of a solid is the temperature at which the solid is converted to a liquid state at atmospheric pressure and the heat absorbed during the melting is termed as latent heat of fusion.

Polymorphism

Elements may exist in more than one crystalline form and are said to be allotropic (eg. carbon, sulphur etc). When compounds exist in more than one crystalline forms and/or amorphous forms, they are said to be polymorphic. This phenomenon is termed as polymorphism. However this word polymorphism is often applied both for elements and compounds.

A solid substance may exhibit various polymorphic forms. These forms have different melting points, x-ray diffraction patterns and different solubilities. Many organic substances exhibit polymorphism. Theobroma oil (coco butter) exhibits four different forms α, β, β' and γ. The other substances that exhibit polymorphism are aspirin, cortisone acetate, novobiocin etc. (Refer Page 29).

Solid dispersion

Solid dispersion is solid solution. In this, a solid phase contains both the components. In other words, a solid is dissolved (i.e. dispersed as molecules) in another solid to give a mixed crystal. Using this technique, solubility of slightly soluble substances can be increased. For example, the solubility of a drug such as trimethoprim or griseofulvin can be increased by dispersing the drug in some soluble substance such as urea, polyvinyl pyrrolidone etc.

Liquid crystals

Apart from the common three phases (states) some asymmetric molecules often exhibit a fourth phase - ***liquid crystalline state***. Liquid crystals have the property of mobility and rotation (a property of liquid molecules) and the property of being *birefringent* (a property of solid crystals). When light passes through a crystal, it is divided into two components (*right-circularly polarised light and left circularly polarised light*) with different velocities and hence different refractive indices. This property is termed ***birefringence***.

The two main types of structure of liquid crystals are *smectic* (soap or grease like) - the molecules of which are mobile in two directions and show rotation about one axis and *nematic* (thread like) - the molecules of which are mobile in three directions and can rotate about one axis.

The liquid crystalline phases are believed to be involved in the stabilisation of emulsion and solubilisation of water insoluble materials. The liquid crystalline state is found in nature - in nerve, brain tissue and blood vessels.

Glassy state

Glass is a type of solid matter. It represents neither a typical solid or liquid. It differs from solid in not being structurally ordered. But they may have some short range order. They do not have specific melting points as the solids do.

The uniqueness of glassy state can be explained with its cooling curve. When a glassy former (in its liquid state) is cooled, it does not show a large drop in volume or density or in refractive index (Solids show a large drop in volume or density or in refractive index) at any particular temperature and when it passes through the freezing point (melting point) to form glassy state, it does not show a rapid drop in its volume as that of a super cooled liquid. With the supercooled liquid, the cooling curve is a simple continuation of the liquid cooling curve itself.

Atomically, the structure of the glassy state is composed of a random selection of polyhedral molecules probably linked together at their corners. Formation of glass is easy with certain materials and with others glassy state can be formed with difficulty and still with others, it is not possible. Glassy forming materials have a high viscosity at their melting point and this high viscosity prevents the formation of an ordered structure.

Most of the glass formers are the metal oxides. Steel can be cast into glassy state if it is cooled very very rapidly. Due to the nature of the material and due to the technique in crystallisation process, the material during crystallisation undergoes incomplete or imperfect crystallisation and this leads to the formation of crystallites (which is also different from crystals), glasses or liquid crystals.

6 Eutectic Mixture

When a pure liquid such as water is cooled to form ice, the temperature remains constant until all the water taken has been converted into ice. You know the water is converted to ice at 0°C. Once the ice has started to form ice at this temperature (i.e 0° C), the temperature remains at 0°C until all the water taken has been converted into ice. The same fact is applied to boiling point also, that is, once the water reaches the boiling temperature, the temperature remains constant until all the water taken is converted to vapour state. At the boiling point, the vapour pressure above the boiling water is equal to the atmospheric pressure. This applies to any liquid. It can be inferred that by increasing or decreasing the pressure above a liquid, the boiling point of the liquid can be raised or lowered respectively.

The boiling point of water can also be raised by adding soluble solutes. This property is known as colligative property and it depends on the number of solute particles present. A solute molecule may constitute a particle. Sometimes two or more molecules may associate to form a single particle or a single molecule may dissociate to form two particles (eg: Sodium Chloride forms NH^+ and Cl^-. However it must be born in mind that the degree of association or dissociation may vary.)

When a pure substance such as water is cooled to transform it from liquid state to solid state, the slope of the curve obtained by plotting temperature versus time is continuous and the curve becomes horizontal (or reaches a plateau region). That is, from the start of formation of ice to the point where all the water has been converted to ice, the curve will be horizontal.

When a solution of solute in water is cooled, the slope of the curve is continuous and it becomes horizontal from the temperature point at which the solute begins to crystallize into a solid. The change of the slope (i.e of cooling curve) to horizontal plateau indicates the precipitation (i.e crystallisation) of one of the components (i.e of dissolved component, the solute)

However, when a binary solution is cooled, the formation of plateau indicates that both the components of the binary solution are coming out together as precipitate. The temperature at which both the components are coming out as precipitate is called as eutectic temperature (or eutectic point) and the composition of the two components is generally called the eutectic mixture or simply eutectic. At this eutectic point, the composition of the precipitate formed is the same as that of the solution from which it is precipitated or separated. Thus at this point both the components come out together in a constant proportion.

The eutectic mixture is not a chemical compound but it is an intimate physical mixture of constant proportion. This can be termed as a simple two phase mixture with a very fine grained structure and such a mixture imparts to it different properties such as better solubility than of a gross mixture of the same composition. Further explanation of this system is given under Phase Rule (page no.)

Complexes

A complex refers to a species formed by the interaction of two or more interacting molecules or ions. Some solutes may form some sort of structure within a solvent.

A solution of benzocaine in water forms a complex with caffeine and this complex shows a much reduced rate of hydrolysis. The drug chlorpromazine hydrochloride is light sensitive and it is decomposed in presence of light. The light stability of the drug in water solution is improved in the presence of saccharin. Complexation technique can also be used to prolong the action of a drug. For example, hydroxy-propyl β-cyclodextrin forms a complex with certain drugs which dissolves slowly in body fluids. See under complexation for more details.

Aerosols

Liquids obtained by liquefying the gases revert to the gaseous state when the pressure above the liquid is reduced i.e liquid molecules expand and revert to gaseous state. Aerosols are based on this simple principle of reversible change of state on the release of pressure.

In aerosols liquified gas (also called liquified gas propellant) i.e liquid propellant is sealed within an aerosol container with the product concentrate drug dissolved or suspended). Within the container, an equilibrium is quickly established between the gaseous propellant (occupying the space above the liquid in the container) and the liquid propellant. The gaseous propellant forming the vapour phase exerts pressure in all directions. If this pressure is reduced by pressing the aerosol valve (only a momentary reduction in pressure occurs), it will force the liquid up the dip tube in the aerosol container and out of the orifice of the valve into atmosphere. As a result, the product concentrate is sprayed as airborne liquid droplets in the case of drug in solution or as drug particles in the case of drug in suspension. As the liquid phase is expelled from the container, equilibrium is reestablished rapidly. Thus the pressure remains virtually constant until the liquid in the container is depleted.

Inhalalers: These are drugs or solutions of drugs that may be administered though the nasal or respiratory route. They are mainly administered for their local action on the bronchial tree and sometimes, they are used for their systemic effects through absorption from lungs. Ether is administered for its anaesthetic action. **Finely powdered drug substances and solutions of drugs are administered as fine mists.**

A number of drug substances are administered through what is called as inhalation aerosols. The instrument capable of producing fine particles for inhalation therapy is called nebuliser.

9. Humidity

It is important to know air-water vapour system i.e about the mixture of air and water vapour. The humidity of the air refers to the concentration of water vapour in air. In other words it refers to the moisture content of the air. Actual amount of water vapour present in a given quantity of dry air can be given in terms of humidity and there are different terms such as absolute humidity, saturation humidity and relative humidity (R.H.)

Absolute humidity in defined as the amount of water vapour in kg present in 1 kg of dry air. The saturation humidity is the absolute humidity at which the partial pressure of water vapour in the air equals the vapour pressure of pure bulk water at a particular temperature. The relative humidity is, however, the most familiar expression of moisture content in the air. It is usually expressed as the ratio of actual concentration of water vapour in the air to the saturation concentration of water vapour in the air under the same conditions of temperature and atmospheric pressure. Mathematically, it is expressed as

$$\text{R.H} = \frac{\text{Measured vapour pressure of water in air}}{\text{Saturation vapour pressure of water in air}} \times 100$$

$$\text{or, } \frac{\text{Absolute humidity}}{\text{Saturation humidity}} \times 100$$

Relative humidity is an important factor to be considered and controlled

1. in drying of pharmaceutical products

2. in air conditioning

3. in the manufacture and filling of hard gelatin capsules

4. in the stability study of pharmaceuticals under controlled conditions.

5. in the production of effercescent products.

Thermal Analysis

Many physical and chemical properties of matter are temperature dependent. Density, refractive index, surface tension etc. have significant temperature coefficients. But the measurement of these properties does not provide analytical information. However, there are certain other alterations in the physical and chemical properties produced by temperature changes. Thus the methods for characterising such alterations upon heating or cooling a sample of a material is referred to as thermal analysis.

The methods used to produce such alterations are differential scanning colorimetry (DSC), differential thermal analysis (DTA), thermogravimetric analysis (TGA) and thermomechanical analysis (TMA).

These methods have been used to characterise and identify compounds and to determine purity, polymorphism, solvent and moisture content, stability and compatibility with excipients. These methods are also used widely in pharmaceutical research and in quality control.

In these methods, the sample is heated under controlled conditions and the physical and chemical changes that occur are observed. The properties that are measured are the melting point, heat capacity, heats of reaction, kinetics of decomposition and changes in rheological properties.

Differential Thermal Analysis (DTA)

In DTA technique, phase transitions or chemical reactions can be followed by observing the heat absorbed or liberated. In actual practice, the temperature difference (ΔT) between the test sample and an inert reference material under controlled and identical conditions of heating or cooling is recorded continuously as a function of temperature.

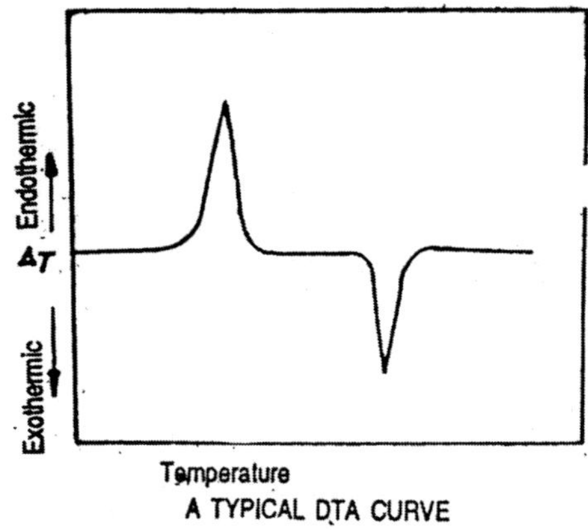

A TYPICAL DTA CURVE

Fig. 8

Fusion, changes in the crystalline state and other physical changes of the sample give up endothermic peaks. In endothermic change, the temperature of the sample lags behind the temperature of the reference since heat is absorbed during the transition. Once the transition is complete, the thermal diffusion brings the sample to zero ΔT, leaving behind a depression in the DTA curve. An elevation in the DTA curve is observed (for exothermic process). Certain chemical changes such as oxidation aided by oxygen show exothermic peaks. (Fig. 8)

In this apparatus, the thermocouples are placed in contact with an inert reference material and the sample. Both the sample and the reference material are heated by a common heat source at a constant rate. The reference does not change in any manner through the temperature range and the sample undergoes transition or thermally induced reaction during heating and this may be recorded as a peak or dip in an otherwise straight line.

Dual thermocouples are used to measure the differences in temperature between the sample and the reference material both of which heated in a furnace operated by a temperature programmer and controller (a constant heat rate). The outputs from the differential thermocouples are amplified and fed to a recorder as shown in Fig. 9.

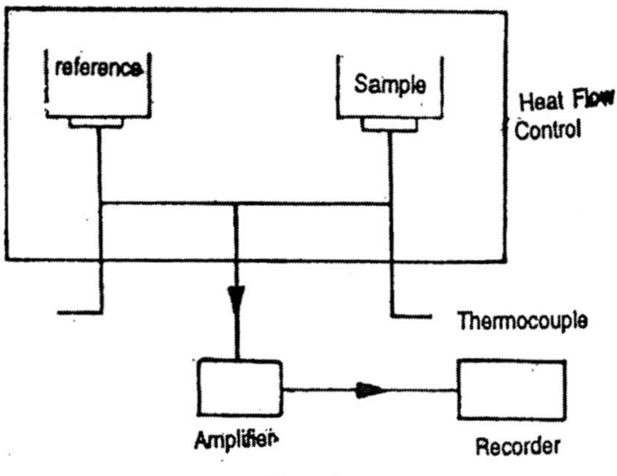

Fig. 9

Differential Scanning Colorimetry (DSC)

In DTA, the sample and the reference material are heated by a common heat source whereas in DSC, individual heaters are used.

The sample and the reference (with a higher melting point) are heated at a predetermined rate. A temperature difference exists when the sample undergoes melting (endothermic process). A second temperature circuit is used to overcome the temperature difference. Thus the temperatures are maintained for the sample and the reference at the same value. The difference in heat input to the sample and the reference per unit time is fed to a recorder and plotted as dH/dt versus the average temperature to which the sample and the reference are being raised. The differential heat input is recorded (Fig. 10) with a sensitivity of ± 0.1 millicalorie per second. The DSC operates with a temperature range of –175° to 725°C.

DSC is used to obtain heat capacities and heats of fusion, to prepare phase diagrams, to study the polymorph, and to carry out the kinetics of decomposition of solids. It has also been used in the standardisation of lyophilisation process and in the identification of eutectic formation in the frozen state.

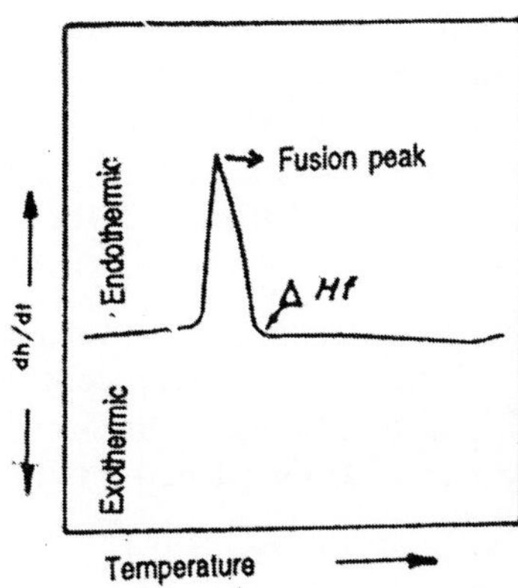

Fig. 10

Thermogravimetric analysis (TGA)

It consists of a recording thermobalance with a sensitivity of 0.1μg, a furnace and a recorder. It operates under low pressures of 10^{-4}mm to 760 mm Hg. It is used to follow the changes in hydrated salts.

The temperature of the sample and the corresponding weight are accurately and precisely noted continually. An automatic recorder is included in modern instruments. In this technique, the change in weight of a substance (sample) with temperature over a period of time is followed. The temperature is increased at a constant rate and the changes in weight are accurately recorded at different times. The weights are plotted against temperatures to obtain a curve (thermo- gravimetric curve or thermogram). (Fig. 11)

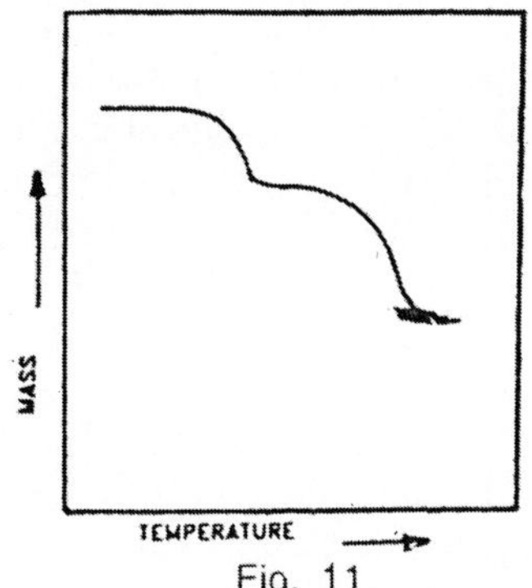

Fig. 11

Thermo Mechanical Analysis (TMA)

This instrument measures changes in mechanical properties (such as changes in viscoelastic properties and heat distortions such as shrinking).

Any physical change is converted into an electrical signal and fed into a recorder. The temperature may be programmed over a range from –150° to 700°C.

The apparatus serves also as a penetrometer, dilatometer, tensile tester over a wide range of temperatures at a predetermined rate.

II. PHASE EQUILIBRIA

Phase rule relates to the principles that govern the equilibria between solid, liquid and gas and is applicable to heterogenous systems.

1.1. Phase (*P*)

A ***phase*** may be defined as a homogeneous physically distinct part of a system separated from other parts of the system by bounding surfaces. Each of solid, liquid and gas forms a separate phase. Each of a liquid such as water, two miscible liquids together (eq. water and alcohol), or a solution (For example, sodium chloride in water) forms a single phase. A gas or mixture of gases forms a single phase.

Two immiscible liquids such as water and castor oil together form a two phase system as there exists a bounding surface between the two immiscible liquids. A system containing water and its vapour in equilibrium is a two phase system. Gas, liquid and solid together in a closed container or an equilibrium mixture of water, ice and vapour is a three-phase system. A liquid together with an insoluble solid is a two phase system.

1.2. Components (*C*)

The ***number of components*** of a system is the smallest number of independent chemical constituents necessary to represent the composition of all the phases present in the system.

In the case of an equilibrium mixture of ice, water and water vapour (a three phase system), all the phases can be expressed in terms of the chemical formula H_2O and hence it is a one component system. A solutic of salt in water is a two component system since it has two chemical species NaCl and H_2O and each of the chemical species is independent of the other.

1.3. Degrees of freedom (*F*)

The ***number of degrees of freedom*** is the minimum number of variables such as temperature, pressure and concentration that can be varied without changing the number of phases or components. In other words, it is the minimum number of variables that must be fixed to define a system completely. For example, to define a given mass of gas it is necessary to give any two of the variables volume, pressure, and temperature. That is, we should know any two of the variables to represent a given mass of gas. Therefore the system is said to have two degrees of freedom.

The relationship between the number of phases (*P*), the components (*C*), and the degrees of freedom (*F*), is given by the **Gibb's phase rule**

$$F = C - P + 2 \qquad \ldots (1)$$

Gibb's phase rule governs the number of intensive variables such as temperature, pressure, volume and concentration which can be varied in any equilibrium system without changing the number of phases (*P*) or the number of components (*C*) that will be present in the system.

Phase equilibria can be indicated by graphs called phase diagrams. It would require a three dimensional model to represent the simultaneous effect of three variables. However if one variable is fixed, ordinary planar diagram is enough to explain the effect of the other two variables.

2. One-component system

The ice, water, and water vapour system is a *typical one component system* and is represented by the chemical formula H_2O.

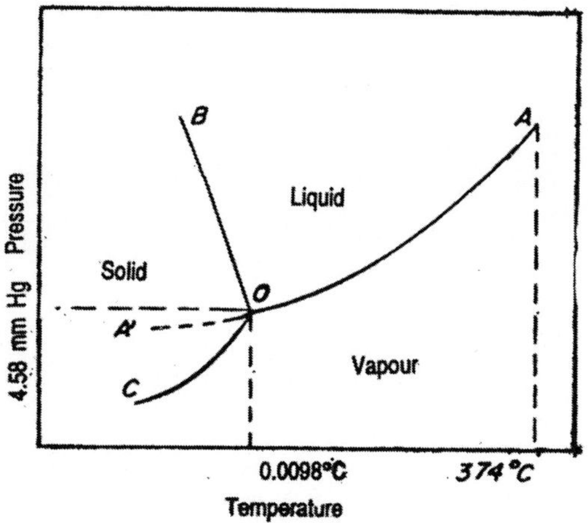

Fig. 12 Phase diagram of one component system

The following $P-T$ (Pressure Temperature) diagram (Fig. 12) represents a phase diagram for one component system of ice, water and water vapour

In the phase diagram, the curves OA, OB, and OC represent *vapour pressure curve (or boiling point curve), melting point curve and sublimation curve* respectively. The point at which these three curves meet is called **triple point.** At this point all the three phases co-exist. The temperature and pressure corresponding to this point are 0.0098°C and 4.58 mm of Hg respectively. On the curve *OC*, solid and vapour co-exist; on the curve *OB*; solid and liquid co-exist; and on the curve *OA*, liquid and vapour co-exist. The upper limit for the vapour pressure curve is at 374°C and it represents the ***critical temperature*** of water.

The area indicated in the diagram as solid, liquid or vapour corresponds to a single phase. The degree of freedom within any of these areas represented as solid, liquid or vapour phase is given by the phase rule

$$F = C - P + 2$$

$$F = 1 - 1 + 2 = 2$$

It means the temperature and pressure can be varied within these areas without any change of the existing phase (or appearance of any other phase). That is within the liquid (water) phase area, one can alter two variables pressure and temperature independently of each other without any change in the liquid phase i.e. without the appearance of any other phase such as vapour and/or solid ice. Conversely, it is not sufficient to state only the temperature *to define a given quantity of water at a point within the liquid area* but also the pressure. Therefore, we say that any of the phases represented as solid, liquid, or vapour within its respective region exhibits two degrees of freedom.

2.1. Boiling Point Curve

The curve *OA* is the boiling point curve or vapour pressure curve. It represents the co-existence of liquid water and water vapour in equilibrium under various temperatures and pressures. It gives the effect of pressure on the boiling point of water. That is, as the pressure is increased, the boiling point also increases. The upper limit is at the critical temperature of water. Above this critical temperature water and water vapour become indistinguishable.

The degree of freedom along the curve *OA* where two phases co-exist in equilibrium is given by

$$F = 1 - 2 + 2 = 1$$

Thus only one variable is required to be fixed or specified to define the system completely along the curve. For example, if we want to define the system in which liquid water and water vapour are in equilibrium at 100°C we need not mention the pressure because the vapour pressure at 100°C is 760 mm Hg and it can have no other value than 760 mm Hg. Or else, it is enough to state the liquid and vapour are in equilibrium at 760 mm Hg and we need not specify the temperature as it can have no other value than 100°C at 760mm Hg pressure.

Metastable Equilibrium: The vapour pressure curve *OA* terminates at *O*, when the liquid freezes. However, by careful cooling of the liquid below the freezing point without forming crystals, the liquid can be supercooled (curve *OA'*). This liquid is metastable, that is, a slight disturbance or addition of a seed crystal causes the entire liquid to solidify immediately.

2.2. Melting Point Curve

The curve *OB* is the melting point curve and it is also the freezing point curve. It represents the coexistence of liquid water and solid ice at equilibrium. It indicates the effect of pressure on the melting point of ice. That is the melting point decreases as the pressure is increased. This effect is represented by the negative slope of the line *OB*. Skatting on ice is possible because of this effect.

The degree of freedom along the curve *OB* where two phases (liquid water and solid ice) coexist in equilibrium is given by

$$F = 1 - 2 + 2 = 1$$

Thus, only one variable is required to be fixed to define the system along the curve. That is, in order to maintain equilibrium conditions between the two phases, the temperature and the pressure can not be varied independently of each other. If we change any one of the variables, the other variable also gets changed and hence there is only one degree of freedom.

2.3. Sublimation curve

The curve *OC* is termed sublimation curve and it represents the coexistence of solid ice and water vapour at equilibrium under various temperatures and pressures. It gives the effect of pressure on sublimation of solid ice directly into vapour.

2.4. Significance of Triple point

The three boundary lines between vapour and liquid *OA*, liquid and solid ice *OB*, and solid ice and vapour *OC*, meet at a point *O* where the three phases (solid ice, liquid water, and water vapour) coexist in equilibrium.

Applying the phase rule, the degree of freedom at the triple point '*O*' is given as

$$F = 1 - 3 + 2 = 0$$

The system having solid ice, liquid water, and water vapour in equilibrium has no degree of freedom. It is an invariant system. That is, the system can be defined by saying as ice, water and vapour in equilibrium. It indicates it can have only one temperature and one pressure. Any attempt to bring about a change in pressure or temperature will result in the disappearance of one or two of the phases and hence the system has no degree of freedom.

The triple point for water occurs at a temperature of 0.0098°C and a pressure of 4.58 mm Hg (or 610 N/m^2). The triple point temperature occurs at 0.0098°C above the normal freezing point of 0°C. This is due to the change in pressure from 760 mm Hg to 4.58 mm Hg. (This change in pressure produces a depression in the freezing point by 0.0075°C) and to the presence of dissolved air in water. (This dissolved air produces a further depression in the freezing point by 0.0023°C). Thus there is a total depression of freezing point by 0.0098°C (0.0075+0.0023)

This sublimation curve occurs below the triple point and it indicates that ice can be converted directly into vapour by supplying heat if pressure is kept below the triple point pressure. This transition of state from solid ice to water vapour is applicable in drying substances that are highly heat sensitive. Drying refers to removal of water and this removal of water by means of sublimation is termed **sublimation drying** or **freeze drying**. The other term used for freeze drying is **lyophilization.**

2.5. Polymorphism

When a substance exists in more than one crystalline form, it is said to exist in different polymorphic forms. Such a phenomenon is called **polymorphism**. When an element (such as sulphur and carbon) exists in different crystalline forms, then the phenomenon is termed *allotropy.*

One polymorphic (crystalline) form changes into another polymorphic (crystalline) form at a definite temperature. The temperature at which such a change occurs is termed as *transition temperature.* At transition temperature both the forms exist in equilibrium. Crystalline forms exhibiting this type of behaviour are said to be *enantiotropic.* For example rhombic sulphur (stable at ordinary temperature) is transformed into the monoclinic form at the transition temperature of 368.5°K. The transition can be reversed by cooling (that is monoclinic to rhombic). These enantiomorphs co-exist as separate phases and the number of degrees of freedom at equilibrium is restricted to one as in the case of melting point curve, boiling point curve or sublimation curve in one component system of water. Therefore this transition temperature is affected by pressure.

There are some substances in which one polymorphic form to another polymorphic form is like one-way traffic. That is transition occurs in one direction only and the reversion is not possible in a direct manner. Such substances exhibiting this type of polymorphism are called *monotropic.* For example diamond can be transformed directly into graphite but not the graphite into diamond.

The polymorphic changes between different forms of fatty acids and glycerides are generally monotropic. One such example is theobroma oil (otherwise called cocoa butter). It exists in four different polymorphic forms. They are metastable γ, α and β' forms and stable β form. Theobroma oil is used in the preparation of suppositories. During the preparation, one must be careful to preserve the stable β form which melts at 34.5°C. All the other forms γ, α and β' melt at 18°, 22°, and 24°C respectively. If the temperature is raised greatly above the melting point of stable β form, the stable form will be destroyed.

Polymorphism is possible in liquids also. For example cholesterol acetate exists as *clear* and *turbid* solution. These two polymorphic forms have different optical properties. The turbid form is termed as liquid crystals.

Different crystalline polymorphic forms have different solubilities and therapeutic effects because of difference in thermodynamic activities of the polymorphs and hence it is pharmaceutically important to take into consideration the properties of these different polymorphic forms during formulation of dosage forms. Some drug substances which exhibit polymorphism are novobiocin sodium, methyl prednisolone, sulphathiozole and chloramphenicol palmitate.

3. Two - component system

In the case of one component system, the maximum number of degrees of freedom is two whereas for a two component system, a maximum of three degrees of freedom is possible (temperature, pressure and concentration or composition).

The degrees of freedom in a two component system may be given with respect to number of phases as:

P	F
1	3
2	2
3	1
4	0

When only one phase is present in a two component system, there are three degrees of freedom (temperature, pressure and concentration). In order to represent the effect of these variables upon phase equilibrium of such a system, one would require a three dimensional model. In other words, the behaviour of a two component system may be represented completely only by a three dimensional diagram.

3.1. Condensed systems

We are only concerned with liquid and/or solid phases in most systems under consideration. Hence we can disregard the vapour phase and work under normal condition of one atmosphere. The system in which the vapour phase is disregarded and only solid and/or liquid phases are considered is termed condensed system. To represent such condensed systems it is enough to make use of planar figures on rectangular co-ordinate graph paper to show the relation between two of the variables while the third is kept constant. For example, we make use of diagrams showing the variation of pressure with concentration at constant temperature or the variation of concentration with temperature at constant pressure. Usually the variation of concentration with temperature is studied under constant pressure. Thus ***any system in which the vapour phase is disregarded is known as condensed system*** and in such cases, the reduced phase rule is often used and is given by

$$F' = C - P + 1 \quad \ldots (2)$$

3.2. Liquid - Liquid systems of two components

Liquid – liquid systems may be conveniently put into three types according to the degree of miscibility of two liquids with each other. They are:

1. Completely miscible liquids
2. Partially miscible liquids
3. Immiscible liquids.

A liquid-liquid system in which one liquid is miscible (or soluble) with the other in contact with their vapour forms a two phase system of two components Applying the phase rule, the degree of freedom of such a system will be two (2)

$$F = 2 - 2 + 2 = 2$$

To define such a system at equilibrium, two variables have to be fixed. The variables temperature and concentration must be fixed keeping the pressure constant or the variables pressure and concentration must be fixed keeping the temperature constant.

A liquid – liquid system in which each liquid is immiscible with the other in contact with their vapour in equilibrium forms a three phase system (liquid, liquid and vapour phases) of two components. Applying the phase rule the degree of freedom of such a system will be

$$F = 2 - 3 + 2 = 1$$

In this system, only one variable has to be fixed to define the system (either the pressure or temperature).

A liquid – liquid system in which one liquid is partially miscible with the other is phenol-water system. This system will be considered in some detail.

3.3. Phenol-water system

A condensed phase diagram for phenol-water system is shown (Fig. 13). The curve *gbhci* represents the boundary line between one liquid phase and two liquid phases. The area within the curve indicates a two phase system of two mutually saturated liquids and the area outside this curve shows a single phase system. The area within the curve *gbhci* (binodal curve) gives the limits of temperature and concentration within which two liquid phases co-exist in equilibrium.

The point '*h*' on the curve gives the critical solution temperature or upper consolute temperature. For phenol water system *the critical solution temperature is 66.8°C for a composition of 34.5% phenol in water.* All combinations of phenol and water above this temperature are completely miscible producing one phase liquid system and it indicates an increase in miscibility with rise in temperature. For phenol

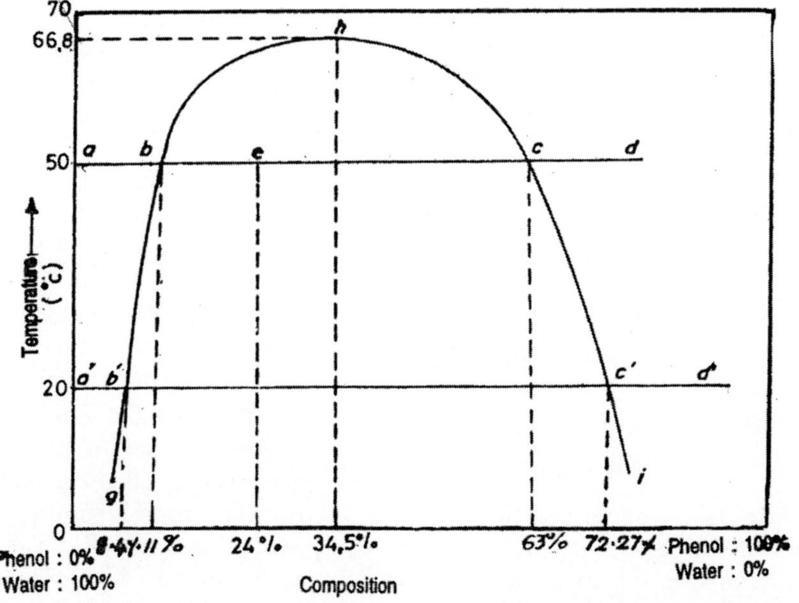

Fig. 13 Temperature composition diagram of Phenol-Water system

water system, the critical solution temperature occurs at a composition of 34.5% phenol in water. This means 34.5% phenol in water will remain separated into two layers (i.e. two phases) upto a higher temperature of 66.8°C.

By drawing a line *ad* (called the tie line) parallel to the abscissa at 50°C, we find that we can actually prepare two sets of single phase systems one containing 0 to 11% of phenol in water corresponding to *a* to *b* on the line *ad* and the other containing 63% of phenol in water and above corresponding to *c* to *d* on the line *ad*. The systems at different points on the line *ad* in between the point *b* (corresponding to 11% of phenol in water) and the point *c* (corresponding to 63% of phenol in water) will have two liquid phases (i.e. two conjugate phases) at equilibrium. Of these two phases, one phase will be water rich containing 11% of phenol (corresponding to the system at the point *b*) and the other phase will be phenol rich containing 63% of phenol (corresponding to the system at the point *c*). However, the proportion of phenol rich layer increases as one moves from point *b* to *c*. For example at the point corresponding to 20% phenol (on abscissa) at 50°C, there will be more of water rich layer than of phenol rich layer and at 50% phenol in water there will be more of phenol rich layer than of water-rich layer.

Outside *b* and *c*, there is only one liquid phase and applying the phase rule, the number of degrees of freedom will be given as

$$F = 2 - 1 + 2 = 3$$

For the condensed system, the number of degrees of freedom is (two) 2. This means temperature and concentration must be specified to define the system.

For the systems on the line between *b* and *c* where two phases coexist, the number of degrees of freedom is given as

$$F = 2 - 2 + 2 = 2$$

For the condensed system, the number of degrees of freedom is 1. Thus any system on the tie line between *b* and *c* is completely defined if the temperature is specified.

The relative proportion of the two conjugate phases may be calculated from such a tie line at any temperature and composition and also the amount of phenol present in each of the two phases.

If a tie line is drawn at 20°C parallel to the base line (abscissa), the percent of phenol corresponding to point *b′* will be 8.4. (8.4% of phenol in water) and the percent of phenol corresponding to the point *c′* will be 72.2 (72.2% of phenol in water). These two will form the two conjugate solutions on the tie line drawn at 20°C within the binodal curve.

Consider the tie line drawn at 50°C parallel to base line (abscissa). The composition and the amount of phenol present in each of the two phases corresponding to any point on the tie line between *b* and *c* can be calculated. For example, the composition of the two conjugate phases (one is water rich and the other is phenol rich) at the point *e* on the tie line may be given as

$$\frac{\text{Weight of water rich phase } (A)}{\text{Weight of phenol rich phase } (B)} = \frac{\text{length } ce}{\text{length } eb}$$

Instead of measuring the length '*ce*' and '*be*' it will be convenient to use percent weights of phenol given on the abscissa in the figure. In the figure, point *b* corresponds to 11%, the point *c* corresponds to 63% and the point *e* corresponds to 24%. Then the ratio *ce*/*eb* is given as

$$\frac{63-24}{24-11}=\frac{39}{13}=\frac{3}{1}=3:1$$

Suppose we prepare a mixture containing 24 grams of phenol and 76 grams of water (total 100 grams) and heat it to 50°C. Now we will have two conjugate solutions co-existing. As this mixture corresponds to point *e* on the tie line the phenol in the two conjugate phases will be 11% and 63%. As the proportion of these two conjugate solutions is 3:1 (already calculated) the proportion of *A* and *B* is 3:1 i.e. 75:25. The weight of phenol in phase *A* (i.e weight of phenol in water rich phase) will be

$$\frac{11}{100}\times 75 = 8.25 \text{ g}$$

and in phase *B* (i.e. weight of phenol in phenol rich phase) will be

$$\frac{63}{100}\times 25 = 15.75 \text{ g}$$

The total weight of phenol in both the phases *A* and *B* will be $8.25 + 15.75 = 24$ g of phenol. This is the amount of phenol originally added.

The phase diagram is useful in arriving at a solution containing a large proportion of phenol at ordinary room temperatures. Phenol in solution form is preferable in dispensing practice since phenol in solid form is difficult to handle (highly corrosive) and to weigh (deliquescent). Phenol being necrotic, it is convenient to handle in solution form. From the phase diagram, it may be arrived at that the most concentrated stock solution of phenol that remains as solution without the separation of phenol as crystals even at a temperature of around 3.5°C is 76% *w/w* of phenol in water equivalent to 80% *w/v*. It should be noted that the liquefied phenol USP contains 90% *w/w* of phenol in water and it freezes at 17°C.

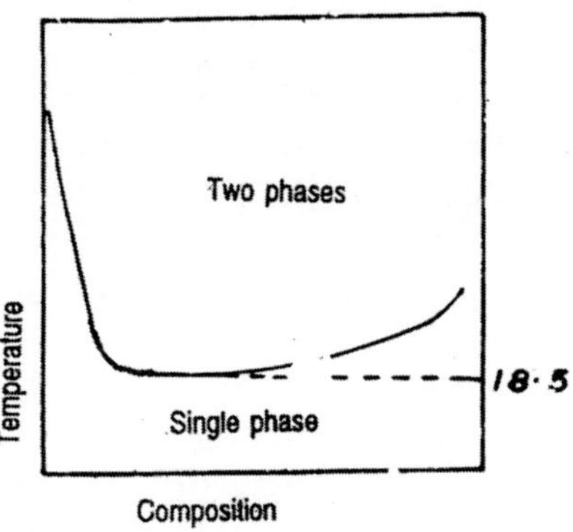

Fig. 14. Temperature composition diagram of triethanolamine-wate, system

Phenol has upper consolute temperature. But there are systems which have *louer consolute temperature (Fig. 14). Triethanolamine – water* is such a system which has lower consolute temperature. The two liquids are miscible in all proportions below this temperature. But above this temperature, two liquid phases exist.

Paraldehyde-water system also exhibits a lower critical solution temperature (or lower consolute temperature). Miscibility increases as the temperature is lowered.

In the preparation of paraldehyde enema (a solution of paraldehyde in normal saline) cooling produces rapid solution. Storage in a cool place is also em-

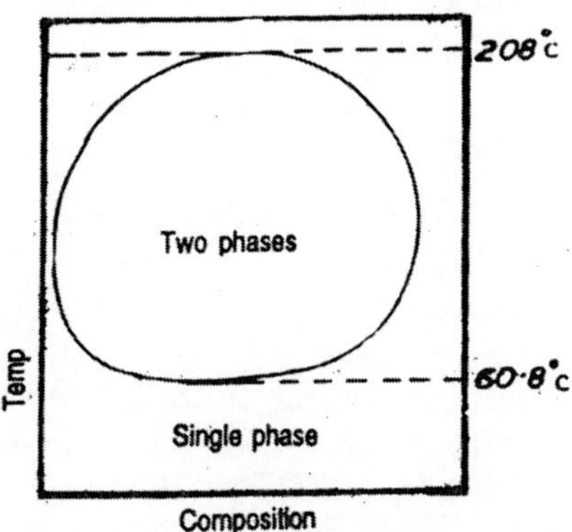

Fig. 15. Temperature composition diagram of nicotine-water system

phasized for this preparation. Thus, the effect of temperature is taken advantage of in the preparation of this enema. However, when this enema is administered, it should be warmed to the body temperature (37°C).

Some other systems show both upper and lower consolute temperatures. For example *nicotine – water system* shows *both upper and lower consolute temperatures* (Fig. 15). Between these two temperatures, the system is a two phase system. Above the upper consolute temperature and below the lower consolute temperature the nicotine and water mix with each other in all proportions.

3.4. Liquid-gas systems of two components

Liquid-gas system of two components is obtained when a saturated solution of a gas in a liquid is in equilibrium with the gas above the liquid. The solubility of the gas depends on the pressure and temperature under the condition of no reaction between the gas and the liquid.

The effect of pressure on solubility of a gas in a liquid at constant temperature is given by **Henry's law**

$$x = kp. \quad \ldots (3)$$

where x = mole fraction of dissolved gas

p = partial pressure of the gas above the solution

k = a constant called Henry's constant.

The effect of pressure is made use in the preparations of effervescent solutions containing carbon-dioxide. It should be borne in mind that carbon-dioxide reacts with water to form carbonic acid i.e. $CO_2 + H_2O \Leftrightarrow H_2CO_3$. In this case, the equilibrium is influenced by the solubility of carbon-di-oxide which in turn depends on pressure.

Henry's law applies mostly to systems at high temperatures and low pressures. The solubility of most gases in liquids is decreased with rise in temperature. This fact is taken advantage of in the preparation of carbon-dioxide free water by heating. Addition of electrolytes will also decrease the solubility of gases in liquids. This is called **salting out**. This occurs as a result of more attraction between electrolytes and water molecules than between gas and water molecules.

3.5. Solid-vapour system of two components

The pressure of water vapour in the atmosphere is about 13.33×10^2 N/m^2 at 293°K. A hydrated salt which exerts greater vapour pressure than this will tend to lose water to form a lower hydrate or an anhydrous salt. This phenomenon is called *efflorescence*. For example, hexahydrated sodium carbonate will tend to lose its water of crystallisation to form the monohydrate. As this monohydrate still exerts a greater vapour pressure, it tends to form the anhydrons salt. However further apparent loss of water does not take place as the anhydrous form which exerts a lower vapour pressure gets hydrated instantly and hence there exists an equilibrium between the monohydrate and the anhydrous form of sodium carbonate.

The rate of efflorescence can be enhanced by heating. Acceleration of the rate of efflorescence by raising the temperature to get rid of water of crystallisation from a hydrated salt is termed *exsiccation*. For example anhydrous form of copper sulphate ($CuSO_4$) may be obtained by this process.

$$CuSO_4 \cdot 5H_2O \xrightarrow{303°K}$$

$$CuSO_4 \cdot 3H_2O \xrightarrow{373°K}$$

$$CuSO_4 \cdot H_2O \xrightarrow{473°K} CuSO_4 \text{ (anhydrous)}$$

3.6. Deliquescence and Hygroscopicity

Certain substances take up water vapour from the atmosphere and become hydrated. A *hygroscopic* substance is one which takes up water but remains in the same physical state whereas a deliquescent substance which will, after taking up water, eventually form a liquid phase. In both the cases, the hydrated forms must still exert a lower vapour pressure than that of the water vapour in the surrounding atmosphere. Otherwise, (i.e., if it exerts greater vapour pressure), it will lose water by efflorescence.

Some hygroscopic substances are *exsiccated sodium sulphate, ammonium chloride* etc. Deliquescent substances include *potassium hydroxide, sodium lactate, potassium carbonate etc.*

Semisolids such as wool fat and liquids such as glycerin are hygroscopic.

In storing the efflorescent, deliquescent and hygroscopic substances, a moisture free atmosphere within the container must be ensured. Hence they must be stored in well closed containers that will prevent the access of water vapour. A further protection may be obtained by including a drying agent which takes up moisture in preference to the material. Silica gel is often used for this purpose. Whether the drying agent has been saturated with moisture (i.e. it can act no more as a drying agent) can be known by including an*hydrous cobaltous chloride*. The cobaltous chloride which is *blue* in colour turns *pink* when the silica gel has taken up (adsorbed) maximum amount of water vapour it can. Thus, the pink colour shows that it can no longer act as drying agent.

3.7. Solid-liquid system of two components

As the solids and liquids are practically incompressible, the effect of pressure on solid-liquid system is expressed by the reduced phase rule in which the vapour phase is disregarded.

$$F' = C - P + 1$$

The behaviour of two components solid-liquid system may be given as follows.

1. Systems that show the formation of eutectic mixture.
2. Systems that produce a compound with a *congruent melting* point (i.e. a compound in which one of the components is solvated by the other). The composition of the compound remains unaltered in the liquid obtained by melting.
3. Systems that produce a compound with an *incongruent melting* point. This compound yields a liquid and a new solid phase on melting. The composition of the new solid phase is different from that of the original compound.

We will consider only the first system which produces eutectic mixture as it is pharmaceutically significant.

Formation of Eutectic Mixtures

eg: Ice-potassium chloride system.

The behavior of the above system is represented by a phase diagram as shown in Fig. 16.

In this the point A represents the melting point of ice and the point B represents the melting point of potassium chloride. Curve AC indicates that the freezing point of water is depressed

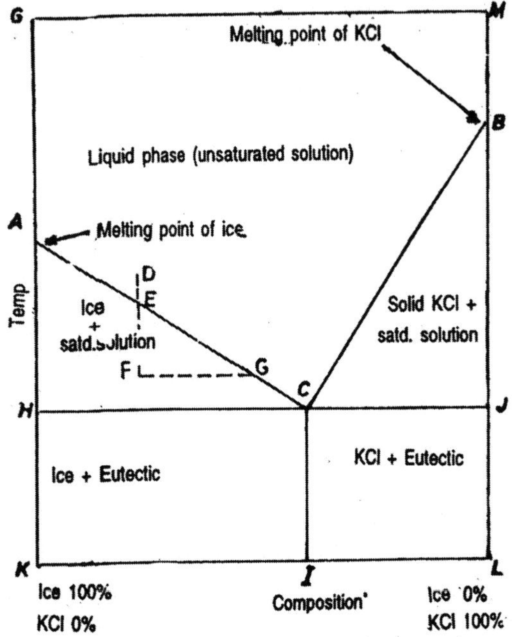

Fig. 16. Temperature-composition diagram for KCl-water system

gradually as the concentration of potassium chloride increases in water. Curve *BC* indicates that the melting point (or freezing point) of potassium chloride is depressed gradually as the amount of water increases in the potassium chloride solution. Thus the curve *AC* represents the effect of potassium chloride on temperature at which ice separates from the system. The curve *BC* represents the effect of ice on temperature at which solid KCl separates from the system.

The point *C* is the critical point at which both the solid components separate which will be in equilibrium with a liquid of definite composition. The system is invariant at point *C* since there is no degree of freedom. Applying the reduced phase rule

$$F = C - P + 1$$

$$= 2 - 3 + 1 = 0$$

In this, the components (*C*) are two, i.e., KCl and water, and the phases (*P*) are three, i.e., *solid KCl, solid ice,* and *the solution*. The reduced phase rule is applied since its vapour phase is not taken into account.

To understand the system better, take a point *D* on the diagram which represents a solution of KCl in water of known composition. On cooling the system to the point 'E' on the freezing point curve *AC*, some ice will separate out.

Further cooling to the point '*F*' will produce more ice and the remaining solution will become more concentrated since it will contain all the original KCl. The composition of '*F*' will correspond to the point '*G*'. Thus as the temperature falls, the composition of the remaining liquid moves along AC. A limit is reached when the remaining solution is saturated with KCl. On colling this solution further below the critical temperature, ice and KCl separate out together in the same ratio in which they exist in the saturated solution and the temparature remains constant at '*H*' (called eutectic temparature which is less than the melting point of the component having the less melting point) until all the saturated solution is solidified having the composition corresponding to the point *I* (i.e., ***eutectic composition***).

Although the eutectic has a definite melting point, the following evidence suggests that it is only a mechanical mixture.

(a) the component can be separated mechanically
(b) addition of each component raises the melting point of eutectic
(c) a heterogeneous structure can be seen under a microscope
(d) X-ray analysis reveals the existence of two phases.

The various parts of the diagram can be summarised as follows:

- Area *NACBM* indicates liquids phase of unsaturated solution
- Area *ACH* indicates ice + saturated solution
- Area *BCJ* indicates solid KCl + saturated solution
- The point *C* indicates eutectic point
- The point *H* or *J* indicates eutectic temperature which is less than melting point of the component having the lower melting point
- The point *I* indicates eutectic composition
- Just below the temparature point *H* on the line *CI*, eutectic solid will be formed immediately
- The line *CI* indicates only eutectic mixture
- The area *HCIK* indicates eutectic + solid ice
- The area *CJLI* indicates eutectic + solid KCl

Mixture of ice and salt will give a freezing mixture to generate tamparature as low as – 15°C (very much below the freezing point of water). The effect of freezing mixture can be explained as follows:

Adding salt to ice and a little water, some of the salt will dissolve in water to give a system composed of ice, salt and solution. Such a system will be stable only at eutectic point. The system therefore tends to move towards this point and ice will melt and the salt will continue to dissolve in water. Both of these processes are accompanied by absorption of heat and the temperature therefore falls until one of the solid components has been used up completely. By choosing suitable proportions of ice and salt, eutectic temperature will be reached. Mixtures of any two of the substances such as *camphor, salol, chloral hydrate, thymol, menthol* and *beta naphthol* form similar eutectic mixtures.

Substances forming eutectic mixture produce a solution on mixing. In order to dispense such substances in a dry powder form, it is necessary to add an absorbent powder such as kaolin or light magnesium oxide or carbonate.

True phemaceutical examples of eutectic formation are with aspirin - acetaminophen (37% and 63% respectively) and urea - acetaminophen (46% and 54% respectively) mixtures. They are rapidly soluble.

3.8. Solid dispersion

Eutectic mixtures are considered to be solid dispersions. Another group of solid dispersions is the solid solution. It is a solid solute dissolved in a solid solvent to give mixed crystals.

Solid dispersion is a technique by which the dissolution of poorly soluble drugs can be enhanced. Solid dispersion of a drug is usually fomed with a freely soluble substance (carrier substance) such as urea. The increase in dissolution rate is attributed to reduction in particle size, increase in wettability, reduced aggregation and agglomeration in the pressence of water soluble carrier substance such as urea, povidone etc.

A solid dispersion of a poorly soluble drug may be prepared by distributing the drug throughout a soluble solid carrier. This may be achieved either by melting the drug and the carrier substance together and then stirring to cool to a solid dispersion or by dissolving the drug and the carrier substance in a common solvent for both the solids and then evaporating the solution to co-precipitate the drug and the carrier. Sometimes, a combination of the two methods is used. Some carrier substances which are freely soluble in water are *polyethylene glycol 4000, urea, dextrose, succinic acid, and povidone (polyvinyl pyrrolidone, PVP).*

4. Phase equilibria in three component system

For a system containing three components but only one phase, the number of degrees of freedom may be given as

$$F = 3 - 1 + 2 = 4$$

The four degrees of freedom are the variables temperature, pressure, and two concentrations i.e. concentrations of two of the three components. The concentration of the third component may be obtained by subtracting the sum of the two concentrations from the sum of the three concentrations. For example, if we have three components *A*, *B* and *C*, it is enough to give the concentrations of any of these two (*A* and *B*, *B* and *C*, or *C* and *A*) and the third concentration can be obtained from the sum of the two and total concentration. If we disregard the vapour phase, the system becomes a condensed system and the number of degrees of freedom is 3 instead of 4. Again, if we consider the system at constant temperature, F becomes 2. In such circumstances, we can make use of a planar diagram to explain the phase equilibria. The system being a three component system, it will be appropriate to use triangular co-ordinate graph paper instead of rectangular coordinate graph paper.

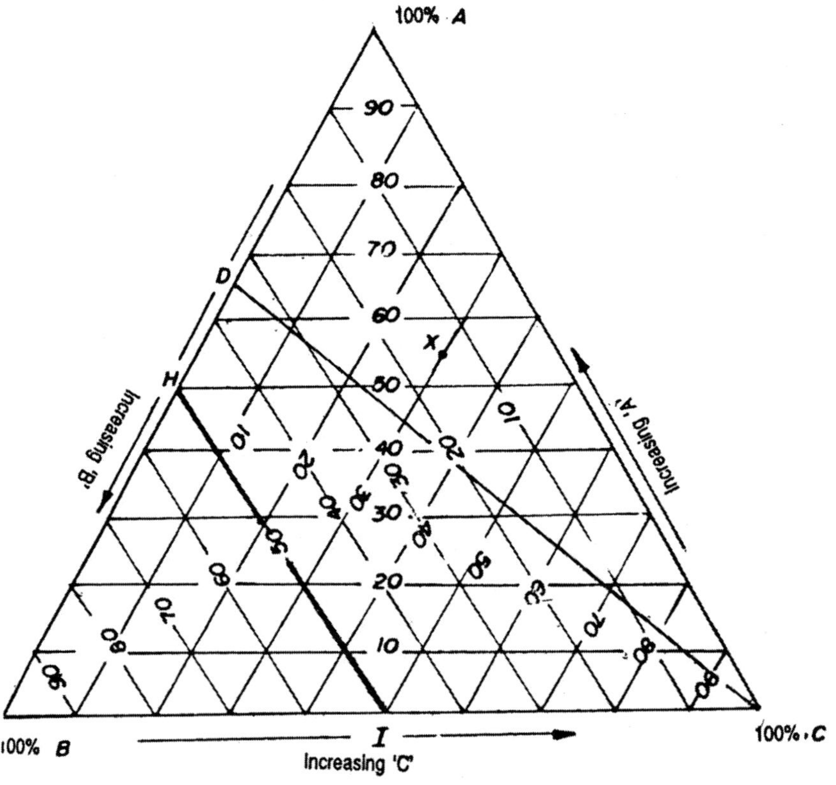

Fig. 17. Triangle diagram for a three component system

It is necessary for the student to become familiar with certain rules relating the use of triangular coordinates before we discuss the phase equilibria in ternary systems. It is convenient to **express concentrations of the components in** terms of W/W as it **facilitates expressions** in terms of mole **fraction and** molality.

The rules relating the triangular coordinates may be given with reference to Fig. 17.

1. Each corner of the triangle represents 100% by weight of one of the components and 0% by weight of the two other components. For example, considering three components *A*, *B*, and *C* if one apex represents 100% of *A*, then the same apex represents 0% of *B* and *C*. The top apex in the figure represents 100% of *A* and 0% of *B* and *C*. In the figure, three apexes are the three corners of the triangle and they are represented as *A*, *B*, and *C*.
2. The line joining the corner points *A* and *B* represents a two component system of *A* and *B*, the line joining *B* and *C*, the two component system of *B* and *C* and the line joining *A* and *C*, the two component system of *A* and *C*. As we move from *A* to *B*, the concentrations of *A* will be decreasing and the concentrations of *B* will be increasing. The center point on the line represents a 50:50 concentrations of *A* and *B*. The same explanation applies if one moves along *BC* from *B* to *C* and along *AC* from *A* to *C*.
3. The region within the triangle represents all the possible combinations of *A*, *B* and *C*. For example, if we consider the point x within the region, the point x gives the concentration of *A* as 55% and *C* as 30%. Then the concentration *B* will be $100 - (55 + 30) = 15\%$
4. If a line is drawn through any apex to a point on the opposite side, all the systems represented by points on the line will have a constant ratio of two components. For example, if a line is drawn from the corner *C* to the opposite side *AB*, systems corresponding to different points on the line will have a constant proportion of *A* and *B* and increasing concentrations of *C* as one proceeds on the line towards the corner *C*. We notice the ratio of *A* and *B* is constant and identical to that existing in the original mixture on the line *AB* at the point *D* and on moving from point *D* to *C* along the line *DC*, the amount of *A* and *B* will be decreasing and the amount of *C* will be increasing. Though the amount of *A* and *B* is decreasing, the ratio of *A* and *B* corresponding to the point *D* remains constant along the line.
5. When a line is drawn parallel to any one side of the triangle, we have varying concentrations of two components and a fixed concentration of the other component. For example, if a line *HI* is drawn parallel to the line *AC*, the concentration of *B* is constant along the line but the concentrations of *A* and *C* will be varying.

4.1. Ternary systems with one pair of partially miscible liquids and the temperature effect

A ternary system consisting of three components benzene, water and alcohol is shown in Fig. 18.

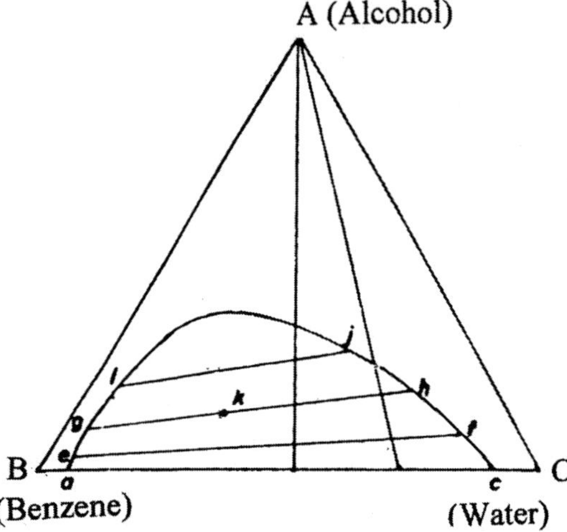

Fig. 18. A system of three liquids with one pair of partially miscible liquids

Each of the corners indicated as *A*, *B* and *C* represent alcohol, benzene, and water respectively. Of these three, the alcohol is completely miscible with water and benzene and water form partially miscible liquids with benzene. The alcohol added to the binary liquid phases (benzene and water) acts in a similar manner as that of temperature in the case of phenol – water system. Alcohol produces a solvent effect in the place of temperature bringing about miscibility as the concentration of alcohol is increased.

By gradually increasing the amounts of alcohol added to this binary system corresponding to the line *BC*, we reach a point and above this point we observe a single phase system. That is, as the amount of alcohol added is increased, the mutual solubility (or miscibility) increases and finally we reach the region with one liquid phase.

The line *BC* represents a binary mixture of *B* and *C* along the line and the point *a* is the limit of solubility of *B* in *C* and the point *c* is the limit of solubility of *C* in *B* at the particular temperature used. Between *a* and *c* we have two conjugate solutions i.e. *B* in *C* (i.e. a saturated solution of *B* in *C*) and *C* in *B* (a saturated solution of *C* in *B*) corresponding to point *c*.

If the temperature is fixed i.e. at isothermal conditions, the number of degrees of freedom reduces to 2. We need to specify only two concentrations. This means we have to fix two concentrations in order to define a particular system outside the binodal curve.

The curve *aegijhfc* is termed the binodal curve or simply binodal. Within the region of this binodal curve, two phase system exists and outside the binodal curve a single phase system exists. The tie lines drawn within the binodal curve are not parallel to the base line (abscissa) and this is due to the shape of the binodal curve which in turn actually depends on the relative solubility of alcohol in the other components benzene and water. The binodal curve will be perfectly symmetric and the tie lines parallel to the base line when the third component produces equal solubility effect on the other two components.

The relative amounts by weight of the two conjugate phases of a system at a particular point on the tie line depends on the position of the system on the tie line. The composition of the two conjugate solutions along the tie line *gh* are denoted by the points *g* and *h*. The ratio of the two conjugate phases at a point (for example at the point *K*) on the tie line and also the amount of one of the two liquids in the two conjugate solutions can be obtained as has been discussed under *phenol water system*.

The number of degrees of freedom considering it as a condensed system outside the binodal curve where the liquid phase exists is given by

$$F' = C - P + 1$$

$$F' = 3 - 1 + 1 = 3$$

4.2. Temperature effect on the miscibility of one pair of partially miscible liquids in a ternary system

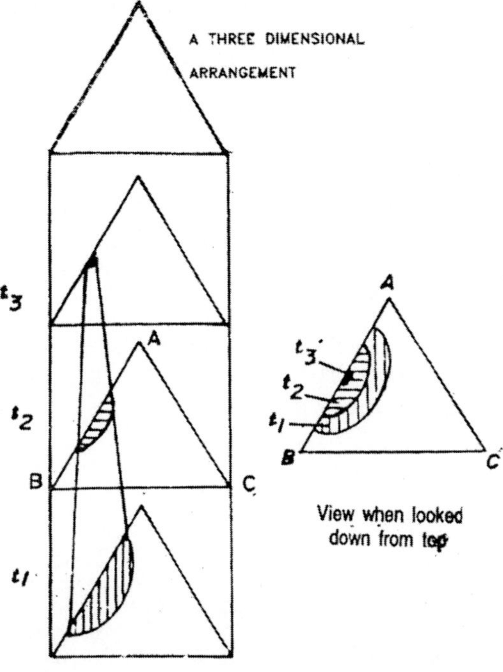

Fig. 19: Temperature effect on the miscibility of one pair of partially miscible liquids

The figure shown under benzene, alcohol, and water system gives the phase equilibria under isothermal conditions for the three component system. Changes in temperature produce changes in miscibility of benzene and water. This means the area bounded by the binodal curve may increase on decreasing the temperature or decrease on increasing the temperature.

Thus there is a gradual decrease in the area of binodal as the temperature is being increased. Ultimately there occurs complete miscibility and the binodal curve vanishes. In order to represent such an effect, a triangular prism (three dimensional figure) may be used. The figure (Fig. 19) shows that as the temperature is raised, there is gradual decrease in the shaded area (shaded area indicates the binary system) containing one pair of partially miscible liquids, *A* and *B*. Finally the binodal vanishes producing a homogeneous single phase system.

4.3. Ternary systems with two pairs of partially miscible liquids and the temperature effect

When two pairs of partially miscible liquids are produced, we have two binodal curves. For example, in the case of liquids *A*, *B* and *C*, suppose two pairs of partially miscible liquids between *B* and *C* and *C* and *A* are formed. This means *A* and *B* are completely miscible in all proportions at the temperature being considered. This may be represented in Fig. 20.

On increasing the temperature, the area of binodal curve decreases and may be represented in the Fig.20-A

When the temperature is reduced, the areas of two binodal curves gradual-

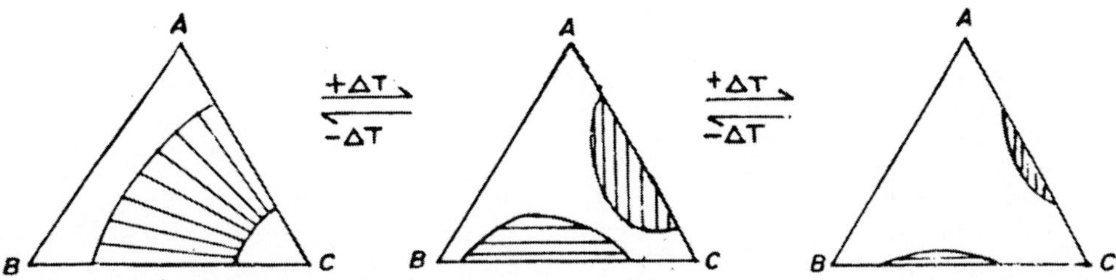

Fig. 20. Temperature effect on the miscibility of two pairs of partially miscible liquids

ly expand and merge at a significantly low temperature and this effect is shown in Fig. 20-B.

4.4. Temperature effect on the miscibility of three pairs of partially miscible liquids in a ternary system

When three pairs of partially miscible liquids are produced. We have three binodal curves. Suppose three pairs of liquids are produced with three liquids *A*, *B* and *C*. Then the three pairs of partially miscible liquids would be *A* and *B*, *B* and *C* and *C* and *A*. This may be represented in Fig. 21.

When the temperature is increased, the area of binodal curves shrink as shown in Fig 21. On further heating, all the shrunk binodal curve would disappear.

On the other hand, if the temperature is reduced, we observe the areas of binodal curve expand and ultimately meet yielding a central region. This effect may be represented as shown in Fig. 21. The central region is triangular and it yields three conjugate liquid phases in equilibrium. Within this area, under isothermal conditions for a condensed system, the number of degrees of freedom is zero. (i.e. $F = 0$). The composition of the three conjugate liquid phases is given by the points x, y and z as shown in Fig. 21.

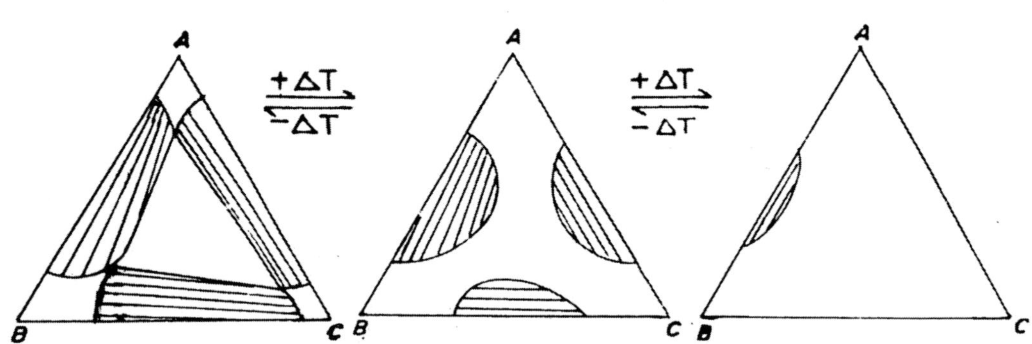

Fig. 21. Temperature effect on the miscibility of three pairs of partially miscible liquids

III. THERMODYNAMICS

Thermodynamics deals with the transformation of heat into other forms of energy such as mechanical, chemical, electric and radiant energy and vice versa. It concerns with the changes in energy that occur when a system undergoes transformation and it is the quantitative treatment of the equilibrium state of the various forms of energy rather than the kinetics of heat flow.

Thermodynamics does not delve into atomic nature of matter under consideration but it deals with macroscopic observable properties of matter like pressure, volume, temperature, etc and it is a subject of general applicability and immense reliability. Since energy changes are involved in *solution, diffusion, complexation, interfacial phenomena, kinetics etc*, thermodynamic principles have been applied to understand those processes and also to derive various equations relating temperature, vapour pressure and heat of vapourisation and solution processes.

The various forms of energy are considered to be a product of ***intensity factor*** which does not depend on the quantity of the material and ***capacity factor*** which is dependent on the quantity of the material.

Energy	Intensity factor (Intensive property)	Capacity factor (Extensive property)
Heat energy $T\Delta S$	temperature $T°$ (deg)	entropy change ΔS (cal/deg)
Surface energy $\gamma\Delta A$	Surface tension γ (dynes/cm^2)	Area ΔA (cm^2)
Chemical energy μn	Chemical potential μ (Cal/mole)	number of moles (n)
Expansion (mechanical energy) PV	Pressure P (dynes/cm^2)	Volume change V (cm^3)

1. First law of Thermodynamics

The first law refers to conservation of energy. That is, the total energy of a system and its surroundings remains constant during any operation. When one form of energy disappears an equal amount of another form of energy must appear and hence, various forms of energy are equivalent.

The first law of thermodynamics may be expressed mathematically as

$$Q = \Delta E + W \qquad \text{... (1)}$$

Consider a gas inside a cylinder fitted with a movable frictionless, non-conducting piston (P). Let the cylinder be thermally insulated except the bottom. When the gas inside the cylinder is heated with a burner, a part of the heat is used up in increasing the

energy is increased) and the remaining heat energy in lifting the piston (i.e. in doing work) because of expansion of the gas.

If Q is the heat energy supplied to the gas, ΔE, the increase in internal energy and W, the work done by the system, then,

$$Q = \Delta E + W$$

It has been already stated that thermodynamics concerns with the changes in energy and considering the changes in internal energy, the finite change in internal energy can be written as

$$\Delta E = E_2 - E_1$$

Where E_2 indicates the internal energy of the system in its final state and E_1, the energy in its initial state.

Internal energy is the total energy a substance possesses as a result of the presence of molecules and atoms and their translational, rotational and vibrational motions, as well as the attractions and repulsions between each atomic part of the substance. Although the total absolute internal energy of any substance can not be calculated, the amount of energy relative to arbitrarily selected reference conditions can be calculated. The internal energy E of a system is a state property and depends only on the conditions of temperature and pressure.

For a finite increase in internal energy ΔE, the first law is written as

$$\Delta E = Q - W$$

It is customary in writing the first law to give *heat input a positive quantity* (+ Q) *and work output a negative quantity* (– W). *Conversely, the heat output is given a negative quantity.* (– Q) *and the work input a positive quantity* (+ W).

1.1. Thermodynamic property

A thermodynamic state refers to a condition in which the measurable (or variable) properties such as pressure, volume and temperature have a definite value. The variables of a thermodynamic state are known as thermodynamic properties. E, V, P and T are all thermodynamic properties. A thermodynamic property depends on the initial and final conditions and not on the manner it is varied.

For an infinitesimal increase in the internal energy dE, the first law of thermodynamics is written as

$$dE = q - w$$

$$\text{or } dE = \delta q - \delta w \qquad \text{... (2)}$$

Where dE is the differential change in the internal energy, δq is the differential change in absorbed heat and δw is the differential change in the work expended.

Consider a system where a change in internal energy occurs and it goes from a state A to a state B. Thus, it is given as

$$\Delta E = \int_A^B dE \qquad \text{... (3)}$$

From the equation it is observed that the internal energy is a state function. It implies that the change in internal energy is dependent only upon the initial and final states and is not dependent on the manner or way the change was brought about*. The **Carnot cycle** discussed under heat engine is a cyclic change. Thus the differential change in internal energy is an ***exact differential.***

From the first law, it is understood that the change in internal energy is related to heat flow and work done. In contrast to the internal energy, the differential change in heat or work is

* Since the energy does not depend on the path taken, it may be said that there is no change in the energy for any system that undergoes a cyclic change i.e. $\oint dE = 0$. This fact is used in calculating changes in the properties of the system that is involved in a cyclic change.

not exact differential. That is, heat and work are ***inexact differentials*** and they are not state functions because their differentials do not depend on the manner the change is brought about.

Considering a change in going from state '*A*' to state '*B*', in the case of heat or work, the change will depend on the path taken from going form state '*A*' to '*B*'. This implies that heat or work may be determined only if more information is available on the manner in which the change in the system was brought about.

The types of work are mechanical (force × distance), gravitational (gravitational potential × mass), electrical (potential difference × quantity of electricity or charge), surface energy (surface tension × area increase) and the volume of expansion (pressure × volume) which is discussed in this chapter elaborately.

1.2. System

A system is that part of the universe which is under consideration and is separated from the surroundings by a boundary. A boundary separates the system from its surroundings and it may be movable allowing changes in the volume of the system or rigid restricting the system to a specified volume.

Closed, open, and isolated systems

A ***closed system*** is one that may exchange *heat and work and not matter* with its surroundings. An ***open system*** refers to a system in which there is an *exchange of heat, work and matter with its surroundings.*

Consider a closed container consisting of two immiscible solvents in which iodine is distributed. If this, as a whole, is considered it is a closed system because this system can exchange only heat and work with its surroundings. If only one of the two immiscible solvents (phases) is considered as a system, the system is open as it exchanges iodine (matter) with the other phase. In this case the other phase itself becomes the surrounding.

In the figures (Fig. 22 and 23) shown, if both the carbontetrachloride (organic phase) and the water (aqueous phase) are together considered as a system, there is no exchange of matter (iodine) with the surrounding and hence it is a *closed system.* (Fig. 23). If CCl_4 (carbon tetrachloride) alone is considered as a system, there is exchange of matter (i.e. iodine) with the aqueous phase water and hence it is an open system. (Fig. 22)

A system and its surrounding put together is an **isolated system** and the boundary between the system and the surrounding may be diathermal that allows free exchange of heat. Conversely, the isolated system as a whole is adiabatic where no heat flow is allowed.

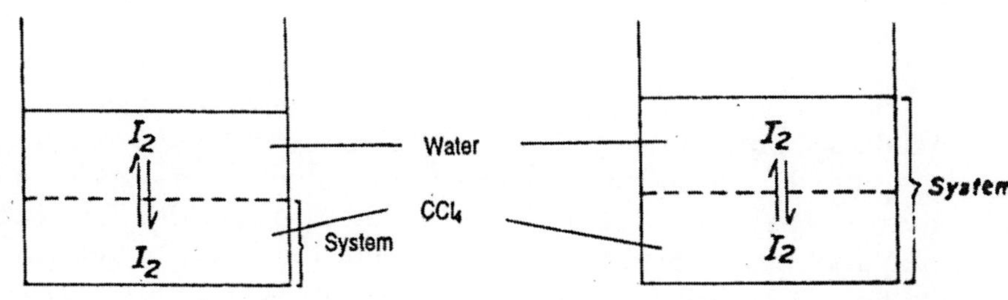

Fig. 22. Open system

Fig. 23. Closed system

1.3. Isothermal and Adiabatic Processes

If a process is conducted in a system which is kept under constant temperature, the process is said to be conducted *isothermally*.

An isothermal process may be carried out by placing the system under consideration in a large constant temperature bath so that heat is drawn from or returned to it without affecting the temperature significantly

When a process is conducted in a system in such a manner that no heat enters or leaves the system, it is said to occur adiabatically. Thus, a reaction that is carried out inside a vessel that is thermally insulated so that no heat enters or leaves, is said to be ***adiabatic.*** In an adiabatic process, $Q = 0$

The first law under adiabatic conditions, can be written as

$$dE = q - w$$

$$dE = 0 - w$$

$$dE = -w$$

$$\text{or,} \quad -dE = w \qquad \dots (5)$$

When work is done by the system adiabatically, the internal energy decreases and hence the temperature falls. Under this condition the work done becomes a thermodynamic property that is dependent on the initial and final states of the system.

Adiabatic process may also be brought about, though not so efficiently, by conducting the process at a greater speed so that sufficient time is not available for the system to attain thermal equilibrium with the surrounding by exchange of heat.

1.4. Reversible process

In a system if the *mechanical process* is reversed, the *thermal process* also gets reversed and the system is restored to its initial state, then, it is called a ***reversible process.***

Thus a system that has been displaced from equilibrium very slightly by an infinitesimal force (may be pressure) may be restored to its original state of equilibrium by applying infinitesimal force (pressure) in the opposite direction.

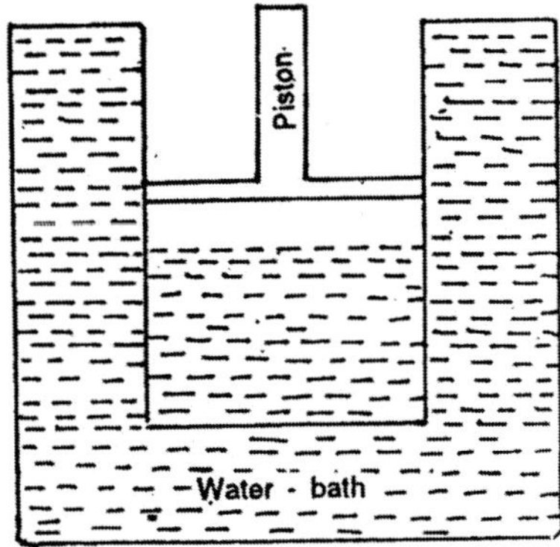

Fig. 24. Reversible process (Representation)

Consider a *hypothetic case* of water in equilibrium with its vapour in a cylinder fitted with a frictionless and weightless piston (Fig. 23). Let the whole system is placed in a constant temperature bath maintained at the same temperature as the water contained in the cylinder. Now, if the external pressure is decreased minutely, the volume of the system (above the water) increases and as a result vapour pressure falls. In order to reestablish the equilibrium vapour pressure, some water evaporates by extracting heat from the bath. In the same way if the external pressure is increased minutely, the system gets compressed (i.e. volume decreases) and the vapour pressure rises. To reestablish the equilibrium vapour pressure, some of the vapour condenses to water giving back the liberated heat which is absorbed by the constant temperature bath. Thus, this process is always in a state of *virtual thermodynamic equilibrium* being reversed by an infinitesimal change of pressure and such a process is said to be reversible.

The process cannot be reversible if the pressure is increased or decreased rapidly or if the temperature of the bath cannot adjust instantaneously to the changes in the system.

The concept of a reversible process used in a thermodynamic sense is quite different from that of a reversible reaction in the kinetic sense. In kinetic sense, a certain time after the reaction has started the rates of forward and reverse reactions become equal and a state of chemical equilibrium sets in. Whereas in thermodynamic sense, the rate of forward reaction should differ from that of the reverse reaction by an infinitely small amount and consequently, the process as a whole should proceed infinitely slowly. In other words if a system is displaced from equilibrium by some small vanishing force, equilibrium may be restored by applying an equal force in the opposite direction.

1.5. Maximum work

No work is done when an ideal gas expands into vacuum where the pressure is zero. Hence any work done depends on the external pressure. Therefore, as the external pressure becomes greater, the system does more work. The work done will be maximum when the external pressure is infinitesimally less than the pressure of the gas. Such a condition indicates the process is reversible. Therefore, when a system in an isothermal process does work reversibly, the work done is maximum.

1.6. Work of expansion against a constant pressure

Consider a *hypothetic case* of a given mass of gas enclosed in a cylinder fitted with a movable weightless and frictionless piston of area A (Fig. 25). If a constant pressure P is applied on the piston, the total force is given as

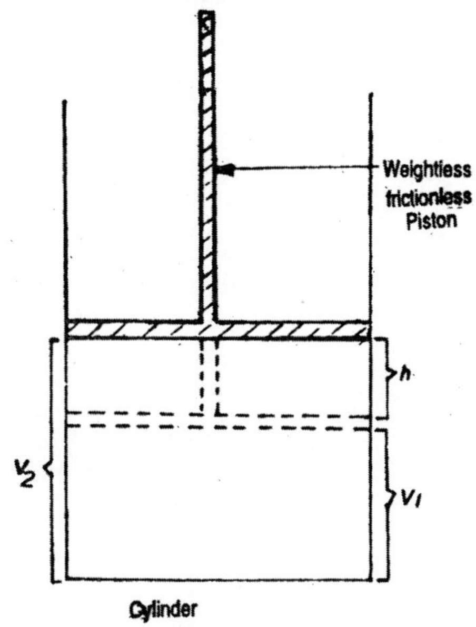

Fig. 25.

$$F = P \times A \text{ since } P = F/A$$

If the cylinder is heated, the gas in the cylinder expands and as a result, the piston is lifted upwards. Let the distance moved by the piston be 'h'. Then the work done by the opposing constant pressure is given by

$$W = P \times A \times h$$

i.e. force × distance ($\because P \times A$ = force).

But $A \times h$ is increase in volume ΔV.

$$\therefore \; W = P\Delta V$$

where $\Delta V = (V_2 - V_1)$, V_1 being the initial volume and V_2 the final volume.

1.7. Ideal gas and first law

Ideal gas molecules exhibit no cohesive forces of attraction. If there is a change in pressure or volume while the temperature remains constant, the internal energy of the ideal gas does not change.

Therefore, when the ideal gas expands, no work is expended for the expansion. We can write

$$\left(\frac{\partial E}{\partial V}\right)_T = 0$$

It indicates the volume coefficient of internal energy is zero at constant temperature and the internal energy of an ideal gas is a function solely of temperature.

If an ideal gas is involved in an isothermal process ($dt = 0$), the change in internal energy (dE) is equal to zero and the first law becomes

$$dE = q - w$$

$$0 = q - w$$

$$\text{or } -Q = -W \text{ or } Q = W \quad \dots (6)$$

It shows that the work done in the isothermal expansion is equal to the quantity of heat absorbed by the gas and can be obtained against a variable pressure as follows.

Work of expansion in an isothermal reversible process for an ideal gas at a pressure P_1 is given by

$$W = P_1 \Delta V \quad \dots (7)$$

In an isothermal expansion, the external pressure is only infinitesimally less than the pressure of the ideal gas. Therefore, the external pressure P_1 may be replaced by the pressure of the ideal gas P

$$\text{i.e. } W_{max} = P\Delta V$$

where, $P = \frac{nRT}{V}$ for an ideal gas

$$W_{max} = \frac{nRT}{V}\Delta V$$

For an infinitesimal change in volume,

$$dW_{max} = nRT\frac{dV}{V}$$

On integration,

$$\int dW_{max} = nRT\int_{v_1}^{v_2} \frac{dV}{V}$$

then

$$W_{max} = nRT \ln\frac{V_2}{V_1} \quad \dots (8)$$

Converting to common logarithm,

$$W_{max} = 2.303nRT \log\frac{V_2}{V_1} \quad \dots (9)$$

This equation gives the maximum work done by an ideal gas involved in an isothermal reversible process and it also gives the quantity of heat absorbed since $W = Q$.

The maximum work done in an isothermal reversible expansion may be given in terms of pressure also

From Boyle's law $\frac{V_2}{V_1} = \frac{P_1}{P_2}$ at constant T

Therefore,

$$W_{max} = 2.303\, nRT \log\frac{P_1}{P_2} \quad \dots (10)$$

1.8. Enthalpy

The first law is

$$\Delta E = Q - W$$

$$\text{or } Q = \Delta E + W$$

The work involved in the expansion at constant pressure is $P\Delta V$.

Replacing W by $P\Delta V$ at constant pressure

$$Q_p = \Delta E + P\Delta V$$

Q_p indicates that the heat is absorbed at constant pressure

Or simply,

$$Q_P = E + PV.$$

The term $E+PV$ is called the ***heat content*** or ***enthalpy*** *H*.

Enthalpy of a system is the sum of the internal energy E and the product of pressure and volume of the system. Enthalpy is a state property, and it depends on temperature and pressure of the system. The absolute value of the enthalpy of a substance cannot be calculated, but values relative to some arbitrarily chosen reference state can be determined.

The increase in heat content ΔH is Q_P.

i.e. $Q_P = \Delta H$

or,

$$\Delta H = \Delta E + P\Delta V \quad \text{... (11)}$$

For an infinitesimal change,

$$dQ_P = dH$$

The heat absorbed in a reaction carried out at atmospheric pressure (i.e. at constant pressure) depends only on initial and final conditions. Enthalpy is a thermodynamic property and this fact is taken advantage in thermochemistry.

1.9. Heat Capacity

When a hot substance '*A*' is brought in contact with a substance at a lower temperature (or a cold substance) '*B*', an amount of heat ΔQ is transferred from *A* to *B* to come to thermal equilibrium.

i.e. $-\Delta Q_A = +\Delta Q_B$

The transferred heat is the difference in heat content before and after thermal equilibrium. The difference can be measured in terms of temperature also.

$$\Delta Q = Q_2 - Q_1$$

or, $\Delta Q = C_V(T_2 - T_1)$

$$\Delta Q = C_V \Delta T$$

$$\text{or, } C_V = \frac{\Delta Q}{\Delta T} \quad \text{... (12)}$$

Where C_V is the heat capacity at constant volume. Since this C_V is proportional to the quantity of material present, it can be defined as ***heat capacity*** per unit mass of substance. If the unit mass is 1 g, it is *specific heat* and it is *molar heat capacity* if the unit mass is 1 mole. Thus, the molar heat capacity is defined as the quantity of heat, Q required to raise the temperature of 1 mole of substance through 1 degree.

For an infinitely small rise in temperature, the equation is written as

$$C_V = \frac{dq_v}{dT}$$

$$\text{or, } dq_v = C_V dT \quad \text{... (13)}$$

The heat required to rise the temperature of one mole of material from T_1 to T_2 at constant volume is $q_v = \int_{T_1}^{T_2} C_v dT$, and this on integration yields

$$q_v = C_V(T_2 - T_1) \quad \text{... (14)}$$

A system at constant volume does no PV work i.e. $dV = 0$, then the first law

$$dE = q_v - PdV$$

becomes $dE = q_v$ (since $dV = 0$, $PdV = 0$)

Therefore, the heat capacity at constant volume is

$$C_V = \frac{Q_v}{dT} = \left(\frac{\partial E}{\partial T}\right)_V \quad \text{... (15)}$$

When pressure is kept constant, the heat capacity (C_p) is given as

$$C_p = \frac{q_p}{dT} = \left(\frac{\partial H}{\partial T}\right)_P \text{ (since } q_p = dH) \quad \dots (16)$$

In this case, the heat absorbed is used to do *PV* work during expansion and to raise the internal energy.

Thus, when a gas is heated at a constant volume, less heat is required for a given temperature rise than would be necessary at constant pressure because no energy is required for the work of expansion in the former case i.e. $C_V < C_P$.

For ideal gases both C_P and C_V are independent of pressure and therefore $C_P - C_V = R$.

where C_P and C_V are on molal basis. As solids and liquids are practically incompressible, the values of C_P and C_V are almost identical for them.

2. Thermochemistry

Thermochemistry is the study of heat changes accompanying chemical and physical processes.

Heat changes may be measured at constant volume or at constant pressure. When closed calorimeters are used, the volume remains constant and the heat changes corresponds to ΔE (i.e. $Q_V = \Delta E$). When heat changes are measured in open calorimeters, the pressure remains constant (i.e. at atmospheric pressure) and the heat change corresponds to ΔH (i.e. $Q_P = \Delta H$). In solution reactions, conducted at constant pressure, the volume change is insignificant or there is only a slight change in volume so that $\Delta E \cong \Delta H$.

Heat may be absorbed or liberated during chemical or physical processes. If the process is accompanied by the liberation of heat, the process is exothermic i.e. ΔE or ΔH has a negative value. Conversely if the process is accompanied by absorption of heat, the process is endothermic i.e. ΔE or ΔH has a positive value.

2.1. Heat of combustion

Heat of combustion is the heat involved (liberated or absorbed) when 1 mole of a substance undergoes complete oxidation at 1 atm pressure.

Consider the reaction

$$\underset{(s)}{C} + \underset{(g)}{O_2} = \underset{(g)}{CO_2} - 94{,}052 \text{ cal}$$

$$\Delta H^\circ_{298} = -94{,}052 \text{ cal or } 94.052 \text{ Kcal}$$

Subscripts *s* and *g*, appearing in equations represent solid and gas respectively. ΔH°_{298} is the standard heat of reaction for the process at 298°K or 25°C (ΔH°_{25}). When pressure is not specified, it is assumed that the reaction is carried out at 1 atm pressure.

The reactants and products of the combustion are taken to be in the form that they would ordinarily be at 298°K or 25°C and 1 atm. pressure. These conditions are referred to as **standard states** of the substances involved in the reaction. In defining the standard state, the state of matter (*g*, *l* or *s*) should also be specified. The heat contents of all elements in their *standard states* are arbitrarily assigned values of zero.

In the above reaction, – 94.052 cal represents the heat of combustion and the negative sign indicates exothermic reaction. That is 94,052 cal of heat is liberated in the complete oxidation of carbon (graphite) to carbon dioxide.

2.2. Hess Law of Heat Summation

Hess showed that, in reactions, ΔH depends only on the initial and final states of a system whether it involves one step or several steps. Therefore thermochemical equations for several steps in a reaction can be added and subtracted to obtain the heat of overall reaction. This principle is known as **Hess's law of constant heat summation.** It provides a means of calculating heat quantities that cannot be determined directly by experiment.

For example, the heat of combustion of carbon (graphite) to carbon monoxide is difficult to measure experimentally. However it may be obtained from the heats of combustion of carbon (graphite) to CO_2 and CO to CO_2 by subtraction as follows:

$$\underset{(s)}{C} + \underset{(g)}{O_2} = \underset{(g)}{CO_2} \; ; \; \Delta H^{o}_{298} = -94{,}052 \text{ cal}$$

$$\underset{(g)}{CO} + \frac{1}{2}\underset{(g)}{O_2} = \underset{(g)}{CO_2} \; ; \; \Delta H_{298} = -67{,}836 \text{ cal}$$

$$\underset{(s)}{C} + \frac{1}{2}\underset{(g)}{O_2} = \underset{(g)}{CO} \; ; \; \Delta H^{o}_{298} = -26{,}416 \text{ cal}$$

2.3. Heat of Formation

Heat of formation of a substance is the heat involved when 1 mole of a compound is formed from its constituent elements, the reactants and products being taken as in their standard states.

The heat of formation of CO_2 from its constituent elements carbon and oxygen is $-94{,}052$ cal and this is also the heat of combustion.

In calculating the heat of reaction using Hess's law, the following equation is used

$$\Delta H^{o}_{\text{reaction}} = \Sigma H^{o}_{\text{products}} - \Sigma \Delta H_{\text{reactants}} \quad \ldots (17)$$

For example, the heat of formation of CH_4 is $-17{,}889$ cal, the heat of formation of CO_2 is $-94{,}052$ cal and the heat of formation of acetic acid is $-116{,}400$ cal.

The heat of reaction of acetic acid from CH_4 and CO_2 is

$$\underset{(g)}{CH_4} + \underset{(g)}{CO_2} = \underset{(l)}{CH_3COOH}$$

(where (l) indicates liquid)

$$\Delta H^{o}_{298} \text{ of } CH_4 = -17{,}889 \text{ cal}$$

$$\Delta H^{o}_{298} \text{ of } CO_2 = -94{,}052 \text{ cal}$$

$$\Delta H^{o}_{298} \text{ of } CH_3COOH = -116400 \text{ cal}$$

Applying Hess's law

$$\Delta H^{o}_{298} = (-116{,}400 \text{ cal}) - [(-17{,}889 \text{ cal}) + (-94{,}052 \text{ cal})]$$

$$= -4459 \text{ cal.}$$

The heat of formation of acetic acid from CH_4 and CO_2 is $-4{,}459$ cal and it indicates 4459 cal of heat would be liberated if 1 mole of CH_4(g) and 1 mole of CO_2(g) react to give 1 mole of CH_3COOH(l).

2.4. Heat of Solution

When a specified amount of solute is dissolved in a solvent, a heat of solution is involved. This heat of solution is not generally constant for a given solute-solvent system but it varies with the volume of solvent used. Therefore, the heats of solution may be expressed as **integral heat of solution, differential heat of solution and heat of solution at infinite dilution.**

The **integral heat of solution** is the heat effect involved when 1 mole of a solute is dissolved in a solvent to form a solution of definite concentration.

The **differential heat of solution** is the heat effect involved when 1 mole of a solute is dissolved in a large quantity of a solution of definite concentration so that no significant change in the concentration of the solution results. It may also be defined as the heat effect involved when so small a quantity of solute is added to a solution of definite concentration so that there is no change in the concentration of the solution.

The **heat of solution at infinite dilution** is the maximum heat of solution obtained as the volume of solvent is increased.

Heats of dilution and heats of hydration are obtained from the integral heats of solution. Heat of solution is the difference between the integral heats of solution of two specified concentrations of solute-solvent system. The heat of hydration is the difference between the heats of solution of the solvated and nonsolvated solute.

In the case of differential heat, the heat effect depends only on the conversion of the crystalline solute to the dissolved state. In integral heat, both the solute and the solvent are affected during the process.

2.5. Applications

Apart from the applications mentioned above, thermochemistry may be applied to various other purposes. Heat of mixing data can be used to determine whether a reaction proceeds with precipitation or not. When there is no reaction if two dilute solutions are mixed, the heat of solution is zero.

There is constancy in the heats of neutralisation when dilute solutions of strong acids and strong bases are mixed. (about – 13.6 Kcal/mole). This knowledge enables to differentiate between strong and weak electrolytes. In the case of neutralisation of a weak electrolyte by a strong acid or base, the heat of reaction is below – 13.6 Kcal/mole since it involves ionisation (absorption of heat) and then neutralisation (liberation of heat).

It is also applied in the determination of energy in calories derived from various foods.

3. Entropy and the second law of thermodynamics

The first law provides only for calculating the change in energy that is associated with chemical or physical changes in state and when the change occurs, energy is conserved. It does not provide enough information as to the probability that the change will occur.

Consider a system composed of two parts with different temperatures (T_1 and T_2). It is a well known fact that heat will flow from a part at a higher temperature to that part which is at a lower temperature. The first law does not predict this change. Such a change (flow of heat from the part at a higher temperature to the part at lower temperature) occurs without any additional stimulation (i.e. it occurs spontaneously). However it should be noted that the above change involves an increase in the disorder i.e. randomness of the system. This change proceeds until a uniform temperature in both the parts is obtained. The disorder or randomness occuring in the system is termed entropy.

Entropy may be defined as a quantitative measure of randomness, disorderliness, or mixed-upness of a system and is fundamental for predicting the spontaneity of chemical reactions and physical changes.

Entropy is a state function which depends only on the initial and final state of the system and may be defined as the capacity factor of thermal energy (heat energy) that is unavailable for doing work and the entropy change is given as

$$\Delta S = \frac{Q_{rev}}{T} \quad \dots (18)$$

Where, the subscript 'rev', denotes that heat flow occurs in a reversible manner i.e. in any step of a reversible process. Then, for any spontaneous process in an isolated system entropy increases.

It is better for the student to know the background leading to the above definition. When heat is permitted to flow into a system, work may be done by the system.

Let us consider a *hypothetical heat engine* which is capable of converting heat into work. Also consider the engine absorbs an amount of heat q_2 from a heat reservoir at a higher temperature T_2 and converts a part of the heat into work and transfers the remaining amount of heat q_1 to a heat reservoir at a lower temperature T_1

According to first law of thermodynamics, the difference $q_2 - q_1$ is converted into work i.e. W_{max}. The second law dictates that not all the heat can be converted into work even if all the changes occur in a reversible manner. Then the efficiency of the heat engine is given by

$$\frac{W_{max}}{q_2} = \frac{q_2 - q_1}{q_2} \quad \text{... (19)}$$

Heat flow follows the temperature gradient and hence the heat absorbed q_2 and heat rejected q_1 can be related directly to temperatures T_2 and T_1 respectively as

$$\frac{q_2}{q_1} = \frac{T_2}{T_1}$$

Hence, we can write

$$\text{Efficiency} = \frac{W_{max}}{q_2} = \frac{T_2 - T_1}{T_2}$$

$$\text{or, } W_{max} = q_2 \frac{(T_2 - T_1)}{T_2}$$

where $T_2 > T_1$.

The efficiency is proportional to the difference in temperature between the two heat reservoirs and it is observed that the efficiency of the engine becomes greater when $T_2 >> T_1$

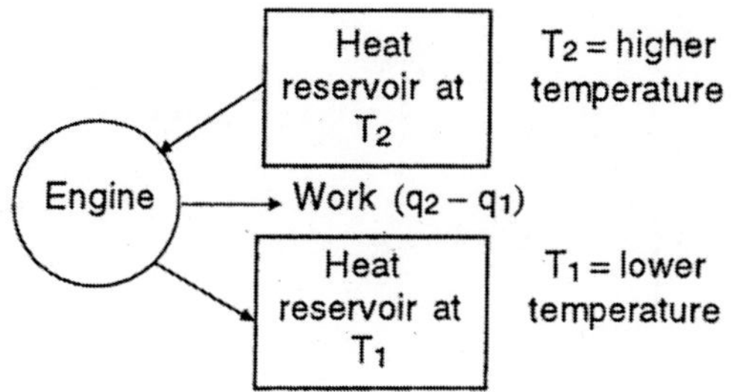

When $T_2 = T_1$, the process is isothermal and the efficiency becomes zero and it confirms that heat is isothermally unavailable for conversion into work. i.e. no work will be done unless there is a difference between the heat reservoirs. The above analysis elucidates the connection between entropy and heat flow. It is also noted that the efficiency of an engine is a function solely of the thermal properties and independent of any substance in the engine.

If $T_1 = 0$ the equation becomes

$$\text{efficiency} = \frac{T_2 - 0}{T_2} = 1$$

The efficiency at this condition becomes unity i.e. 100% efficiency. But $T_1 = 0$ (absolute zero) is considered unattainable as will be noted from the third law and therefore the efficiency is always less than unity. That is, heat can never be completely converted into work.

The impossibility of converting all heat energy into work results from the 'disorderliness' of the molecules existing in the system.

Carnot, a French chemist, established this equation and the equation can be obtained by introducing the Carnot cycle.

Consider an engine, connected to two heat reservoirs, contains an ideal gas which can perform *PV* work. Let the system undergoes cyclic, reversible

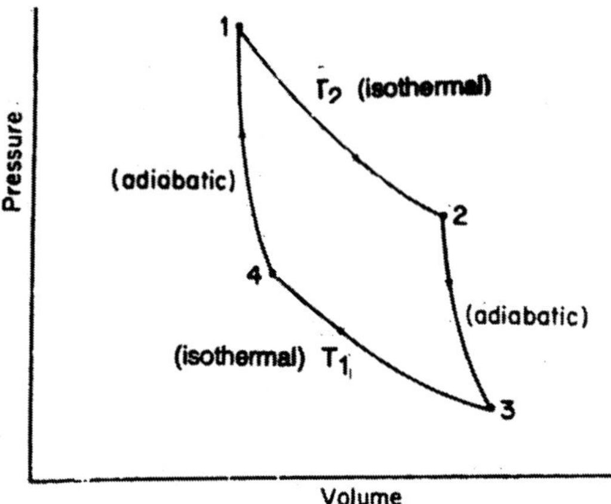

Fig. 26

change as represented in the pressure volume diagram as shown in Fig. 26.

As this one is a cyclic change, the total energy change in the complete cycle is zero (i.e. $\Delta E_{tot} = 0$). The cyclic change comprises four steps. Energy change in each step may be obtained by using first law of thermodynamics, which is given as $\Delta E = q - w$

The first step is an iso-thermal expansion, Let q_2 is the heat absorbed by the system and w_1, the work done by it. The energy is given by

$$\Delta E = q_2 - w_1$$

For an ideal gas involved in isothermal expansion, the energy change is zero and the above equation becomes,

$$0 = q_2 - w_1$$

$$\text{or, } q_2 = W_1 = \int PdV.$$

Substituting for P

$$\left(P = \frac{nRT_2}{V} \text{ for an ideal gas} \right)$$

the above equation is given as

$$q_2 = \int nRT_2 \frac{dV}{V}$$

and integrating between the limits of the initial and final volumes, V_1 and V_2

$$q_2 = nRT_2 \ln \frac{V_2}{V_1} = W_1$$

Second step is an adiabatic process, and for an ideal gas involved in adiabatic expansion, the heat flow is zero i.e. $q = 0$. Thus, the energy change, using the first law is

$$\Delta E = -W_2$$

$$\text{or } W_2 = -\Delta E$$

Obtaining the energy change from the definition of heat capacity at constant volume, the equation may be written as

$$\int C_V dt = \Delta E \text{ where } C_V = \left(\frac{dE}{dT} \right)_V$$

$$\text{or } dE = C_V dT$$

$$\Delta E = \int_{T_1}^{T_2} C_V dt$$

$$\Delta E = C_V (T_1 - T_2)$$

$$\text{or, } -\Delta E_2 = C_V (T_2 - T_1)$$

$$W_2 = C_V (T_2 - T_1)$$

The third and fourth steps are just the reverse of the first and second steps respectively. Thus the mathematical expressions may be given as

$$-W_3 = nRT_1 \ln \frac{V_4}{V_3} \text{ (for isothermal compression)}$$

$$-W_4 = -C_V (T_2 - T_1) \text{ (for adiabatic compression)}$$

The total work for the cycle may be obtained by summing up the results of all the four steps.

i.e. $W_{tot} = W_1 + W_2 + (-W_3) + (-W_4)$

$$W_{tot} = nRT_2 \ln \frac{V_2}{V_1} + C_V (T_2 - T_1) + nRT_1 \ln \frac{V_4}{V_3} + (-C_V (T_2 - T_1))$$

$$= nRT_2 \ln \frac{V_2}{V_1} + C_V (T_2 - T_1)$$

$$+ nRT_1 \ln \frac{V_4}{V_3} - C_V (T_2 - T_1)$$

On simplification,

$$W_{tot} = nRT_2 \ln \frac{V_2}{V_1} + nRT_1 \ln \frac{V_4}{V_3}$$

The heat flow into the system as given by the first step is

$$q_2 = nRT_2 \ln \frac{V_2}{V_1}$$

The efficiency of an engine is given by the ratio of the amount of work extracted to the heat flow into system

$$\frac{W_{tot}}{q_2}$$

W_{tot} is W_{max} for reversible changes and hence the efficiency is

$$\frac{W_{max}}{q_2} = \frac{nRT_2 \ln \frac{V_2}{V_1} + nRT_1 \ln \frac{V_4}{V_3}}{nRT_2 \ln \frac{V_2}{V_1}}$$

or, $$\frac{W_{max}}{q_2} = \frac{nRT_2 \ln \frac{V_2}{V_1} - nRT_1 \ln \frac{V_3}{V_4}}{nRT_2 \ln \frac{V_2}{V_1}}$$

It may be shown that $\frac{V_3}{V_4} = \frac{V_2}{V_1}$

and substituting this, we get,

$$\frac{W_{max}}{q_2} = \frac{nRT_2 \ln \frac{V_2}{V_1} - nRT_1 \ln \frac{V_2}{V_1}}{nRT_2 \ln \frac{V_2}{V_1}}$$

$$= \frac{nR \ln \frac{V_2}{V_1} (T_2 - T_1)}{T_2 nR \ln \frac{V_2}{V_1}}$$

$$\text{Efficiency} = \frac{W_{max}}{q_2} = \frac{T_2 - T_1}{T_2} \quad \text{... (20)}$$

3.1. Entropy

An important thermodynamic quantity that measures the increase in the unavailable energy accompanying the spontaneous processes is called entropy.

Entropy may be defined as the capacity factor of thermal energy (heat energy) that is unavailable for doing work and the entropy change ΔS for the absorption of heat in a system at absolute temperature T in any step of a reversible process is given as

$$\Delta S = \frac{Q_{rev}}{T}$$

The unit of entropy change is cal/deg. For an infinitesimal change, entropy change is given as

$$dS = \frac{q_{rev}}{T}$$

Entropy change $\Delta S = 0$ for a system in a reversible cyclic process and for a system and its surroundings or universe undergoing any reversible process

$$\Delta S_{\text{total system}} = \Delta S_{syst} + \Delta S_{surr} = 0$$

or, $\Sigma \Delta S_{total} = 0$, for a reversible process

Entropy change $\Delta S > 0$, for a total system or universe involved in an irreversible process. That is, entropy of the total system or universe involved in an irreversible process is increasing (total system or universe refers to any system and its surroundings).

$$\Delta S_{\text{total system}} > 0$$

or, $\Sigma\Delta S_{\text{total}} > 0$, for an irreversible process

Thus, entropy can serve as a criterion of spontaneity of a process.

The second law of thermodynamics may be stated that a spontaneous reaction involving a system and its surroundings occurs in the direction of increased entropy. When the system reaches equilibrium, the net entropy change undergone by the system and its surroundings is equal to zero. It may also be stated that for any spontaneous process in an isolated system, there is an increase in the value of entropy. Combining the first and second laws the classic statement is that "energy of the universe is constant, the entropy is increasing"

4. Third Law of Thermodynamics

Entropy refers to disorderliness. Crystalline substances show less disorderliness. Pure crystalline substances at low temperature, exhibit still less disorderliness.

The *third law of thermodynamics states that entropy of a pure crystalline substance is zero when its temperature is absolute zero because of perfect crystal arrangement at this temperature.* It is true that every substance at room temperature possesses a certain amount of entropy owing to molecular motions.

When the temperature of a substance is raised without causing any change in the state of substance (i.e. from solid to liquid or liquid to gas), the motion of the molecules within the substance is increased resulting in the increase of entropy. This process may be considered to be composed of a series of steps in which the infinitesimal change of temperature dT, increases the entropy by an infinitesimal amount dS and is given by the equation

$$dS = \frac{q}{T} \text{ But } q = CdT \text{ since } C = \frac{q}{dT}$$

$$\text{Therefore, } dS = C\frac{dT}{T}. \qquad \text{... (21)}$$

where C = molar heat capacity

The integrated form of this equation is applied to a finite process

$$\Delta S = S_2 - S_1 = C\int_{T_1}^{T_2} \frac{dT}{T}$$

$$= C \ln \frac{T_2}{T_1}$$

Converting to common logarithms

$$= 2.303C \log \frac{T_2}{T_1}$$

When $T_1 = 0$, the absolute entropy is given by $S = 2.303C \log T$ ... (22)

Thus the third law of thermodynamics can be applied for calculating absolute values of entropy of pure substances from their heat capacities. From absolute entropies and heats of formation of substances it is possible to calculate their Gibbs free energy values.

5. Free Energy

Entropy, as a criterion of spontaneity, is not convenient one as it requires the calculation of the entropy change both in the system and in the surroundings. That is, it is applicable only to changes carried out in an isolated system. Such a constraint cannot be applied when the change is undertaken in a laboratory. Free energy functions, which will be considered here, do not demand information concerning the surroundings and are used to predict the spontaneity of a chemical reaction or a physical change. The free energy functions introduced are ***Helmholtz free energy*** or work function (A) and the *Gibbs free energy* (G or F) or simply the free energy.

5.1 Helmholtz Free Energy or Work Function

The internal energy E of a system is considered to consist of a part A, isothermally available internal energy for doing work or work function and a part, TS, isothermally unavailable internal energy for doing work.

$$\text{i.e., } E = A + TS \quad \text{... (23)}$$

The above equation may be written for Helmholtz free energy which is defined as the internal energy minus the isothermally unavailable internal energy for doing work as,

$$A = E - TS \quad \text{... (24)}$$

The driving force of any physical or chemical change resides in the part 'A' of internal energy for a system at constant temperature and volume. Consider the system undergoes a change, then the equation may be written as

$$\Delta A = \Delta E - \Delta(TS)$$

Then, at constant temperature

$$\Delta A = \Delta E - T\Delta S$$

or $\Delta A = Q - W - T\Delta S$ (since $\Delta E = Q - W$)

In a reversible process, maximum work is obtained and from the definition of entropy

$$\Delta S = \frac{Q_{rev}}{T}$$

$$T\Delta S = Q_{rev}$$

Substituting this value in the above equation, we obtain

$$\Delta A = T\Delta S - W_{max} - T\Delta S$$

$$\Delta A = - W_{max}$$

$$\text{or, } - \Delta A = W_{max} \quad \text{... (25)}$$

Helmholtz free energy (A) is the energy available to do PV work in a reversible isothermal process or a decrease in A is a measure of capacity of the system to do work and the driving force for the spontaneous change in the direction of diminishing its work capacity or function. Alternatively for systems at constant temperature and volume, spontaneity of a reaction is indicated when A (work function) undergoes a decrease.

If a system at a constant temperature and pressure increases in volume, the capacity of the system for doing work is diminished by an amount equivalent to work of expansion ($P\Delta V$) against the atmospheric pressure. The net work is then given by

$$W_{net} = W_{max} - P\Delta V \quad \text{... (26)}$$

This quantity W_{net} may be correlated with Gibbs free energy G (or F).

5.2 Gibb's Free Energy

Most of the reactions are carried out in the laboratory at constant temperature and pressure and hence Gibbs energy is the most useful function and is defined as isothermally available energy and is equal to the total heat content minus isothermally unavailable energy. It is given by,

$$G = H - TS \quad \text{... (27)}$$

or $G = E + PV - TS$ (since $H = E + PV$)

When a system undergoes a change, the above equation may be written as

$$G = \Delta E + \Delta(PV) - \Delta(TS)$$

At constant pressure and temperature, $G = \Delta E + P\Delta V - T\Delta S$

Substituting $Q - W$ for ΔE and Q for $T\Delta S$ for a reversible reaction.

$$G = Q - W + P\Delta V - Q$$

where ($W = W_{max}$ for a reversible process)

$$G = - W_{max} + P\Delta V$$

Multiplying by –, the equation becomes

$$-G = W_{max} - P\Delta V$$

$$\text{or} \quad -G = W_{net} \qquad \dots (28)$$

$$(W_{net} = W_{max} - P\Delta V) \qquad \dots (29)$$

Thus the decrease in free energy ($-\Delta G$) is a measure of maximum net work at constant temperature and pressure available from the system. It gives a measure both of the net capacity of a system for doing useful work and of the driving force for the spontaneous change in the direction of diminishing its free energy.

If the system undergoes no change in volume, W_{net} equals W_{max} and that ΔA and ΔG must be equal.

If the system undergoes a decrease in volume, the term ΔV becomes negative and W_{net} is larger than W_{max}.

The following ***differential forms of equations*** are useful in the study of reversible processes where the only work done is pressure-volume work.

$$G = H - TS \qquad \dots (30)$$

or $\quad G = E + PV - TS \quad$ (since $H = E + PV$)

On partial differentiation,

$$dG = dE + PdV + VdP - TdS - SdT \dots (31)$$

According to the First law restricted to expansion work $dE = q - PdV$. For a reversible process $q_{rev} = TdS$. Therefore, $dE = TdS - PdV$. Substituting this value in the above equation for dE.

$$dG = TdS - PdV + PdV + VdP - TdS - SdT$$

$$dG = VdP - SdT$$

At constant pressure, where $VdP = 0$, the equation reduces to

$$dG = -SdT$$

$$\text{or} \quad \left(\frac{\partial G}{\partial T}\right)_P = -S$$

At constant temperature, where $SdT = 0$, the equation reduces to

$$dG = VdP$$

$$\text{or} \quad \left(\frac{\partial G}{\partial P}\right)_T = V$$

For an ideal gas $V = n\dfrac{RT}{P}$

$$\text{Therefore} \quad \left(\frac{\partial G}{\partial P}\right)_T = \frac{nRT}{P}$$

$$\text{or} \quad dG = nRT\frac{dP}{P}$$

This on integration between G_2 at P_2 and G_1 at P_1,

$$G_2 - G_1 = \Delta G = nRT \ln\frac{P_2}{P_1} \qquad \dots (32)$$

Converting to common logarithm,

$$\Delta G = 2.303nRT \log\frac{P_2}{P_1} \qquad \dots (33)$$

ΔG is the free energy change of an ideal gas undergoing an isothermal reversible or irreversible change.

5.3. Free energy relationship

In computing free energy changes accompanying a given reaction, it is necessary to refer to some standard free energy state of a substance because of lack of knowledge of absolute Gibbs free energy value. Free energy is obtained by referring differences in G to some standard state. The standard free energy change ($\Delta G°$) for a *hypothetical* reaction is referred to in dealing with chemical reactions.

The standard free energy ($\Delta G°$) can be defined as the free energy change that occurs when one mole of a compound in its standard state is formed from its elements in their standard state. The standard free energy of all elements is taken as zero.

When the equilibrium constant (K) for a reaction is known, the standard free energy change is given by

$$\Delta G^\circ = -2.303RT \log K \quad \text{... (34)}$$

The equilibrium constant for the reaction ($CH_3COOH + C_2H_5OH = CH_3COOC_2H_5 + H_2O$) is 4.00 at 25°C. Compute ΔG° for the reaction at the same temperature

$$\Delta G^\circ = -RT \times 2.303 \log K$$

$$= -1.987 \times 298 \times 2.303 \times \log 4.00$$

$$= -821 \text{ cal/mole}$$

5.4. Criteria of Spontaneity and Equilibrium

Criteria for spontaneity and equilibrium are given in the following table.

Thermodynamic function	Conditions Total system	Spontaneous	Equilibrium
ΔS	$\Delta E = 0$, $\Delta V = 0$ isolated system	+ or > 0	0
ΔG	$\Delta T = 0$, $\Delta P = 0$ isothermal and isobaric	– or < 0	0
ΔA	$\Delta T = 0$, $\Delta V = 0$ isothermal and isochoric	– or < 0	0
ΔE	$\Delta S = 0$, $\Delta V = 0$ constant entropy and isochoric	– or < 0	0

5.5. Chemical potential (or Molar Free Energy)

Closed systems exchange heat and work whereas open systems exchange heat, work and also matter with their surroundings.

Thus in open systems, there is exchange of matter in addition to heat and work among phases. Consider a system that consists of two components. Then, any one of the extensive properties such as free energy becomes a function of temperature, pressure and also of the number of moles of the various components.

$$\text{i.e. } G = f(P, T, n_1, n_2) \quad \text{... (35)}$$

Changes in free energy of a system resulting from the variation of number of moles because of exchange of matter with surroundings can be obtained.

Considering a system consisting of two components (1 and 2) for an infinitesimal reversible change of state, the free energy change is

$$dG = \left(\frac{\partial G}{\partial T}\right)_{P, n_1, n_2} dT + \left(\frac{\partial G}{\partial P}\right)_{T, n_1, n_2} dP + \left(\frac{\partial G}{\partial n_1}\right)_{T, P, n_2} dn_1 + \left(\frac{\partial G}{\partial n_2}\right)_{T, P, n_1} dn_2$$

where n_1 and n_2 represent the number of moles of the components 1 and 2 respectively.

Replacing $\left(\frac{\partial G}{\partial n_1}\right)$ by μ_1 and $\left(\frac{\partial G}{\partial n_2}\right)$ by μ_2, the equation is written as

$$dG = \left(\frac{\partial G}{\partial T}\right)_{P, n_1, n_2} dT + \left(\frac{\partial G}{\partial P}\right)_{T, n_1, n_2} dP + \mu_1 \, dn_1 + \mu_2 \, dn_2$$

μ_1 and μ_2 are the chemical potentials (introduced by Gibbs) of the components 1 and 2 respectively.

This equation for a closed system may be given as follows since $\left(\frac{\partial G}{\partial T}\right)_P = -S$ and $\left(\frac{\partial G}{\partial P}\right)_T = V$.

$$dG = -SdT + VdP + \mu_1 dn_1 + \mu_2 dn_2$$

This relationship also applies to an open system and at constant pressure and temperature (i.e. when $VdP = 0$ and $-SdT = 0$)

$$dG_{T,P} = \mu_1 dn_1 + \mu_2 dn_2$$

When n_2 is also constant

$$dG_{T,Pn_2} = \mu_1 dn_2$$

$$\text{or} \left(\frac{\partial G}{\partial n_1}\right)_{T,P,n_2} = \mu_1 \qquad \text{... (36)}$$

This partial differential expression states that the chemical potential of component 1, at constant temperature and pressure is defined as the change in free energy brought about by an infinitesimal change in the number of moles of component 1 (n_1) provided the number of moles of the other component 2 (n_2) is held constant. Chemical potential is otherwise called as *partial molar free energy*.

The product $\mu_1 dn_1$ represents the change of free energy produced by dn_1 moles of component 1.

For a closed system at equilibrium and at constant temperature and pressure, the free energy change is zero. $dG_{T,P} = 0$

In a heterogeneous system, the chemical potential of a component A is identical in all phases when all the phases are in equilibrium at a fixed temperature and pressure.

That is, $\mu_{A_\alpha} = \mu_{A_\beta} = \mu_{A_\gamma}$ ... (37)

where α, β, γ are various phases among which the substance (A) is distributed.

When two phases are not in equilibrium at constant temperature and pressure, the substance from the phase of higher chemical potential passes spontaneously to one of lower chemical potential until the chemical potentials are equal in the two phases. Hence the chemical potential can be used as a measure of the escaping tendency of the component from its phase.

For a phase consisting of a single pure substance, the chemical potential is the free energy of the substance per mole.

$$\mu = \frac{G}{n} \qquad \text{... (38)}$$

For a two phase system consisting of a single component (eg. liquid water and water vapour in equilibrium at constant temperature and pressure) the molar free energy or chemical potential $\frac{G}{n}$ is identical in both the phases.

5.6. The Clapeyron Equation

Consider liquid water (l) in equilibrium with its vapour (v) at a temperature T and pressure P, then, the free energies of the liquid and the vapour must be equal

$$\text{i.e. } G_l = G_v$$

If the temperature is raised by a small increment dt that is $(T + dt)$, the pressure is also increased to $P + dP$ to correspond to the vapour pressure at the raised temperature to maintain equilibrium. The free energy of both the liquid and the vapour is also increased by an equal amount since both the phases are at equilibrium so that

$$dG_l = dG_v$$

The change of free energy of a pure substance with pressure and temperature is given by

$$dG = VdP - SdT$$

Then the change in free energy for 1 mole of vapour is

$$dG_v = V_v dP - S_v dT$$

and the change in free energy for 1 mole of liquid is

$$dG_l = V_l dP - S_l dT$$

At equilibrium

$$V_v dP - S_v dT = V_l dP - S_l dT \text{ (since } dG_v = dG_l \text{ at equilibrium)}$$

$$V_v dP - V_l dP = S_v dT - S_l dT$$

$$dP(V_v - V_l) = dT(S_v - S_l)$$

$$\frac{dP}{dT} = \frac{S_v - S_l}{V_v - V_l} = \frac{\Delta S}{\Delta V}$$

The heat absorbed at constant pressure in the reversible process is equal to the molar heat of vaporisation

$$\text{i.e., } \Delta S = \frac{\Delta H_v}{T} \text{ (since } \Delta H_v = Q_{rev})$$

Substituting this value for ΔS in the above equation yields

$$\frac{dP}{dT} = \frac{\Delta H_v}{T\Delta V} \qquad \text{... (39)}$$

where $\Delta V = (V_v - V_l)$, the difference in the volume of the two phases.

This is *Clapeyron equation.*

This equation is applied to the equilibrium between a liquid and its vapour in the process of vaporisation. With suitable modifications, this may also be applied to the equilibrium between solid and gas, solid and liquid and between two crystalline forms.

5.7. Classius - Clapeyron Equation

Classius assumed that the vapour obeys Boyle's ideal gas law (especially when the temperature is far enough away from the critical point) and that the molar volume of the liquid V_l is insignificant when compared with molar volume of the gas V_v Based on the above assumptions, the Clapeyron equation becomes

$$\frac{dP}{dT} = \frac{P\Delta H_v}{RT^2} \qquad \text{... (40)}$$

$$\left(V_v = \frac{RT}{P} \text{ when vapour obey's ideal gas law} \right)$$

This equation is known as *Classius-**Clapeyron** equation*

Integrating this equation between the limits of vapour pressures P_1 at T_1 and P_2 at T_2 after rearrangement to

$$\frac{dP}{P} = \frac{\Delta H_v}{R} \cdot \frac{dT}{T^2}$$

$$\int_{P_1}^{P_2} \frac{dP}{P} = \frac{\Delta H_v}{R} \int_{T_1}^{T_2} \frac{dT}{T^2}$$

$$[\ln P]_{P_1}^{P_2} = \frac{\Delta H_v}{R} \left[\left(-\frac{1}{T_2} \right) - \left(-\frac{1}{T_1} \right) \right]$$

$$\ln \frac{P_2}{P_1} = \frac{\Delta H_v}{R} \left[\frac{1}{T_1} - \frac{1}{T_2} \right]$$

Converting to common logarithms

$$\log \frac{P_2}{P_1} = \frac{\Delta H_v (T_2 - T_1)}{2.303 R T_1 T_2} \qquad \text{... (41)}$$

The Classius-Clapeyron equation may be used to calculate the heat of vapourisation of a liquid if its vapour pressures at two temperatures are available. Or, if the heat of vapourisation and vapour pressure at one temperature are known, the vapour pressure at another temperature can be obtained.

The equations (Clapeyron and Classius-Clapeyron equations) are used to calculate the *theoretical* values of the *molal boiling point elevation constant* and the *molal freezing point depression constant* for dilute solutions.

IV. SURFACE AND INTERFACIAL PHENOMENA

An interface is a boundary between two distinct phases, while a surface is strictly a boundary between a solid or a liquid phase and a vacuum or air. Interfaces occur in a variety of heterogeneous dosage forms such as suspensions (insoluble solid dispersed in liquid), emulsions (liquid dispersed in another liquid both being immiscible with each other), foams (air dispersed in liquid) etc. Surface and interfacial phenomena refer to the properties exhibited at the surface or the interface. The various properties are

(i) Surface and interfacial tensions

(ii) Adsorption

(iii) Electrical properties at the interfaces

1. Surface and Interfacial tensions

Let us consider water in a beaker. (Fig. 27) The boundary between water and air is the surface. The water molecules within the bulk of the liquid are attracted to one another equally in all directions (i.e. there is a balance of forces of attraction) whereas those molecules at the surface experience very little attraction from the vapour phase above the liquid and are attracted only laterally and downwards. As a result, the molecules at the surface are subjected to a net inward pull into the liquid. To satisfy this inward pull which is unbalanced, there is spontaneous movement of molecules from the surface into the bulk of the liquid. This withdrawal of molecules from the surface increases the intermolecular distances between the molecules within the surface slightly. This results in the surface acting as a stretched membrane. It may be said that the surface is under tension in a tangential direction and the surface tends to contract spontaneously.

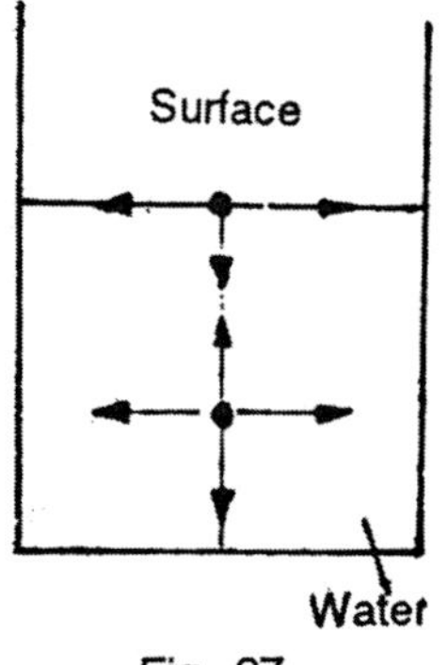

Fig. 27

The tension that is exhibited because of the unbalanced forces at the surface is termed surface tension and is ***defined as the force per unit length acting parallel to the surface of the liquid to counterbalance the net downward pull. The unit of surface tension is dynes per cm or ergs per meter.***

Let us consider two immiscible liquids such as water and mineral oil in contact with each other. The boundary separating the two liquids is the interface. As already mentioned, the molecules within the bulk of each of the liquid experience equal forces from all sides. At the interface where the two immiscible liquids meet, the molecules of each of the liquid are subjected to different forces of attraction. The molecules of one liquid at the interface are attracted away into another liquid less strongly than they are into themselves. In otherwords, the cohesive forces (forces of attraction between like molecules) are more than the adhesive forces (forces of attraction between unlike molecules). This leads to imbalance of forces at the interface. Such unbalanced forces cause some molecules from the interface to move into the bulk of the liquid leaving fewer number of molecules per unit area at the interface and at the same time reducing the actual contact area between the molecules of the two immiscible liquids. To reverse this process i.e. to increase the contact area between the two phases, we have to bring more molecules to the interface expanding the interfacial area. But there is resistance for this attempt and because of this the interface is under tension and ***the tension per unit length of the interface is called interfacial tension.***

At the interface between oil and water, the net attractive force into bulk of the water leads to a reduced number of molecules in the interfacial region. So is the case with the oil. At the interface there is a gradual decrease in density as one moves from water to oil. i.e. density decreases gradually from 1 (density of water) to that of oil density

Interfacial tensions are always less than the surface tensions because the number of air/gas molecules in contact with the liquid molecules are less than the number of liquid molecules in contact with one another at the interface. In otherwords, the adhesive forces between air molecules and liquid moleules are less than the adhesive forces between the two immiscible liquid molecules at the interface and that results in an interfacial tension that is less than that of surface tension.

The interfacial tension serves as a measure of the degree of interaction between two immiscible liquids in accordance with the adhesive forces and this is evident from different interfacial tensions between different liquids. For example the interfacial tension is less between water and octanol than between water and octane. This is because of more adhesive forces between water and octanol due to hydrogen bonding.

The interfacial tension may be expressed as force per unit length or as energy per unit area.

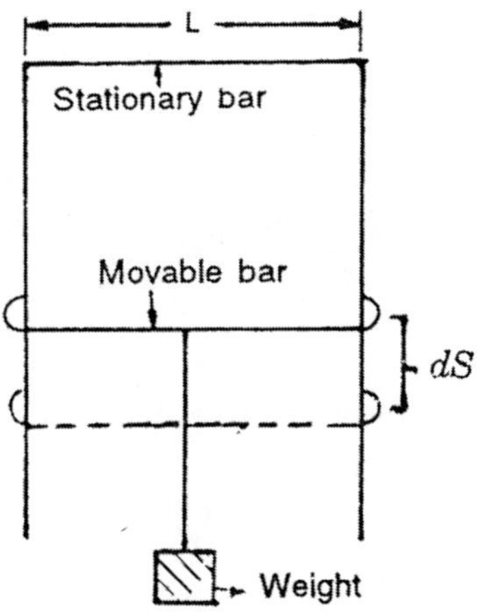

Fig. 28.

1.1. Interfacial tension – *Force per unit length*

Let us consider a three sided wirerame with a movable bar. If this wireframe is dipped into a soap solution and taken out of it, a film of soap solution is formed as shown in Fig. 28. This soap film tends to contract in an attempt to reduce surface area and pulls the movable bar towards the stationary bar. This pull due to surface tension can be counterbalanced by adding weight to the movable bar. This applied force (weight, multiplied by acceleration) is equal to the interfacial tension γ multipled by twice the length of the movable bar as the soap film forms an interface on both the sides of the movable bar

i.e. $w \times a$ or $F = \gamma \times 2L$

where L = length of the movable bar,

a = acceleration due to gravity and

F = Force

$$\text{i.e. } F = 2\gamma L \quad \dots (1)$$

$$\text{or } \gamma = \frac{F}{2L} \quad \dots (2)$$

Thus, the interfacial tension is force per unit length.

1.2. Interfacial tension - *Energy per unit area increase*

Interfacial tension may be expressed as energy per unit area increase if we consider the work needed to increase the surface area of the film.

The work (dW) (or surface free energy) needed to displace the movable bar in the above Fig. 28 by a small distance dS can be given by

$$dW = F \times dS$$

But $F = \gamma \times 2L$

Therefore, $dW = \gamma \times 2L \times dS$

or $dW = \gamma dA$ (since $2L \times dS = dA$)

where dA = increase in area

For a finite work

$$W = \gamma \Delta A \quad \dots (3)$$

$$\text{or } \gamma = \frac{W}{\Delta A} \quad \dots (4)$$

Thus, the surface tension may be defined as surface free energy per unit area increase.

Surface or interface possesses free energy and this energy increases as the surface area is increased. According to thermodynamics all systems will tend to react spontaneously to reach a state with the lowest total free energy (i.e. react in the direction of decrease in free energy). Thus, one of the methods by which a system reduces its surface free energy is by contracting its surface area. This is evident in liquids when a liquid is suspended in air (or in a gas) or in an immiscible liquid, it assumes a minimum surface area to the volume i.e. a spherical shape.

Most interfaces that we come across in pharmaceutical systems are curved. Hence, it is worthwhile to express surface tension in terms of pressure difference across a curved interface.

Interfacial tension — Pressure difference across curved surface

Consider a soap bubble with radius 'r' Fig. 29. Then, the total surface free energy is surface area × surface tension

i.e. $W = 4\pi r^2 \gamma$ ...(5)

where $4\pi r^2$ = surface area of the bubble

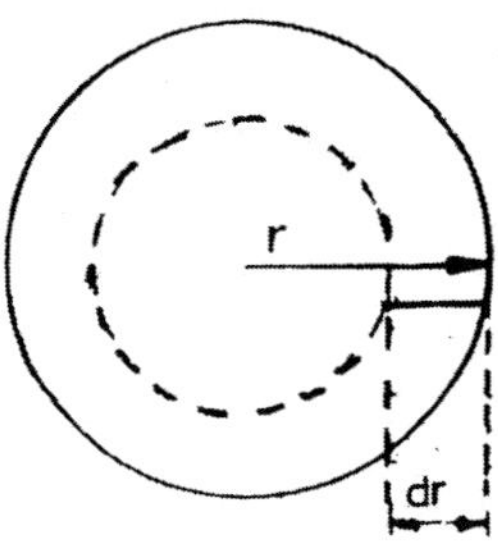

Fig. 29. Representation of pressure difference across curved surface of a soap bubble

If the radius is decreased by dr (caused by shrinkage of the bubble) the surface free energy is given by

$$W = 4\pi\gamma(r - dr)^2$$
$$= 4\pi\gamma(r^2 - 2rdr + (dr)^2$$
$$= 4\pi\gamma r^2 - 8\pi\gamma rdr + 4\pi\gamma(dr)^2 \quad \dots (6)$$

The dr is very small when compared to 'r'. Therefore, the term $4\pi\gamma r(dr)^2$ may be disregarded. The surface free energy change is then given by, as difference of equations 5 and 6.

$$= 4\pi r^2\gamma - (4\pi r^2\gamma - 8\pi\gamma rdr)$$
$$= 4\pi r^2\gamma - 4\pi r^2\gamma + 8\pi\gamma rdr$$
$$= 8\pi\gamma rdr.$$

Due to decrease in radius by dr, the surface free energy changes by the amount $8\pi\gamma rdr$. However this change is opposed by the pressure difference (ΔP) across the wall of the bubble.

Pressure is force per unit area or force is pressure multiplied by area

$$F = \Delta P \times 4\pi r^2$$

The free energy change due to decrease in radius by dr is

$$W = \Delta P \times 4\pi r^2 \times dr$$

where $\Delta P \times 4\pi r^2$ = force, dr = distance

At equilibrium,

$$\Delta P 4\pi r^2 dr = 8\pi\gamma rdr$$

$$\Delta P = \frac{8\pi\gamma rdr}{4\pi r^2 dr} = \frac{2\gamma}{r} \quad \dots (7)$$

$$\text{or, } \gamma = \frac{\Delta Pr}{2} \quad \dots (8)$$

This equation predicts that as the radius of a bubble decreases the pressure inside the bubble increases relative to that outside. That is, the smaller bubble or droplet has greater internal pressure.

1.3. Effect of temperature on Surface tension

When the temperature of a liquid is increased, there is decrease in its surface tension. This decrease in surface tension (due to thermal expansion of liquid) continues as the temperature reaches critical temperature of the liquid (critical temperature is the temperature at which the interface between the liquid and its vapour disappears) at which the surface tension becomes zero.

The relationship between temperature and surface tension is

$$\gamma = \gamma_0 \left(1 - \frac{T}{T_c}\right)^{1.2} \text{ Newtons/metre} \quad \dots (9)$$

where γ = surface tension at temperature T

γ_0 = surface tension at thermodyn zero

T_c = critical temperature

Therefore, one of the conditions in the measurement of surface and interfacial tensions is the control over temperature of the experiment.

2. Measurement of Surface and Interfacial Tensions

The most frequently used methods for the measurement of surface and interfacial tensions are

1. Capillary Rise Method
2. Maximum Bubble Pressure Method
3. Drop-Method
4. Wilhelmy Plate Method
5. Ring-detachment Method (Du-Nuoy tensiometer)

Of the five methods, the ***latter three methods*** are used for determining ***both surface and interfacial tensions*** and the ***first two methods*** are used only to determine ***surface tensions.***

2.1. Capillary Rise Method

When a capillary tube is placed in a liquid such as water contained in a beaker, the liquid immediately rises up the tube to a certain height (Fig. 30).

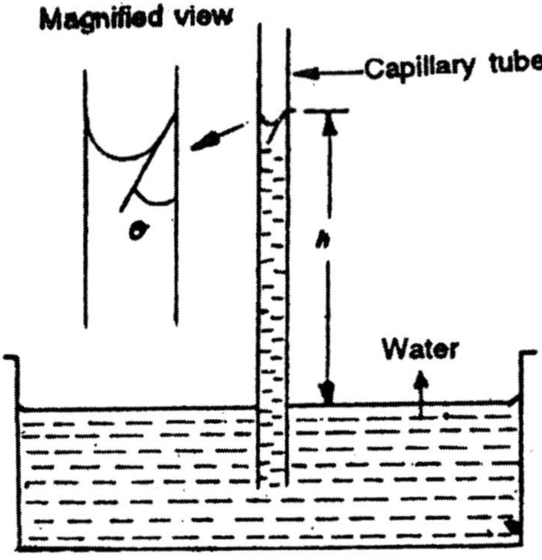

Fig. 30. Measurement of surface tension using capillary method

This rise of the liquid in the tube is due to the surface tension (This occurs when the forces of adhesion between water molecules and glass are greater than the cohesive forces between water molecules). This upward movement stops when the downward force of gravity due to the weight of the liquid just balances it.

Thus, there are two forces one is the upward force due to surface tension and the other is the counteracting force due to the weight of the column of liquid in the tube.

Force due to surface tension

The surface tension at any point on the circumference of the capillary tube is given by

$$\gamma \cos \theta$$

where θ is the angle between the surface of the liquid and the capillary wall. Then the total upward force along the inside circumference of the capillary is given by

$$2\pi r\gamma \cos \theta$$

When a liquid such as water wets the surface of the capillary tube, the θ is taken as unity. Then, the upward force is given by

$$2\pi r\gamma.$$

Counteracting force due to weight of the liquid column

The counteracting force of gravity is given in terms of the weight of the liquid column and is given by

$$\pi r^2 h(\rho - \rho_o)g + w.$$

where πr^2 = cross sectional area of the capillary tube

h = height of liquid column upto the lowest point of the meniscus

ρ and ρ_o = densities of the liquid and its vapour respectively

g = acceleration due to gravity

w = weight of the liquid above h in the meniscus

The density of the liquid is much greater than the density of its vapour and the weight of the liquid in the meniscus above 'h' is negligible as compared to the weight of the liquid column in the capillary. Hence the terms ρ_o and w may be disregarded

Thus the term $\pi r^2 h(\rho - \rho_o)g + w$ reduces to $\pi r^2 h\rho g$

At equilibrium, the upward force due to the surface tension and the counteracting force due to the weight of the liquid column are equal.

$$2\pi r\gamma = \pi r^2 h\rho g$$

$$\gamma = \frac{\pi r^2 h\rho g}{2\pi\gamma}$$

$$\text{or, } \gamma = \frac{1}{2} rh\rho g \quad \text{... (10)}$$

For more accurate result, the equation used for calculation is

$$\gamma = \frac{\left(h + \frac{r}{3}\right)(\rho^l - \rho^V) gr}{2 \cos \theta}$$

For the determination of surface tension, a capillary tube of known diameter is dipped to a desired depth into water contained in a vessel having large diameter. The '*h*' of the liquid column within the capillary tube is determined with the help of a travelling microscope. The other parameter density of the liquid is determined using a density bottle. These values are, then substituted in the formula given below to obtain the surface tension of water

$$\gamma = \frac{1}{2} rh\rho g$$

Precautions

1. The outer vessel should have a larger diameter
2. The capillary tube should have uniform diameter throughout its length
3. It is better to allow the meniscus to fall than to allow it to rise.
4. The height of the column should be measured accurately (with a cathetometer).
5. Temperature must be maintained constant throughout the experiment

2.2. Maximum Bubble Pressure Method

Two capillary tubes of radii r_1 and r_2 are immersed to the same depth in a liquid. The pressure required to liberate bubbles from each of the tube is measured. The surface tension can be calculated from the difference of these pressures. If r_1 is less than 0.01 cm and r_2 is not greater than 0.2 cm, the surface tension is given by

$$\gamma = AP\left(1 + 0.67 r_2 g \frac{D}{P}\right) \quad \text{... (11)}$$

where A is an apparatus constant determined with a standard liquid. D is the density of the liquid and P is the difference in pressure.

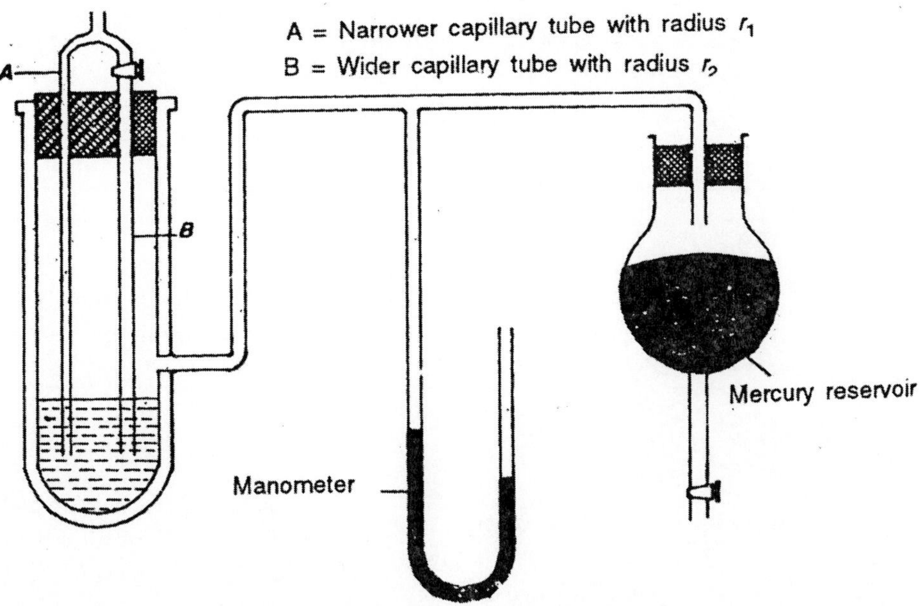

Fig. 31. Measurement of surface tension by maximum bubble pressure method

The apparatus is assembled as shown in Fig. 31.

The stopcock is opened. The mercury is allowed to drop down from the reservoir slowly till the bubbles come out from the wider capillary (B). The maximum pressure required for this is noted from the manometer. The apparatus is reset and the stopcock of capillary B is closed so that bubbles will form only from the smaller (thinner) capillary. The pressure is noted. The experiment is repeated. The difference between these pressures will give the value of P. Substituting these values in the formula, the surface tension is obtained.

2.3. Drop Method

When a liquid is allowed to fall through a capillary tube, it forms a drop which increases in size and detaches from the tip of the tube when the weight of the drop of the liquid just equals the total surface tension at the circumference of the tube (Fig. 32).

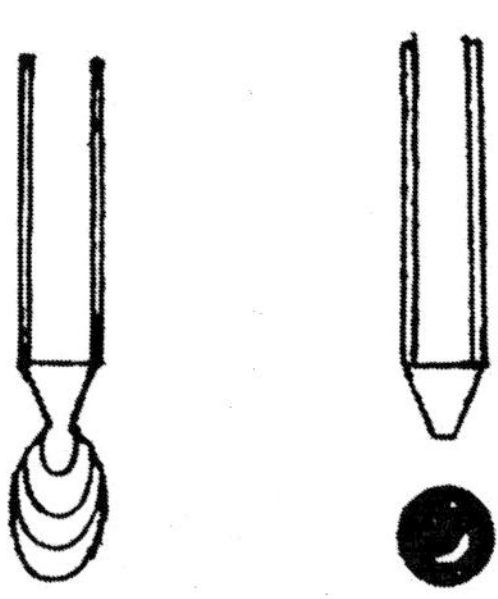

Fig. 32. Formation of a drop from the tip of capillary tube

Expressing mathematically

$$w = 2\pi r\gamma \qquad \text{... (12)}$$

where w = weight of one drop of the liquid

r = radius of the capillary

γ = surface tension of the liquid.

Determination of surface tension can be undertaken in two ways by using a drop pipette **(Stalagmometer)**

1. Drop weight method
2. Drop count method

Drop weight method

The stalagmometer (Fig. 33) consists of a glass tube with a bulb blown approximately in the middle of the tube. There are two markings A and B as shown in the figure. The tip of the stalagmometer is capillary.

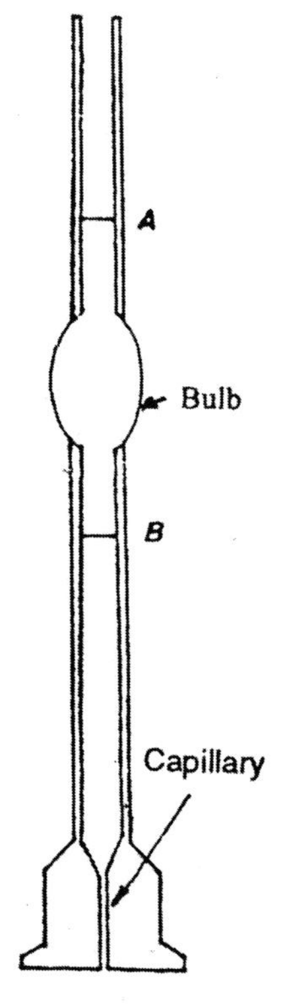

Fig. 33. Stalagmometer (or) Drop pipette

The given liquid is sucked into the drop pipette upto the marking A. Then the liquid is allowed to drop slowly from the tip of the pipette. Twenty to thirty drops are collected from the pipette kept vertically into a clean tarred beaker and the weight of one drop of the liquid is found out (w). The surface tension of the liquid is, then given by

$$w = 2\pi r\gamma$$

$$\gamma = \frac{w}{2\pi r}$$

It is usual to report relative surface tension of a liquid with respect to water. For this, the liquid is first taken in the pipette. The weight of one drop of the the liquid (w_l) is found out as decribed above. Similarly water is taken in the pipette and the weight of one drop of water (w_w) is obtained. The relative surface tension of the liquid

$$= \frac{\text{Surface tension of the liquid}}{\text{Surface tension of water}}$$

$$= \frac{w_l/2\pi r}{w_w/2\pi r}$$

$$= \frac{w_l}{w_w} \quad \text{... (13)}$$

Drop count method

In this method, the given liquid is sucked into the drop pipette upto the mark *A*. Keeping the pipette vertically, the number of drops formed when the liquid level falls from mark *A* to *B* is noted.

We know that

$$\gamma = \frac{\text{weight of one drop of liquid}}{2\pi r}$$

$$= \frac{mg}{2\pi r \times n}$$

where m = mass

g = gravitational force

n = number of drops

$$\text{Also, } \gamma = \frac{vdg}{2\pi r \times n}$$

where vd = volume × density = mass (m)

For relative surface tension of a liquid, the number of drops of water (n) formed for the same volume (*A* to *B*) is found out. Then, the relative surface tension of the liquid is given by

$$= \frac{\text{Surface tension of liquid}}{\text{Surface tension of water}}$$

$$= \frac{vd_l g/2\pi r n_l}{vd_w g/2\pi r n_w}$$

$$= \frac{d_l/n_l}{d_w/n_w}$$

$$= \frac{d_l}{d_w} \times \frac{n_w}{n_l} \quad \text{... (14)}$$

When the interfacial tension is determined, the drops are formed within the other immiscible liquid. It is important to make sure that the tip of the pipette is completely wetted by one of the two immiscible liquids.

Precautions

1. The tip of the pipette should have no imperfections in the outer circumference.
2. The drops should be formed slowly.
3. About 20 to 30 drops should be collected and from this average weight is determined.
4. Temperature should be maintained constant.

2.4. Wilhelmy Plate Method

It provides for the direct measurement of force exerted on a piece of thin platinum foil at the interface between two immiscible liquids or surface of a liquid. The force exerted is equal to the

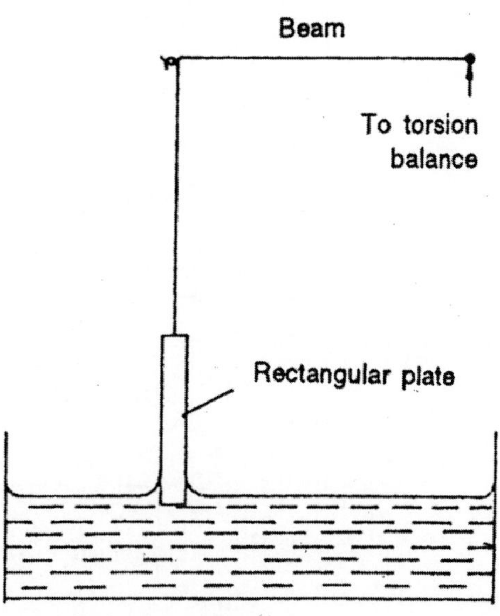

Fig. 34. Wilhelmy plate

surface tension multiplied by the perimeter of the foil.

A thin rectangular plate of platinum (or mica) is suspended vertically from a beam attached to a torsion balance (Fig. 34). The liquid whose surface tension is to be measured is taken in a dish and this is raised under the plate until the bottom edge of the plate just comes in contact with the surface of the liquid. When the plate touches the surface, the surface forces will drag the plate downwards and this force exerted around the perimeter of the plate is measured by the rotation of the torsion wire required to restore the plate to its original position (i.e. when the edge of the plate is coincident with the plane of the free liquid surface).

If the liquid completely wets the plate, the force exerted in terms of weight is given by

$$W = 2(L + T)\gamma$$

$$\gamma = \frac{W}{2(L + T)} \quad \ldots (15)$$

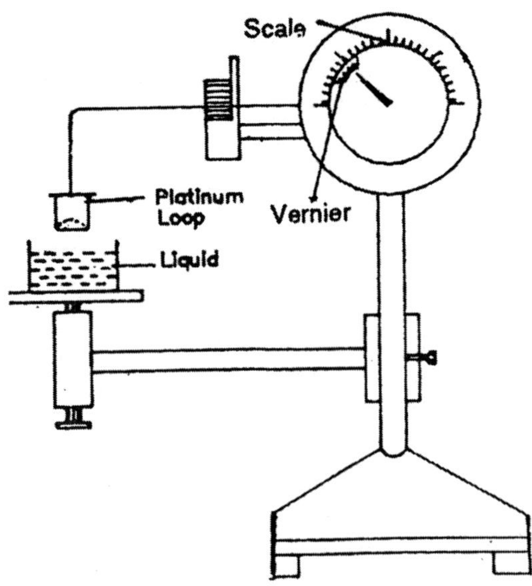

Fig. 35. Du Nuoy ring tensiometer

where L and T are the length and thickness of the plate on the horizontal plane respectively and $2(L + T)$ represents the perimeter of the rectangular plate.

2.5. Ring detachment method (Du Nuoy Ring Tensiometer)

The principle involved in *Du Nuoy* tensiometer is that the force needed to lift a wire ring from the surface or between two immiscible liquids is proportional to the surface or interfacial tension respectively.

The apparatus is also called *Torsion balance* or *Du Nuoy*'s balance which is shown in Fig. 35.

A platinum wire ring of about four centimeter in circumference is suspended from the loop attached to a scale through a torsion wire. The liquid is taken in the pan and the position of the pan is adjusted so that ring just touches the surface of the liquid. The torsion on the wire is increased gradually so that the ring just detaches from the surface of the liquid. The force required (to detach) is read in dynes on the graduated disc which is directly proportional to the surface tension

$$P = w = 2\pi(r_1 + r_2)\gamma$$

$$\text{or } \gamma = \frac{P}{2\pi(r_1 + r_2)} \quad \ldots (16)$$

where P is the pull exerted through torsion wire on the ring and is read on the scale, where $w =$ force in terms of weight and r_1 and r_2 are inner and outer radii of the ring

Introducing a correction factor (c.f), the equation becomes

$$\gamma = \frac{P}{2\pi(r_1 + r_2)} \times \text{c.f.} \quad \ldots (17)$$

If the radius of the wire is small and that $r_1 = r_2$

$$\gamma = \frac{P}{4\pi r} \times \text{c.f.} \quad \ldots (18)$$

The correction factor (c.f.) is introduced to compensate for variables in the radius of the ring, radius of the wire used to form the ring and for the volume of the liquid raised out of the surface.

For the determination of interfacial tension, the ring is detached from the interface between two immiscible liquids. The ring should be preferentially wetted by the denser liquid.

Experimental Precautions

1. The ring should lie in a flat plane
2. The plane of the ring must be horizontal
3. The vessel (pan) containing the liquid should have wider diameter.
4. Temperature control should be adequate.

3. Spreading coefficient:

When oleic acid is dropped on to water, it spreads immediately on the surface of water. In this case, oleic acid is considered as the spreading liquid (L) and the water as the sublayer liquid (S).

In general, spreading occurs when the adhesive forces exceed the cohesive forces.

The work of cohesion (w_c) may be considered as the surface free energy increase produced by separating a column of pure liquid into two halves (Fig. 36).

The free energy increase on increasing the surface area has already been given as $\gamma \Delta A$

Then,

$$w_c = \gamma_L \Delta A + \gamma_L \Delta A$$

$$= \gamma_L (\Delta A + \Delta A)$$

Considering a column of liquid with a cross sectional area of 1 cm^2, the equation is

$$w_c = \gamma_L (1 + 1)$$

$$w_c = 2\gamma_L \quad \text{... (19)}$$

(When these two newly created surfaces are brought together to form a column of liquid, again an equal and opposite amount of energy will be released)

The work of adhesion (w_a) may be considered as the free energy increase produced by separating a column of two immiscible liquids at the boundary (at the interface) into two sections (Fig. 37).

The work of adhesion is

$$w_a = \gamma_L \Delta A + \gamma_S \Delta A - \gamma_{LS} \Delta A$$

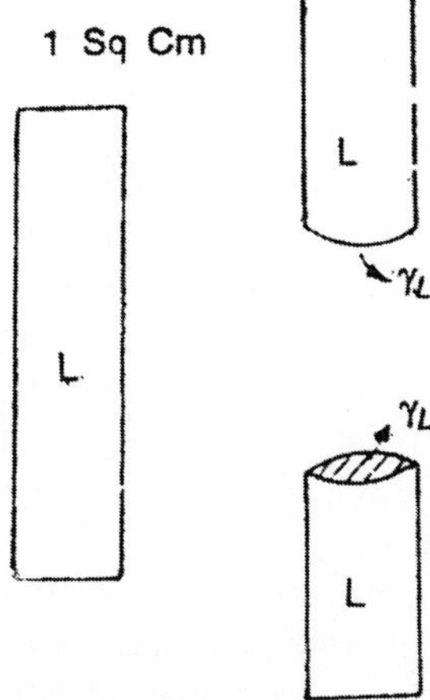

Fig. 36. Work of cohesion

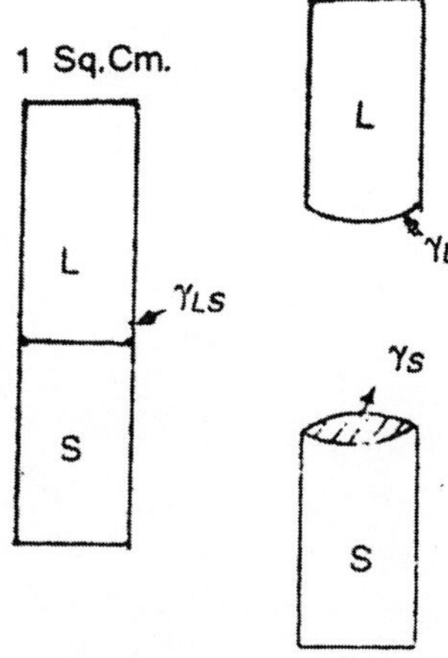

Fig. 37. Work of adhesion

As the two sections of the immiscible liquids are already separated by a boundary (because of more of cohesive forces than of adhesive forces), the energy required to separate into two sections is less by an amount equal to γ_{LS} and hence the term γ_{LS} in the equation.

Considering a column with a cross sectional area of 1 cm^2

$$w_a = \gamma_S \cdot 1 + \gamma_L \cdot 1 - \gamma_{LS} \cdot 1$$

$$= \gamma_L + \gamma_S - \gamma_{LS} \quad \text{... (20)}$$

When the two newly created surfaces in the two sections are brought together to form a single column of liquid again with the interface, an equal and opposite amount of energy will be released.

The **spreading coefficient (S) is the difference between the work of adhesion and the work of cohesion ($w_a - w_c$)**. That is, if the work of adhesion is more than the work of cohesion, spreading will occur

Then, $w_a - w_c = \gamma_S + \gamma_L - \gamma_{LS} - (2\gamma_L)$

$$\text{or } S = \gamma_S + \gamma_L - \gamma_{LS} - 2\gamma_L$$

$$= \gamma_S - \gamma_L - \gamma_{LS}$$

$$S = \gamma_S - (\gamma_L + \gamma_{LS}) \quad \text{... (21)}$$

where γ_L refers to the surface tension of the spreading liquid, γ_S refers to the surface tension of the sublayer liquid and γ_{LS} refers to the interfacial tension.

Spreading occurs when the surface tension of the sublayer liquid is greater than the sum of the surface tension of the spreading liquid and the interfacial tension between the sublayer and the spreading liquid.

If 'S' is negative that is when $(\gamma_L + \gamma_{LS})$ is larger than γ_S, the spreading liquid forms a globule or a floating lens. That is, spreading will not take place.

Under Thermodynamics, we have studied that a process is spontaneous where there is a decrease in free energy. In the same way when the free energy of the spreading liquid and the interfacial tension with the sublayer is less than the free energy of the sublayer liquid, spreading becomes spontaneous in an attempt to reduce the free energy of the sublayer liquid.

However, it is to be understood that what has been discussed so far refers to initial spreading. There may be saturation of one liquid within the other and that there may be a change in the surface tension of the sublayer liquid. In that case, if the spreading coefficient becomes negative after saturation, the spreading liquid coalesces and forms a lens on the surface of the sublayer liquid. The initial spreading may be positive or negative but the final spreading coefficient is always negative in the case of organic liquids.

In the case of **Duplex film** (a multilayer film with a thickness of about 100 Å), if 'S' becomes negative after saturation, the film becomes unstable and it forms monolayer and the excess liquid (spreading liquid) remains as a lens on the surface.

Fatty acids and alcohols have high spreading coefficients as they contain polar groups such as – COOH and – OH respectively. As non-polar character is increased by increasing the hydrocarbon chain of an acid or alcohol, the spreading coefficient gradually decreases. For example, propionic acid and ethyl alcohol have high spreading coefficients while non-polar substances such as liquid petroleum do not spread on water. Benzene spreads on water not because of its polar nature but because the cohesive forces are much weaker than the adhesive forces.

3.1 Applications of spreading coefficient

Spreading coefficient is a factor to be considered in the preparation of lotions. One requirement for lotions is the proper spreading on the skin which has polar-nonpolar character. A lotion with an oily base may need a surfactant to promote spreading on the skin. Spreading coefficient may also be applied to know the proper HLB value (dealt later) for emulsification of an oil. The oil as such may not spread on water. Surfactant blends with various HLB values are added to the oil and a drop of it is placed on water. Then the spreading is related to the required HLB value for emulsification.

4. Adsorption at Liquid Surfaces

4.1. Surfactants

Certain solute molecules and ions when added to a liquid are partitioned in favour of the surface or the interface and this phenomenon is termed *positive adsorption*. Some other solute molecules or ions (eg. glucose and sodium chloride) are partitioned in favour of the bulk of liquid and this is termed *negative adsorption*.

In the case of positive adsorption, there is a decrease in surface tension and with negative adsorption there is an increase in the surface tension.

Solute molecules or ions that are perferentially adsorbed at the surface or interface reduce the surface or interfacial tension and they are termed surface active agents or surfactants. All surfactants are amphiphiles. i.e. they have both polar and non-polar groups. The amphiphile may be hydrophilic if it is predominantly polar in nature (eg. ethyl alcohol) and lipophilic when predominantly non-polar in nature (eg. cetyl alcohol). In some amphiphiles, both polar and non-polar nature may be well balanced.

If a surface active agent with a good balance between polar and non-polar groups is added to water, it gets perferentially adsorbed (or concentrated) at the surface that is, the polar end is oriented towards water and the non-polar end is projected upwards into space (Fig. 38). When the same agent is added to immiscible liquids such as oil and water, the molecules of the surface active agent get adsorbed at the interface between the two immiscible liquids as shown below (Fig. 39).

At low concentration of the surfactant, the surface of the water is not completely filled with the surfactant molecules (Fig. 40). However, the surface gets filled up progressively as the concentration is increased with a marked decrease in the surface tension. At certain higher concentration the energy required to push more molecules into surface approaches the energy that is given up on adsorption. Subsequently

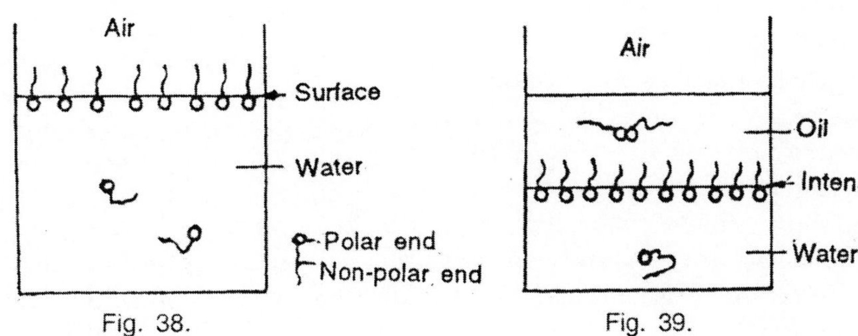

Fig. 38. Fig. 39.

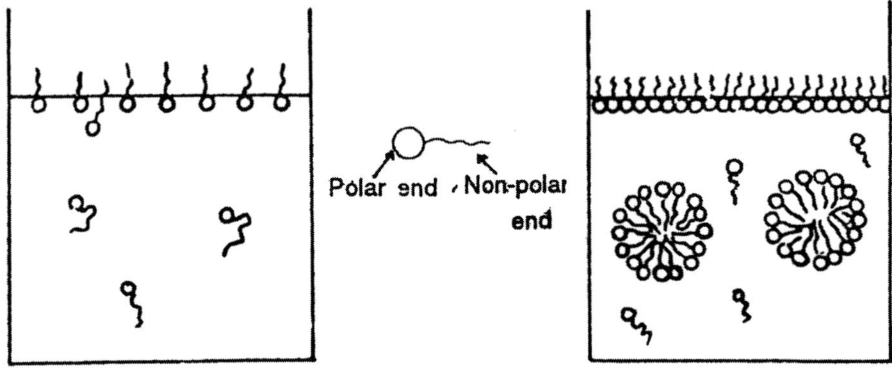

Fig. 40. At low conc.

Fig. 41. At C.M.C.

there is a greater lowering of free energy in the bulk of the liquid because of the association of surfactant molecules into small aggregates called ***micelles*** (Fig. 41). The micelle formed is of colloidal dimension and is believed to contain 50 to 100 molecules (Association colloid). In a micelle, polar groups of the surfactant molecules are oriented towards aqueous phase and the non-polar groups are associated together at the centre into a spherical structure as shown in the diagram. The lowest concentration at which these micelles are formed in appreciable number is called the ***critical micellar concenti ation*** (CMC). It represents effective concentration within the bulk of the solution. Micellation is an alternative mechanism to interfacial adsorption.

These micelles are usually spherical in shape. However at much higher concentrations than the CMC, the spherical micelles are believed to rearrange into lamellar micelles (Fig. 42). The micelles are not static aggregates, but dissociate, regroup and reassociate rapidly.

However, if the surfactant is too hydrophilic, it remains within the bulk of the aqueous phase and produces little effect at the interface and so is the effect with surfactant which is too lipophilic as it remains completely within the bulk of the oil.

The critical micellar concentrations and aggregation number of some surfactants in water at room temperatures are.

(a) $nC_{11}H_{23}COOK$ (potassium laurate) CMC (in mM/L) is 24, aggregation number of the micelle is 50

(b) $nC_{12}H_{25}OSO_3Na$ (sodium lauryl sulfate) CMC (in mM/L) 59.8, aggregation number of the micelle is 60

The critical micellar concentration of a surfactant is the concentration of surfactants in the bulk of the liquid at which the micelles start forming. This concentration will not include the amount of surfactants accomodated at the interfaces. As increasing amounts of a solid surfactant are dissolved in a beaker full of water and as its concentration in solution increases, a

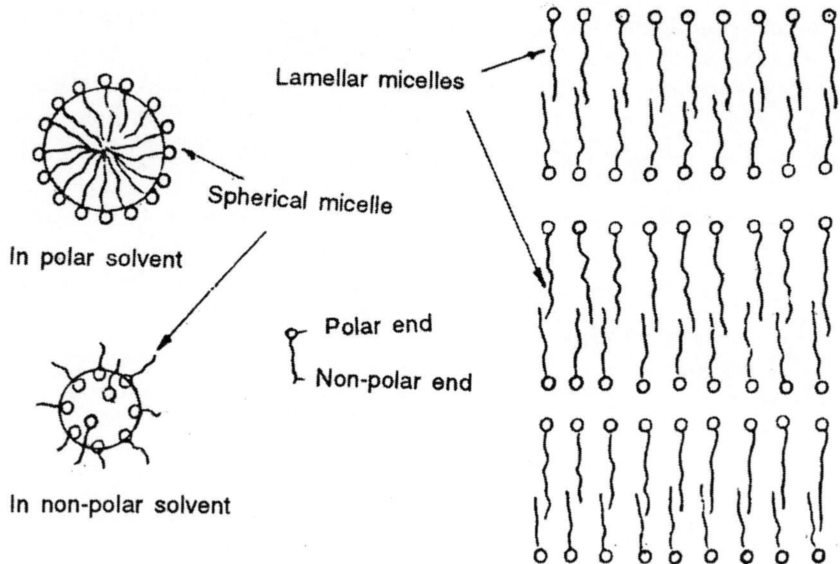

Fig. 42.

monoloyer is adsorbed at the air-water and glass-water interfaces and the molecules become more and more crowded at the adsorbed surfaces until they are so tightly packed that further occupancy requires excessive compression of the surfactant molecules in the two monolayers (one is air-water interface and the second is glass-water interface). It is called saturation adsorption. Further increments in the amount of dissolved surfactant beyond that concentration cause the molecules to aggregate into micelles. The process begins at a characteristic concentration of the surfactant called critical micellar concentration (CMC). From then on, the concentration of the monomeric or non associated molecules hardly increses, but the concentration of micelles or associated molecules increases in direct proportion to the increase in overall surfactant concentration. In dilute solutions, the micelles are approximately of the same size and increments in surfactant concentration merely increase the number of micelles. At CMC, physical porperties of the solution of the association colloids show marked changes which may be used to find out CMC of surfactant (refer suggestions for practicals).

4.2. Surfactant Classification

Surfactants can be classified according to the chemical structure i.e. according to the polar portion. They may be ionic and non-ionic.

The ionic surfactants are further classified into anionic, catonic and ampholytic (or amphoteric).

Anionic surfactants

An anionic surfactant ionises in aqueous solution to yield a large anion which is responsible for its action and a small cation. They are mostly carboxylates (eg. potassium stearate soap), sulphonates (eg. *di(2-ethyl hexyl) sodium sulpho succinate and. sodium cetyl sulfonate)* and sulfates (eg *sodium lauryl sulfate*).

Cationic surfactants

A cationic surfactant ionises in aqueous solution to yield a large cation which is responsible for its action and a small anion. They are amines and quarternary ammonium salts. They are mostly used as anti-microbial preservatives (eg. *cetyl trimethyl ammonium bromide or cetrimide*) That is, it acts both as antimicrobial preservative as well as surfactant.

Amphoteric surfactants

They contain mainly carboxylate or phosphate groups as the anion and amine or quarternary ammonium groups as the cation. They are polypeptides, proteins, lecithins and cephalins (eg. *N-dodecyl alanine*).

Non-ionic surfactants

The widely used class of surfactants in pharmaceutical systems are non-ionic surfactants which do not ionise in aqueous solution. The most widely used compounds are the *polyoxyethylene sorbitan fatty acid esters* in both internal and external pharmaceutical formulations (eg. *polyoxyethylene sorbitan mono-oleate*).

4.3. HLB value of surfactants

Surfactants are amphiphiles which mean they have both polar and non-polar characters. Surfactants with more polar characters are termed hydrophiles and those with more non-polar characters are termed lipophiles. The balance between hydrophilic and lipophilic nature may be given in terms of HLB values. Thus HLB is hydrophile-lipophile-balance. Griffin devised an arbitrary scale of HLB values to indicate the measure of hydrophilic-lipophilic balance of surface active agents. The oil soluble surfactants have low HLB values and the water soluble surfactants have high HLB values. The higher the HLB value, the more hydrophilic is the surfactant. Depending upon the HLB values, the surfactants have different uses.

HLB values of polyhydric alcohol fatty acid esters such as glyceryl monostearate, sorbitan mono-oleate, sorbitan mono-laurate, polyoxyethylene sorbitan mono-oleate, polyoxyethylene sorbitan monolaurate etc. may be estimated by employing the formula

$$\text{HLB} = 20\left(1 - \frac{S}{A}\right) \quad \text{... (22)}$$

where S = saponification number of the ester

A = acid number of the fatty acid

(refer suggestions to practicals)

Another method is given by Davies. In this method the component groups of the surfactant molecules are assigned group numbers. By adding the group numbers of a surfactant, we can arrive at the HLB value of that surfactant. The equation used for this purpose is

$$\text{HLB} = \Sigma\ (\text{hydrophilic group numbers}) - \Sigma\ (\text{lipophilic group numbers}) + 7$$

HLB Group numbers

Hydrophilic groups	Group number	Lipophilic groups	Group number
$-SO_3^- Na^+$	38.7	$- CH -$	0.475
$- COO^- Na^+$	19.1	$- CH_2 -$	0.475
ester (sorbitan ring)	6.8	$- CH_3 -$	0.475
ester (free)	2.4	$= CH -$	0.475
hydroxyl (free)	1.9		
hydroxyl (sorbitan ring)	0.5		

HLB values of some surfactants (Amphiphilic agents)

Oleic acid – 1

Glyceryl mono stearate – 3.8

Sorbitan mono-oleate (span 80) – 4.3

Sorbitan mono-laurate (span 20) – 8.6

Triethnolamine oleate – 12.0

Polyoxyethylene sorbitan mono-oleate (Tween 80) – 15.0

Polyoxyethylene sorbitan monolaurate (Tween 20) – 16.7

Sodium oleate – 18.0

Sodium lauryl sulphate – 40.0

Surfactant Functions on the basis of HLB Value:

	HLB number		Function
Lipophilic	1-3	–	Antifoaming agents
	3-8	–	w/o emulsifying agents
	7-9	–	wetting and spreading agents
Hydrophilic	8-16	–	o/w emulsifying agent
	13-16	–	detergents
	> 16	–	solubilising agents

4.4. Applications of Surfactants

Surfactants are mainly used as *wetting, solubilizing* and *emulsifying agents* and as *detergents.*

In the case of capsules, once the capsule content is released, the rate of dissolution of poorly soluble drugs depends upon wetting. This can be achieved by including surfactants and the rate of dissolution is found to be proportional to the reduction in surface tension of the solution.

Disintegration and dissolution of tablets are affected by binding between the granules, the presence of adsorbed air on the granules and hydrophobic surface which may be due to hydrophobic lubricant. However these defects may be greatly diminished by including a surfactant such as sodium lauryl sulphate.

Wetting with the help of surfactants can be of great help in the dispersion of powders to prepare suspensions, in the use of contact lens and in implants intended for slow release of drugs.

Foaming agents: Solutions of surface active agents produce stable foams when mixed with air intimately and hence surface active agents are called foaming agents. Foams are air pockets enclosed within thin films of liquid. Surfactants are used to stabilise gas in liquid. They are extensively used in shampoos and lathering shaving creams.

Antifoaming agents: When the liquid drains away from the area surrounding the air globules, the foam finally collapses. Surfactants which are used to break the foam are known as antifoaming agents. Other antifoaming agents are octanol, ether, castor oil and silicones. Foams are produced in fermentation processes and is a nuisance. Hence they are prevented or destroyed using antifoaming agents. Foaming in solubilised liquid preparations also poses a problem in formulation.

In addition to applications so far mentioned, surfactants find application as anti-bacterials, protective agents and as aids to the absorption of drugs in the body. A surfactant may itself exert a drug action (eg. procain amide) or may affect the activity of a drug. For example, the activity of hexylresorcinol on pinworm Ascaris is potentiated by the presence of a low concentration of surfactant. The surfactant reduces the interfacial tension between the liquid phase and the cell wall of the organism facilitating the adsorption and spreading of hexylresorcinol over the surface of the organism. However when the concentration approaches CMC, the rate of penetration of the anthelmintic drops nearly to zero as a result of partitioning of the drug between the micelles and the aqueous phase. This leads to a reduction in effective concentration.

Quarternary ammonium compounds, which are surface active agents, in themselves possess antibacterial activity. These agents, getting adsorbed on the bacterial cell surface, increase permeability or leakiness of the lipid cell membrane of the organism. Ultimately death occurs due to the loss of essential materials from the cell. Both gram positive and gram negative organisms are susceptible to the attack of cationic quaternary ammonium compounds. In the case of anionic surfactants, gram positive organisms are more susceptible to the attack than are gram-negative organisms. Non-ionic surfactants are the least effective and they often aid rather than inhibit the growth of micro-organisms. This may be attributed to the presence of long chain fatty acids in a form easily metabolisable by the organism.

Rate of intestinal absorption of some drugs may be increased or decreased by some surfactants. It may possibly be due to alteration of the intestinal membrane by the surfactant.

Many of the surfactants are drugs. For example, phenothiazine and procaine are tranquilizer and local anaesthetic respectively. Some other drugs which are also surfactants are acridines (antibacterial) streptomycin, penicillins (antibiotics), barbiturates (hypnotics), veratrum alkaloids (anticancer drugs) and vitamin A.

5. Monomolecular surface films

The surfactants which get adsorbed at the surface of a liquid (may be water) may be divided into two groups.

1. Those that form *insoluble monomolecular layer* and
2. Those that form *soluble monomolecular layer.*

For example, cetyl alcohol forms an insoluble monomolecular layer and amyl alcohol is said to form a soluble monomolecular layer.

a) Insoluble monomolecular layer or film

The technique used in the study of insoluble film or layer in the film balance (Fig. 43). In this technique the substance (surfactant) to be studied is dissolved in a volatile solvent. The solution is, then, placed on the surface of the substrate (may be water). The solution spreads as a film. The solvent evaporates leaving the molecules of the surfactant on the surface. A movable barrier is moved in the direction of the float against stationary barrier so that it just comes in contact with the film that covers an area. Now the area of the film is noted. Then the movable barrier is further moved against the stationary barrier compressing the film gradually.

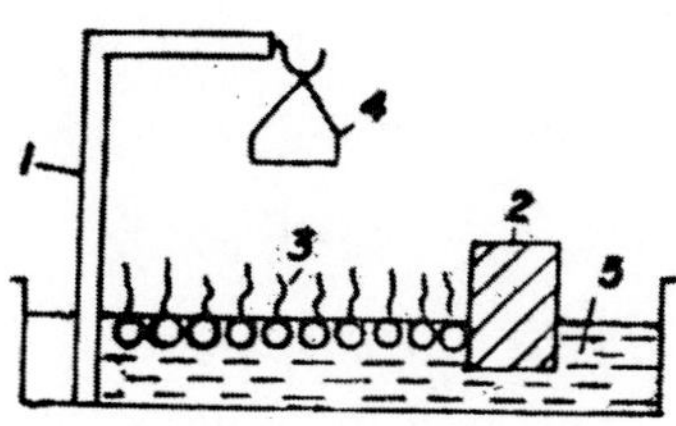

Fig. 43. Film balance
1. Fixed barrier 2. Movable barrier
3. Film 4. Weight 5. Water

The area of the film and the film pressure 'π' at each position are measured. A graph of the area of film against the film pressure 'π' is obtained. This graph is called π–A curve.

The film pressure is the difference between the surface tension (γ_0) of the substrate (water) and the surface tension (γ) of the film covered surface.

$$\pi = (\gamma_0 - \gamma)$$

A typical curve is shown in Fig. 44.

When the area available per molecule is greater than 50 Å^2, it exerts little pressure on the barrier and hence the film behaves like a gas in two dimensions (They act like gas molecules as they are far apart). However as the film is compressed using the barrier a liquid phase that is in equilibrium with the gas phase appears. As the film is further compressed, a liquid phase in two dimensions results followed by a less compressible condensed liquid state region L_2. This leads to a two dimensional solid state. Thus the slope gives information about the nature of packing in the surface film. Finally the film collapses or breaks when it is greatly compressed. The smallest area the molecules occupy before the film collapses is known as *limiting area*. It gives information about the dimensions of the molecules in the film. The film pressure

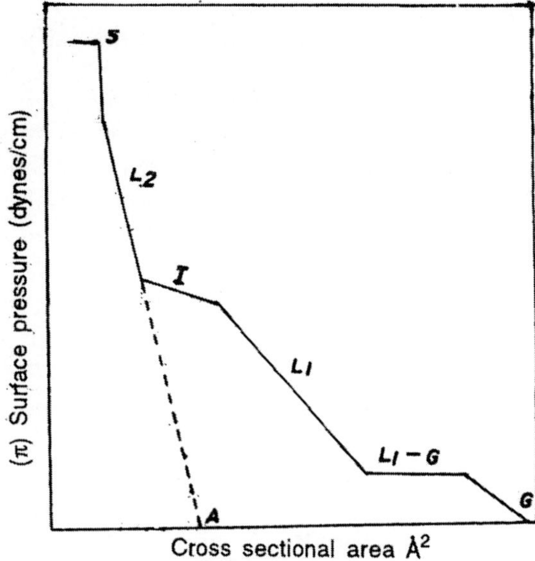

G = Behaves like gas (two dimensional)
L_1-G = Gas-liquid in equilibrium
L_2 = Condensed liquid state
I = Intermediate phase
S = Two dimensional solid phase
A = Areas of close packed molecule

Fig. 44. π-A Curve

that causes the film to collapse is called the *collapse pressure*.

From the graph, it can be understood that the inter-molecular distances of the surfactant molecules get reduced upon moving the barrier. The surface pressure rises as the air-water surface is being covered by the surfactant molecules to a greater extent and it gives the rate of change in π with A and this will depend on the extent of interaction among film molecules. A greater rate of change indicates the film gets more condensed.

The cross-sectional area per molecule when close packed at zero pressure is obtained by extrapolating the linear portion of the curve to the horizontal axis as shown in the figure. Film balance can also be used to study the viscosity of monomolecular films. The molecular weight of high polymers (such as proteins) may be estimated. The relationship between the biologic activity and unfolding of some protein molecules from spherical configuration can also be obtained using film balance technique. The size and shapes of molecules of steroids, hormones and enzymes and the interaction of these with drugs at the interfaces can also be investigated.

b) Soluble monomolecular layer or film

Some surfactants such as amyl alcohol form a soluble monomolecular layer or film on the surface of water on adding directly to water. After the monomolecular layer is formed, if the film is compressed (using movable barrier against stationary barrier), it produces no increase in π as in the case of insoluble monomolecular film. Generally, the more polar the molecule, the higher is the area per molecule where a constant pressure occurs.

This behaviour may be explained by assuming that polar molecules form monomolecular films when placed on water. On compression, the molecules enter the aqueous bulk solution rather than to remain as an intact insoluble film. This constant surface pressure even with increased compression is due to a constant number of molecules per unit area that remains at the surface at equilibrium with dissolved molecules. The extent of such a behaviour will be greater for substances exhibiting weaker intermolecular interaction and greater water solubility.

Since such soluble monomolecular adsorbed film cannot be compressed, there is no simple direct way to estimate the number of molecules per unit area at the surface under a given set of conditions. However, it is possible to estimate this value applying Gibbs equation which relates surface concentration to surface tension change produced at different surface activities.

Gibbs equation is given as

$$\Gamma = -\frac{c}{RT}\frac{d\gamma}{dc} \qquad \dots (23)$$

where Γ = surface excess concentration (the excess surfactant found per unit area at the surface with respect to the amount found in the bulk of the liquid) in moles per unit area

c = concentration of surfactant in the bulk of the liquid.

T = absolute temperature.

R = gas constant.

$\frac{d\gamma}{dc}$ = change in surface tension with change in concentration of the surfactant.

For the study of soluble monomolecular film, a microtome blade may be used. The microtome blade may be fired on the surface of the substrate liquid to which the surfactant has been already added. This operation collects surface layer. This scooped liquid is analysed and the concentration is found and compared with the concentration in the bulk to verify the Gibb's equation. The results have been found to agree well.

A knowledge of surface excess also allows calculation of area occupied by each molecule at the surface.

c) Mixed films

Water soluble surfactants can penetrate into an insoluble monolayer of a surfactant to form mixed monolayers (Fig. 45). There may be molecular association between the two components due to a strong attraction between the polar groups. This is accompanied by a monolayer penetration only if the soluble molecules have large hydrocarbon groups so that they can form interchain cohesion with hydrocarbon chain

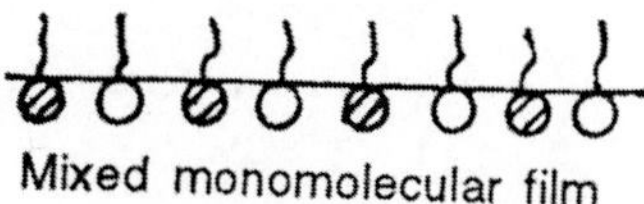

Mixed monomolecular film

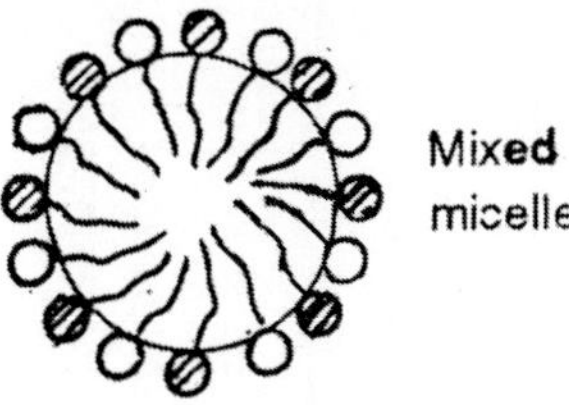

Fig. 45.

of the insoluble monolayer molecules. Sometimes, the association is strong enough to form complexes. But not all surfactants form complexes. The extent of molecular association at a water-oil interface is indicated by the stability of emulsions.

At critical micellar concentration, there may be formation of mixed micelles (micelle containing molecules of two surfactants) (Fig. 45). The mixed micelles (liquid crystals) may contribute for greater stability.

d) Macromolecular films

Like monomolecular layers containing simple molecules, there may be macromolecular films especially in the case of proteins and hydrocolloids. Interfacial tension is greatly reduced with solutions of proteins at isoelectric point. For example, in the case of gelatin, the molecules have large inter- and intra molecular cohesion and also better packing at the interface leading to greater reduction in interfacial tension.

Hydrocolloid molecules such as acacia are adsorbed at oil-water interface and they are said to form multilayers stabilising the dispersions. Branched molecules of acacia form rigid films whereas unbranched sodium alginate molecules form liquid films. Thus the properties of these films have an important role to play in the stability of emulsions. The thickness of an acacia multilayer varies with the type of oil used in the emulsions.

6. Adsorption

The surface tension of solids are difficult to obtain as the solid molecules are immobile and not homogeneous in comparison to liquid surfaces. A molecule within the bulk of a solid is attracted equally by the surrounding neighbour molecules in all directions. However those at the surface experience an imbalance of forces as in the case of liquid surface. Due to this imbalance of forces, the surface molecules attract other molecules (gas or liquid molecules or solute molecules from its solution). This is termed adsorption. Adsorption may be considered as an attempt to reduce the surface free energy of solids.

Adsorption is a surface phenomena whereas absorption refers to uniform distribution of one substance throughout another. The adsorption within highly porous solids, is often termed as ***sorption***.

The degree of adsorption depends on

1. the chemical nature of the adsorbent (that which adsorbs)
2. the chemical nature of the adsorbate (that which is adsorbed)
3. the temperature and
4. the partial pressure of the adsorbed gas in the case of gas molecules adsorption or the concentration of solution in the case of solute molecules adsorption from its solution.

Adsorption may be of two types – physical adsorption and chemical adsorption (chemisorption) Physical adsorption is associated with *van der Waals* forces and hence physical adsorption is also known as *van der Waals* adsorption

Desorption is the opposite of adsorption and is the removal of the adsorbate from the surface of the adsorbent. Desorption of gas molecules from a solid surface may be undertaken by increasing the temperature and by reducing the pressure.

van der Waals adsorption is characterised by low heats of adsorption (20 to 40 kJ per mole of gas). Adsorption of gases is at maximum near the liquefaction temperatures and at partial pressures near to one. It is a reversible process.

Chemisorption is due to chemical combination of adsorbate molecules and the surface molecules of the adsorbent. It involves a high heat of adsorption (740 kJ/mole). It is irreversible. It is of little importance in pharmacy.

6.1. Adsorption at Solid/Gas interface

The results of adsorption processes are usually expressed in the form of a graph showing the relationship between the amount of gas adsorbed on a given mass of adsorbent (solid) with the equilibrium pressure of the gas at constant temperature. Such a relationship yields an adsorption isotherm (isotherm refers to a plot at constant temperature).

In the adsorption isotherm of vapours, it is usual to plot relative vapour pressure instead of equilibrium pressure against the amount of vapour adsorbed per gram.

In obtaining adsorption isotherm, the number of moles, grams or ml. (x) of gas adsorbed per gram (m) of adsorbent at STP is plotted against the equilibrium pressure on the horizontal axis.

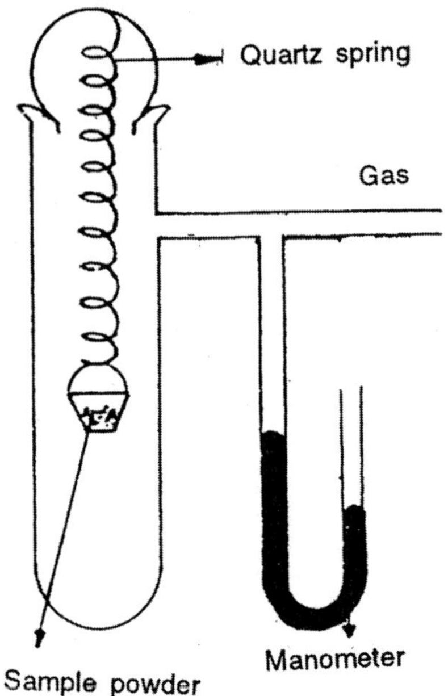

Fig. 46.

The data required may be obtained from an apparatus shown in the figure (Fig. 46). This apparatus consists of a balance within a vacuum system. This is connected to a pressure recorder. The adsorbent to be used is first degassed and placed on the pan of the balance. Known amounts of gas are admitted into the apparatus. The gas will get adsorbed on the adsorbent. This is indicated by the increase in weight. This weight as well as the corresponding equilibrium gas pressure are noted. In the same manner, the weights at different increased equilibrium gas pressures are recorded. From the values obtained, an isotherm may be constructed.

Adsorption isotherms of following types may be obtained depending upon the factors influencing adsorption (at constant temperature) (Fig. 47).

Many equations have been suggested to explain the relationship between the amount of adsorption and the pressure of gas. As these equations quantitatively express the shapes of the

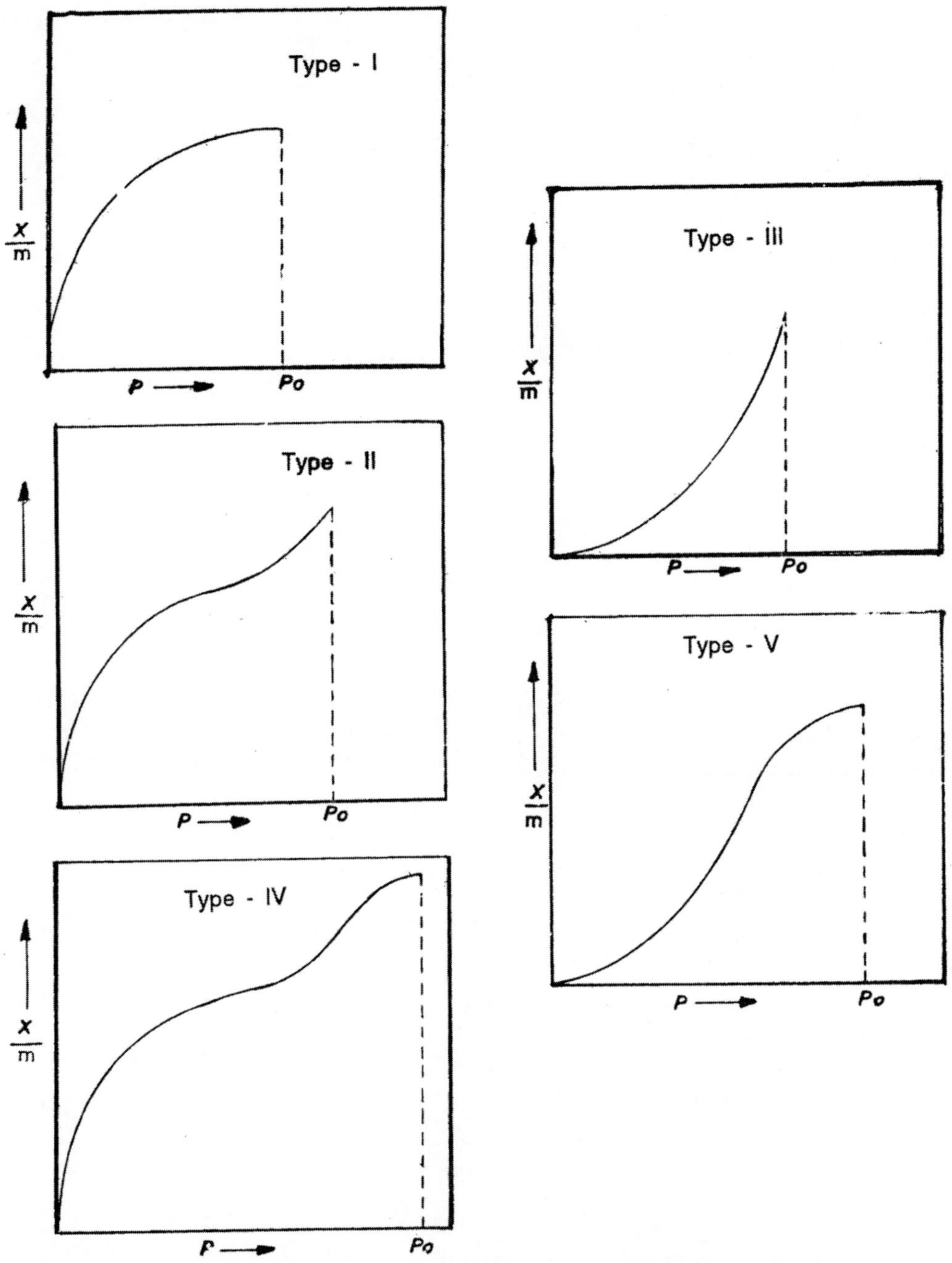

Fig. 47.

graphs, they are referred to as adsorption isotherm. The most common of those equations are of *Freundlich, Langmuir* and *Brunner, Emmett* and *Teller* (BET).

One of the earliest of these equations is the *empirical Freundlich* adsorption isotherm and is given by

$$y = \frac{x}{m} = Kp^{1/n} \qquad \dots (24)$$

where x = mass of gas adsorbed
m = mass of adsorbent
K and n are constants that depends on temperature and nature of adsorbent and adsrobate
p = equilibrium gas pressure
y = mass of gas adsorbed by unit weight of adsorbent.

A plot of $\frac{x}{m}$ (or y) against p, the equilibrium pressure, yields the curve shown (Fig. 48).

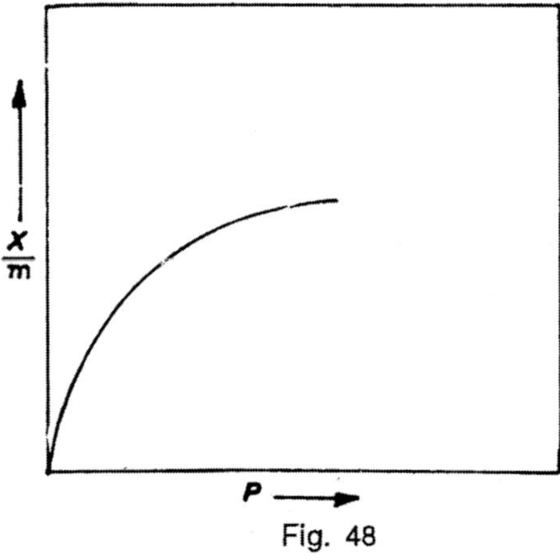

Fig. 48

The logarithmic form of Freundlich equation is

$$\log y = \log K + \frac{1}{n} \log p$$

This permits the graphical solution for the constants K and n. A plot of $\log y$ against $\log p$ yields a straight line. The $\log K$ is the intercept on the ordinate and $\frac{1}{n}$ is the slope of the line (Fig. 49).

Freundlich equation is only empirical. Langmuir derived an equation on the theory that

1. adsorbed gas molecules form a layer, one molecule thick
2. gas molecules are adsorbed on fixed active sites on the adsorbent surface

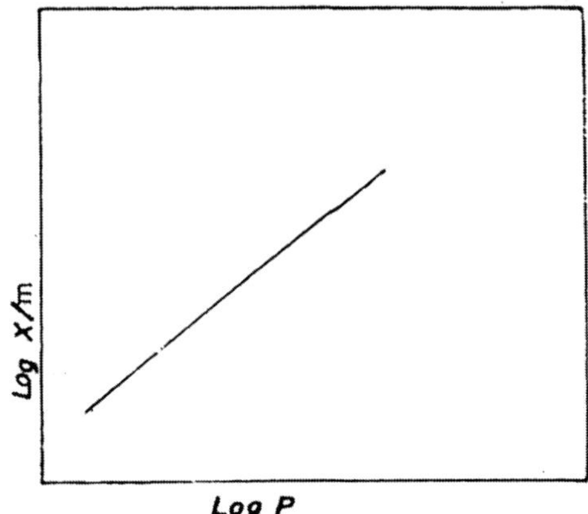

Fig. 49

3. the rate of evaporation (desorption) of adsorbed molecules is related to number of sites occupied and
4. the rate of condensation (adsorption) is related to the number of unoccupied sites.

Let θ be the fraction of sites occupied by gas molecules at pressure p. Then the fraction of sites unoccupied is $1 - \theta$

The rate (r_1) of adsorption (or condensation) of gas molecules on the surface of the adsorbent is proportional to the unoccupied sites and pressure

i.e. $r_1 \propto (1-\theta)p$

or $r_1 = K_1(1-\theta)p$

The rate (r_2) of desorption (or evaporation) of adsorbed molecules on the surface is proportional to the fraction of sites occupied.

i.e. $r_2 \propto \theta$

or $r_2 = K_2\theta$

At equilibrium, the rate of adsorption (r_1) is equal to the rate of evaporation (r_2)

i.e. $K_2\theta = K_1(1-\theta)p$

$$K_2\theta = K_1 p - K_1\theta p$$

$$K_2\theta + K_1\theta p = K_1 p$$

$$\theta(K_2 + K_1 p) = K_1 p$$

$$\theta = \frac{K_1 p}{K_2 + K_1 p}$$

Dividing by K_2

$$\theta = \frac{(K_1/K_2)p}{K_2/K_2 + (K_1/K_2)p}$$

$$= \frac{(K_1/K_2)p}{1 + (K_1/K_2)p}$$

Replacing K_1/K_2 by a constant b and θ by y/y_m, the equation is given as

$$\frac{y}{y_m} = \frac{bp}{1 + bp}$$

θ is the fraction of centers occupied and it can be replaced by y/y_m where y/y_m is the mass of gas adsorbed per gram of adsorbent at pressure p and at constant temperature and y_m is the mass of gas necessary to form a monolayer per gram of adsorbent.

$$\text{or } y = \frac{y_m bp}{1 + bp} \qquad \text{... (25)}$$

This is Langmuir isotherm. For convenience of plotting the experimental data, the Langmuir equation may be obtained in its linear form by inverting the equation and by multiplying through p.

$$\frac{1}{y} = \frac{1 + bp}{y_m bp}$$

Multiplying through p,

$$\frac{p}{y} = p\left(\frac{1 + bp}{y_m bp}\right)$$

$$= \frac{p + bp^2}{y_m bp} = \frac{p}{y_m bp} + \frac{bp^2}{y_m bp}$$

$$\therefore \frac{p}{y} = \frac{1}{y_m b} + \frac{p}{y_m} \qquad \text{... (26)}$$

When p/y is plotted against p, it yields a straight line, b and y_m can be obtained from the intercept on the ordinate and the slope respectively.

Langmuir as well as Freundlich equation describes the type I curve. On observation of the curve, it is inferred that at low pressures the amount of gas adsorbed is proportional to the pressure and at higher pressures the adsorption becomes less and levels off to a contstant value indicating that all the available sites have been filled up. At this stage adsorption is independent of pressure.

The monolayer capacity can be calculated from the value of y where this value reaches a limiting value. Alternatively this monolayer capacity can be calculated from y_m obtained by plotting the data using linear form of Langmuir equation.

Type II isotherms are 'S' shaped and they occur when gas molecules are adsorbed onto nonporous solids of very fine particles to form a monolayer followed by multilayer formation (Fig. 50). There is continued adsorption after first inflection point (which indicates the completion of a monolayer formation) with increasing pressure representing a multilayer formation. This type (II) of curve is explained by BET equation. They found such curves occured at low temperatures and at pressures approaching saturation pressure. They assumed that the molecules were adsorbed on to fixed sites and there was no lateral interaction between molecules and that the heat of adsorption of monolayer is equal to heat of condensation. The BET equation is given as

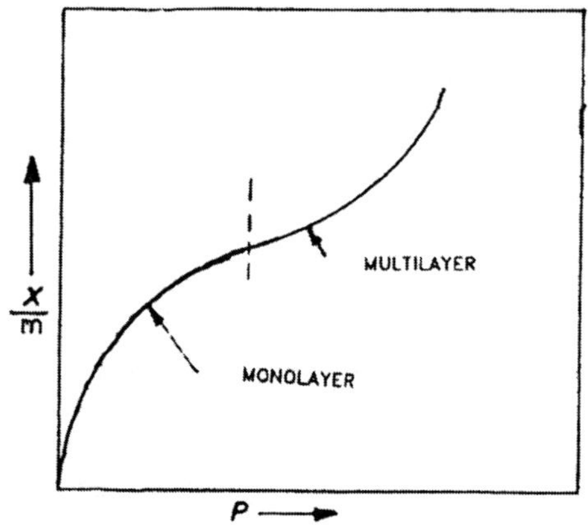

Fig. 50.

$$\frac{p}{y(p_o - p)} = \frac{1}{y_m b} + \frac{(b-1)}{y_m b}\frac{p}{p_o} \quad \ldots (27)$$

where p = the pressure of the adsorbate molecules

y = mass of vapour adsorbed per gram of adsorbent

p_o = saturation vapour pressure i.e. when the adsorbate is saturated with vapour

y_m = mass of vapour adsorbed per gram of adsorbent when the monomolecular layer is complete.

b = a constant that is proportional to the difference between the heat of adsorption of the vapour in the first layer and the latent heat of condensation of successive layers.

For simple monomolecular layer, BET equation reduces to Langmuir equation.

Type IV curve is typical of adsorption onto porous solids. This is somewhat similar to type II. The first inflection point indicates monolayer formation. Then, there occurs multilayer formation and condensation within the pores (capillary condensation) of the solid. It reaches a limiting value before the saturation vapour pressure p_o is attained.

Type III and V isotherms occur when the heat of adsorption of the gas in the first layer is less than the latent heat of condensation of successive layers. Type V curve also shows capillary condensation and that adsorption reaches a limiting value before p_o is reached.

6.2. Adsorption - Solid/Liquid Interface

Solute molecules from its solution may be adsorbed onto solids. The adsorption of solute molecules from its solution is more complicated as there may be competition of the solute and the solvent molecules for the solid/liquid interface. Thus adsorption on solids is a function of the relative adsorption of the solute and the solvent. However at low concentration of solutions, the adsorption of solute molecules onto solids is somewhat similar to that of gas adsorption onto solids. Hence Freundlich, Langmuir or BET equation may be used to describe the adsorption pattern

In adsorption of solute molecules from solution, the pressure term in solid/gas systems is replaced by concentration. The following equation is based on the assumptions that

1. the adsorbate molecules are adsorbed onto specific points on the surface of the adsorbent
2. each point of attachment can take up only one adsorbate molecule and
3. the energy state of adsorbed molecule is not dependent on the presence of adsorbed molecules on neighbouring sites.

$$\frac{c}{y} = \frac{1}{by_m} + \frac{c}{y_m} \quad \text{... (28)}$$

where c = equilibrium concentration of the solute in solution

$y = \frac{x}{m}$, mass of solute (x) per gram of adsorbent 'm' at equilibrium

y_m = adsorptive capacity of the solid i.e. gram of solute per gram of adsorbent when fully covered (i.e. monomolecular layer)

b = adsorption coefficient.

The isotherms for solute adsorption on the adsorbent from solutions have been classified into four main groups at lower concentrations depending on the shape of the initial part of the curve and each of these groups is then subclassified depending on the shape of the curve at higher concentrations (Fig. 51).

S curve

Initial part of the curve shows adsorption becomes easier as the equilibrium concentration is reached. It is characteristic of solute molecules having single point of attachment on to the adsorbent i.e. vertical orientation of adsorbed molecules. It may indicate a strong competition by the solvent for the adsorbent sites.

L curve

It is similar to Langmuir adsorption isotherm. It is obtained for adsorption from dilute solution. In this case adsorption increases as the concentration increases until a limiting plateau value is reached. The adsorbate molecules are likely to be adsorbed flat on the surface of the adsorbent or vertically provided there is little competition from the solvent molecules.

H curve

It is otherwise called "high affinity" curve. It indicates strong interaction between the adsorbed molecule and the adsorbent molecule. It may be indicative of complete removal of solute molecules from solutions of low concentration.

C Curve

This represents a constant partition of solute between the adsorbent and the solution. It is assumed that this type occurs with fibrous materials such as wool. As the concentration in solution increases, the penetration into fibrous materials increases.

6.3 Factors affecting adsorption:

The adsorption of solute molecules from its solution may be influenced by the following factors

1. Surface area of adsorbent
2. Temperature – most of the adsorption processes being exothermic, an increase in temperature will decrease the amount of adsorption.
3. The higher molecular weight solutes are more readily adsorbed than low molecular weight solutes. This is due to *Van der Waals* forces of attraction which increases with the size of molecules.
4. Solutes may be readily adsorbed when they are sparingly soluble in the solvent. In general, it depends on the affinities existing among the solute, the solvent and the adsorbent.
5. There is an increase in the amount of adsorption with an increase in the concentration of solute at equilibrium until it reaches a limiting value. However, the relative amount of solute

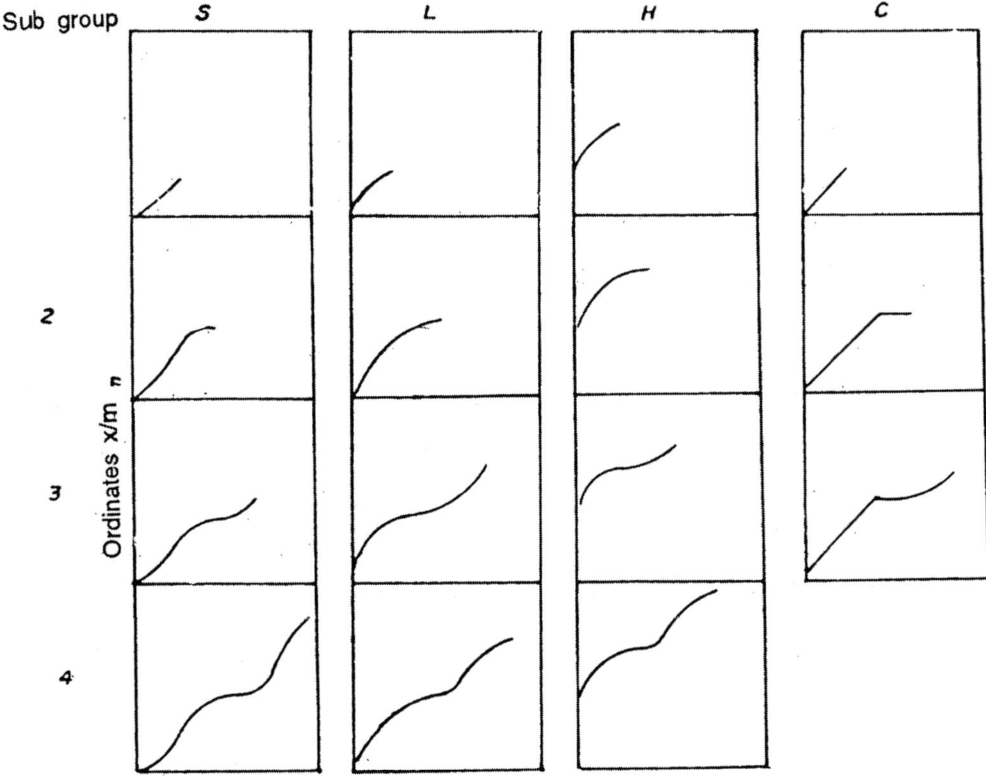

Fig. 51.

removed from solution is greater in dilute solutions.

6. pH of the medium – some drugs are best adsorbed from alkaline solution (high pH). Amphoteric solutes such as proteins are best adsorbed in the region of their isoelectric point.

Some adsorbants which are widely used are activated charcoal, alumina, silica gel, kaolin, kieselguhr and Fuller's earth.

6.4. Applications of adsorption

1. Decolourising agents

Selective adsorption is a term used when an adsorbent adsorbs a particular solute in preference to other solutes present in a solution. This arises due to different affinities exhibited by various substances (solutes) for adsorbents. This principle is taken advantage of in the removal of extraneous colouring matter and impurities from solutions and in the clarification of pharmaceutical preparations.

Removal of colouring matter is usually undertaken by shaking the coloured solution with 1% of activated charcoal or animal charcoal and filtering the solution. Talc is used for clarification of aromatic waters.

2. Desiccants and Drying agents

Traces of water from organic liquids can be removed by shaking with an adsorbent such as alumina or silica gel. These materials contained in small packets are used to provide a dry atmosphere inside the containers of pharmaceutical solid products to protect from high humidity which may adversely affect the product.

*3. Surface area determination of **powders***

Surface area, being the fundamental **property** of powders, influences many **properties of** powders. It may influence the rate of dissolution, flow properties, bulk density, drug activity, packing and adsorption. Determination of surface area may be undertaken from adsorption data of nitrogen on the given powder and substituting the values in BET equation which is given as

$$\frac{p}{V(p_o - p)} = \frac{1}{V_m b} + \frac{(b-1)p}{V_m b p_o} \quad \text{... (29)}$$

where V = volume of nitrogen gas in cm^3 adsorbed per gram of adsorbent at pressure p.

p_o = saturation vapour pressure of liquefied nitrogen at the temperature of the experiment.

b = a constant and is the difference between the heat of adsorption and the heat of liquefaction or condensation.

V_m = volume of nitrogen gas in cm^3 that 1 gram of powder can adsorb when the monolayer is complete i.e. monolayer capacity.

A plot of $\frac{p}{V(p_o - p)}$ against $\frac{p}{p_0}$ yields a straight line. The intercept on the ordinate gives the value of V_m. From this, the specific surface area of the powder is obtained by applying the equation given

$$S_w = \frac{A_m N}{M/\rho} \times V_m \quad \text{... (30)}$$

where A_m = area of a single close packed nitrogen molecule adsorbed as a monolayer on the surface of the powder particles.

S_w = surface area per gram of the powder (i.e. specific surface area)

M/ρ = molar volume of the gas (nitrogen) i.e. 22,413 cm^3/mole at STP.

N = Avogadro's number (6.02×10^{23} *molecules per mole)*

The accurate determination of y_m (monolayer capacity) in the case of adsorption from solution is difficult because it is difficult to obtain close packing of the solute molecules as there may be competition from the solvent molecules. It is also difficult to evaluate A_m as the orientation of the adsorbed solute may vary with the type of solvent. Hence gas adsorption measurements are more reliable than solute adsorption measurements. However adsorption from solution may be applied for quality control on a relative basis.

4. Medicinal uses

Adsorbents such as charcoal and kaolin are used to remove toxic materials from gastro-intestinal tract. Activated charcoal is a valuable emergency antidote for poisoning and overdosing by compounds such as alkaloids, tolubutamide, acetohexamide, acetaminophen and other drugs. However these adsorbents should be used with discrimination since they may adsorb vitamins, drugs, enzymes, etc.

Kaolin is used as poultice for dressing boils, suppurating wounds and ulcers. It is also used in dusting powders.

5. Other Applications

Activated charcoal has been used for the removal of pyrogens from injectable fluids. The stability of colloids is attributed to the adsorption of ions onto their surfaces. The use of protective colloid is based on adsorption. The stability of emulsions is also due to the adsorp-

of emulsions is also due to the adsorption of emulsifying agent at the oil/water interface. Excipients used in pharmaceutical formulations may act as adsorbents which may affect the rate of drug release as well as the rate of absorption. In chromatography, the separation and purification of compounds are based on differences in affinity for an adsorbent for various compounds. In ion exchange chromatography also adsorption principle is utilised. In this, ions are adsorbed on columns of compacted adsorbent. The adsorbent may be the zeolite, analcite ($NaAlSiO_6 \cdot H_2O$) or permutite ($Na_2O \cdot Al_2O_3 \cdot nSiO_2 \cdot H_2O$). Synthetic resinous ion exchangers are also used. This method may be used for the removal of calcium and magnesium ions from hard water.

Adsorption at solid surfaces involves two important phenomena called wetting and detergency.

7. Wetting agent

It is a surfactant which when dissolved in water aids displacing an air phase and replacing it with a liquid phase. The various applications are

1. dispersion of the hydrophobic drugs in water or lipophobic drugs in oil (eg in suspensions)
2. displacement of air from the matrix of cotton pads and bandages so that medicinal solutions may be adsorbed on them
3. displacement of dirt and debris by the use of detergents in washing the wounds.

Wetting agents act by lowering the contact angle between the surface and the wetting liquid. The contact angle is the angle between a liquid droplet and the surface over which the liquid spreads. The angle may vary from 0° to 180° (Fig. 52).

When a drop of water is placed on a clean glass surface, it spreads spontaneously (due to high spreading coefficient of water). In this case, no contact angle exists. However, if a drop of water is placed on a greasy surface, a contact angle results. The contact angle may be reduced drastically by adding a wetting agent to water. Surfactant having HLB values ranging from about 6 to 9 serves as the best wetting agent. To compare relative efficiencies of the wetting agents, *Draver's* test may be performed. In this, time for a weighted skin of cotton yarn to sink through a wetting solution contained in a 500 ml graduated cylinder is used to compare the wetting efficiencies of the wetting agents.

8. Detergents

These are surfactants which are used for the removal of dirt or any other foreign matter from surfaces. The process of detergency involves

(i) initial wetting of dirt

(ii) deflocculation, emulsification or solubilisation of the dirt and

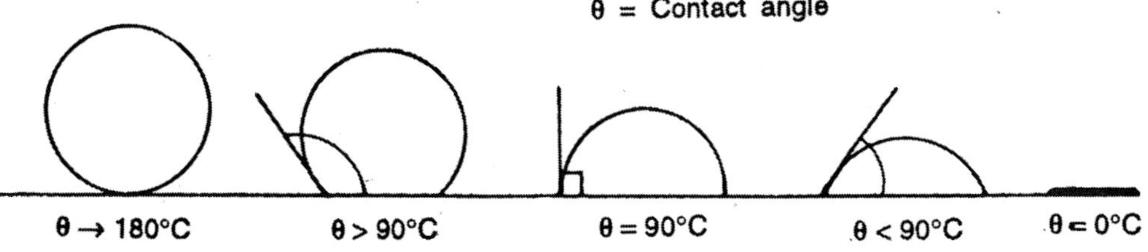

Fig. 52.

(iii) washing away the (dirt) particles.

eg: Surfactants with HLB values of 13 to 16. Its efficiency is better ascertained by actual tests with materials to be cleaned.

9. Electrical Double Layer at Interfaces

Consider a suspension in which the surface of each solid particle preferentially adsorbs positive charges in contact with an aqueous solution containing positive and negative ions (due to dissolved salts).

The positive charges (also called potential determining ions) on the particle now influence the distribution of the ions in the solution (i.e. in the immediate vicinity of the solution surrounding the particle) (Fig. 53 & 54).

The negative ions (or counterions or *gegenions* which mean oppositely charged ions with respect to surface ions) are attracted and held close to the solid surface (Stern layer) and the positive ions are repelled away from its surface. A layer of liquid molecules (solvating layer) is also adsorbed on the solid surface. In addition, thermal motion within the medium will influence the distribution of ions. As a result of these effects, a diffuse double layer of solution (Gouy layer) is created in which the concentration of negative ions gradually decreases and the concentration of positive ions gradually increases upto a certain point in the layer where the number of positive and negative ions are equal (electroneutral region). Thus, the particles are surrounded by a tightly bound layer (Stern layer) consisting of counterions (in this case, negative ions)

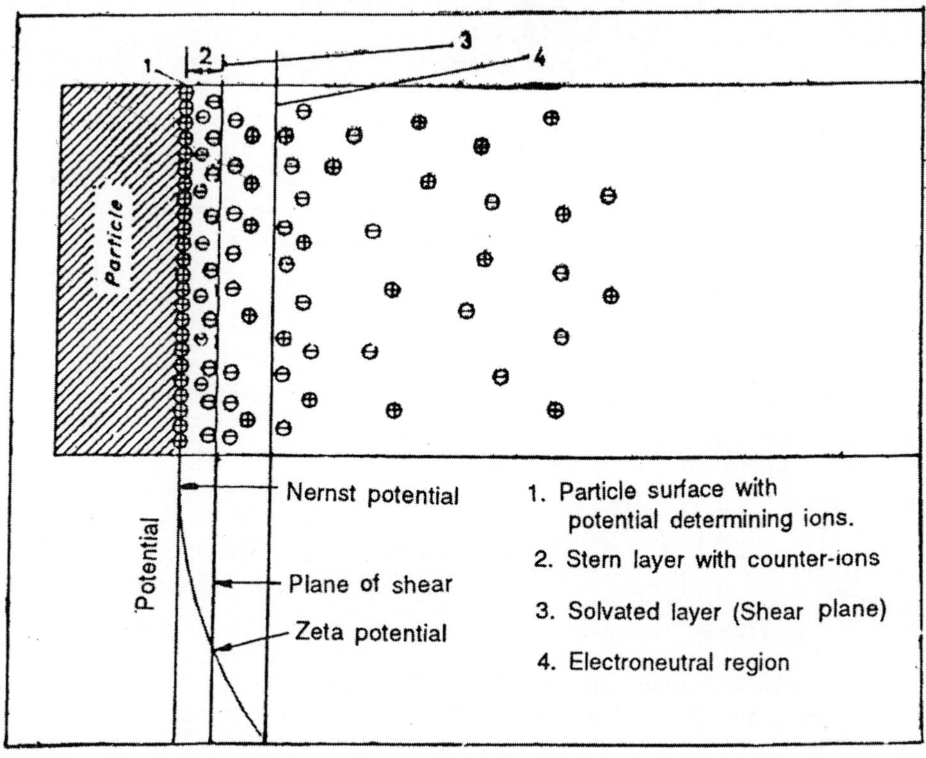

Fig. 53.

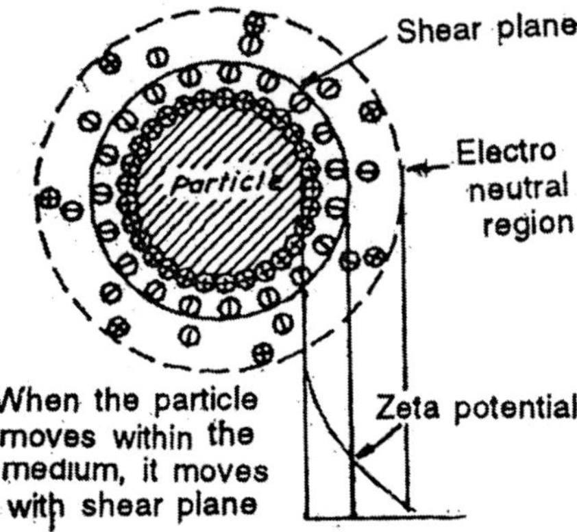

Fig. 54.

sticking to the surface (i.e. positively charged surface) and a diffuse double layer (Gouy layer extenting to the point of electroneutrality). This type of distribution of charges surrounding the particle is called *electrical double layer*.

A decrease in potential occurs across the electrical double layer from its value at the surface of the solid particle (*surface potential or Nernst potential or electro thermodynamic potential*) to zero at the electroneutral region. Thus the potential at the surface of the solid particle is the highest and the potential decreases sharply across the Stern layer and gradually across Gouy layer and then becomes zero at the end of Gouy layer (electro neutral region).

The solvating layer is thicker than the Stern layer. In an electric field, the particles move along with solvating layer. This potential at the surface of the solvating layer is called the zeta potential. Hence ***zeta potential*** is also called ***electro-kinetic potential*** and the surface of the solvating layer is called the surface of shear.

The zeta potential can be found out by using an electrophoretic cell or zeta meter in which the potential just required to make the particles move under a current is found out. The charge across electrical double layer is summarised as follows.

1. Potential at the solid surface (surface potential or Nernst potential) due to potential determing ions
2. Potential at the Stern layer (Stern potential)
3. Potential at the solvating layer (zeta potential or electrokinetic potential)
4. Zero potential at the electro-neutral region.

In the *first situation* just discussed the surface potential is positive, the potential at the solvating layer is still positive (but diminished) and the potential at the end of Gouy layer (i.e. more diffuse layer) is zero.

Two other situations are also possible.

Situation 2: If the positive charge on the solid surface is exactly neutralised by the counterions in the tightly bound solvated layer, the electric neutrality occurs at the surface of the solvating layer itself. In this case the surface potential is positive, the potential at the surface of the solvating layer is zero.

Situation 3: If the total charge of the counterions in the tightly bound solvating layer exceeds the surface charges, (positive charges) it leads not only to neutralisation but also the Stern potential will be reversed and the electric neutrality occurs at the end of Gouy layer (i.e. at the end of diffuse double layer). In this case, the surface potential remains positive, the potential at the surface of solvating layer is negative and the potential at the end of diffuse double layer is zero. All the three situations are represented in Fig. 55.

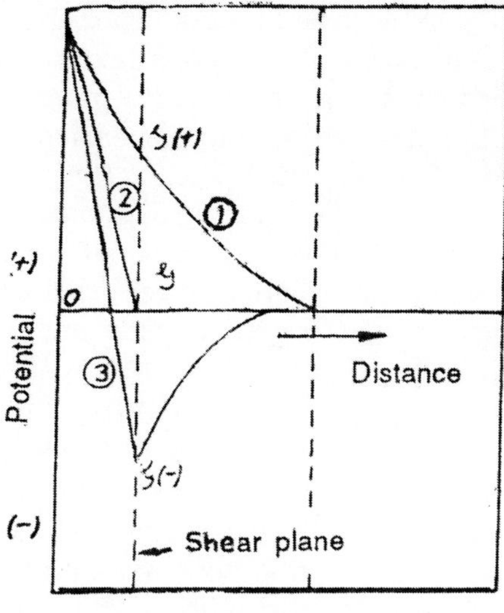

Fig. 55.

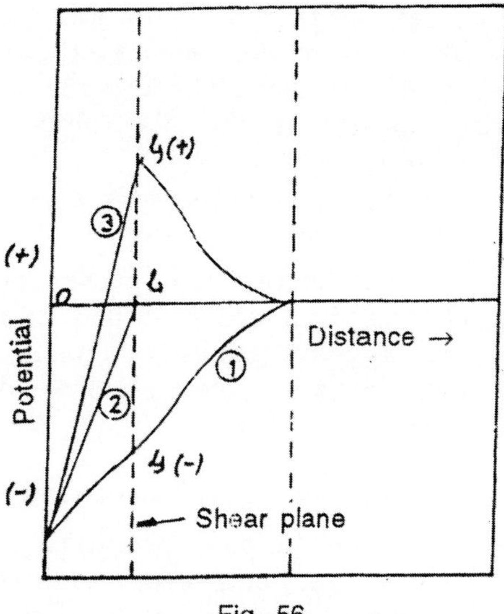

Fig. 56.

In the same way, three other situations will arise if the surface of the particles preferentially adsorbs negative charges in the aqueous solution containing positive and negative ions. All the three situations have been represented in Fig. 56).

9.1. Effect of electrolytes on electrical double layer

If the ionic concentration is increased in the disperse medium of a suspension or a colloid by adding electrolytes, the diffuse part of the double layer is compressed and the

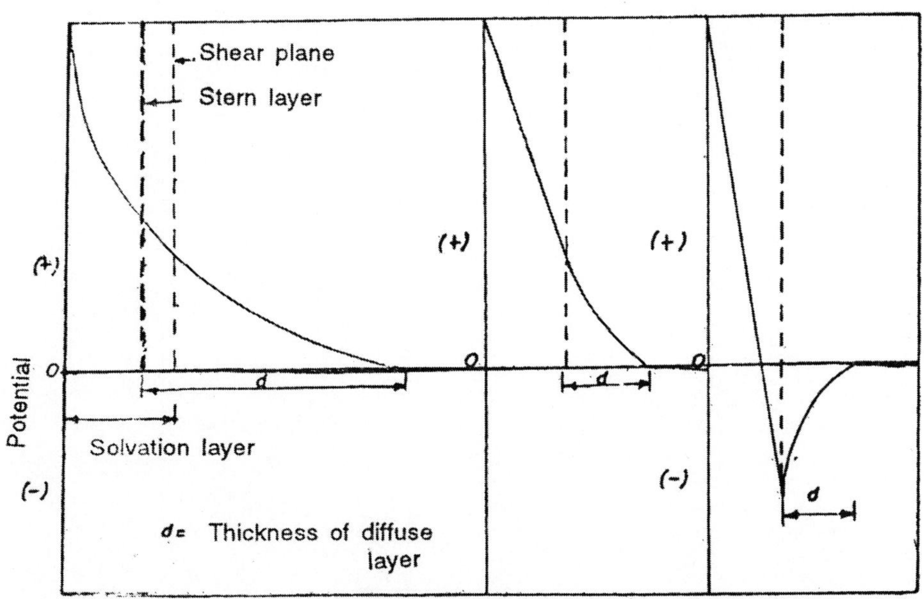

Fig. 57. Effect of electrolytes on the thickness of diffuse layer

potential falls of more rapidly with distance (Fig. 57). A similar situation arises when the valency of the counter ion is increased keeping the total concentration of the electrolyte constant (Hardly Schulze Rule). Due to this effect, Stern potential and zeta potential decrease.

If more and more oppositely charged ions are adsorbed at the surface, it leads not only to neutralisation but the Stern potential also will be reversed.

9.2. Importance of zeta potential

Due to zeta potential, repulsion between particles dispersed in a colloid or in a suspension occurs. The stability of colloids is mainly due to zeta potential of the dispersed particles and may be increased by adding calculated quantity of electrolytes. For example, sodium citrate (one of the ingredients acting as peptizing agent in the prepartion of Calamine Lotion - a suspension) is used to increase zeta potential of the suspended particles in *Calamine Lotion*. The zeta potential acts as an energy barrier for coagulation and this accounts for the stability of colloids and suspensions.

However, the addition of larger amounts of electrolytes decreases the thickness of the diffuse double layer as well as the Stern potential of the particles. Hence the zeta potential is decreased. Because of this effect, the stability of the preparation is decreased. The preparation especially the colloid becomes instantaneously unstable.

Suggestion to Practicals

1. *Determination of density of a given liquid at a given temperature by using specific gravity bottle*

We know that density of a liquid is mass per volume

$$\text{i.e. } D = \frac{M}{V} \text{ gm/ml}$$

where D = density of the liquid

M = mass of the liquid

V = volume

D is also denoted as ρ (rho)

Relative density of a liquid with respect to water is

$$\frac{\rho_l}{\rho_w} = \frac{M_l/V_l}{M_w/V_w} = \frac{M_l}{M_w} \times \frac{V_w}{V_l}$$

When the same specific gravity bottle at the same temperature is used for the determination, $V_w = V_l$

$$\therefore \frac{\rho_l}{\rho_w} = \frac{M_l}{M_w}$$

(Note: The unit of density is gm/ml whereas the relative density has no unit)

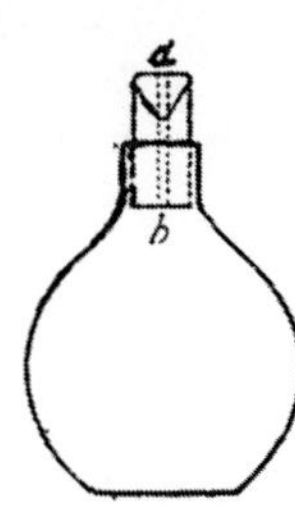

The specific gravity bottle has a definite volume when the lid (the lid has a central hole) is placed correctly into the neck of the bottle. The bottle apparatus is first thoroughly washed and dried. Remove the lid and fill the bottle with the liquid upto the brim of the bottle. The lid is placed with the neck of the bottle. Any excess liquid will drain out through the lid. The excess liquid is removed by absorption with the help of a blotting paper. The outer surface of the bottle is thoroughly cleaned off from the liquid with a dry cloth. The difference between the weight of the bottle and the weight of the bottle with the liquid gives the mass of liquid for the given specified volume on the bottle. In the same way, the mass of water is found out after cleaning and drying the bottle.

The relative density of the liquid with respect to water is then given by

$$\frac{\rho_l}{\rho_w} = \frac{W_l}{W_w}.$$

2. *Determination of surface tension of a given liquid sample by using Stalagmometer (By Drop Count Method)*

Principle: Refer the text

Procedure: Note down the room temperature. Rinse the Stalagmometer (Dropping pipette) with acetone and dry in a hot air oven. Suck water upto the point A on the pipette. Keeping the pipette in a vertical position, count the number of drops when the water level drops from the mark A to B. Clean the pipette, rinse with acetone and dry as before. Repeat the experiment with the given liquid as before. The relative surface tension of the liquid with respect to water is

$$= \frac{\gamma_l}{\gamma_w} = \frac{\text{surface tension of the liquid}}{\text{surface tension of water}}$$

$$= \frac{d_l}{d_w} \times \frac{n_w}{n_l}$$

where d_l = denisty of the liquid

d_w = density of water

n_w = number of drops of water

n_l = number of drops of the liquid

Surface tension of water at

20°C = 71.18 dynes/cm

at 25°C = 71.97 dynes/cm

at 30°C = 72.80 dynes/cm

Absolute surface tension of the liquid = Relative surface tension of the liquid × surface tension of water

Report as follows at room temperature

1. The relative surface tension of the liqud =
2. The absolute surface tension of the liquid =

3. *Determination of surface tension of a given liquid sample by using Stalagmometer (By Drop Weight Method)*

Principle: Refer the text

Procedure: Note down the room temperature. Rinse the Stalagmometer (Dropping pipette) with acetone and dry in hot air oven. Suck water upto the mark A on the pipette. Keeping the pipette vertical, collect atleast 20 drops of water into a tarred beaker. Find out the weight of one drop of water. Clean the pipette, rinse with acetone and repeat the experiment again with the given liquid as before

The relative surface tension of the liquid

$$= \frac{\gamma_l}{\gamma_\omega} = \frac{w_l}{w_w}$$

Where w_l = weight of one drop of liquid

w_w = weight of one drop of water

The absolute surface tension of the liquid = Relative surface tension of the liquid × surface tension of the water

Report the result as follows at room temperature

1. The relative surface tension of the given liquid =
2. The absolute surface tension of the given liquid =

4. *Determination of Critical Micellar Concentration (CMC) of a given surfactant*

Principle

Surface active molecules at and above a certain concentration (characteristic of a particular surfactant) aggregate to form micelles of colloidal dimensions called association colloid and the concentration at which the micelle formation occurs is termed as critical micellar concentration and below this concentration the surfactant will be in true solution. Physical properties such as refractive index, conductance, surface tension, osmotic pressure etc also change markedly at critical micellar concentration. This principle may be applied to find out the critical micellar concentration of a surfactant.

At and above critical micellar concentration of a surfactant, the surface tension remains fairly constant and for the present experiment this principle is applied.

Positive adsorption of surface active agents at the surface of water causes a progressive decrease in surface tension with increase in concentration until CMC is reached. The micelles formed at and beyond this concentration provide an alternative means of removing lipophilic groups from the aqueous environment thus causing a decrease in free energy of the system. Hence above CMC, additional material is used in the production of more micelles and the concentration of the surfactant in the surface layer and in true solution (monomeric units) remains the same. Thus at CMC, surface tension against concentration levels out.

Procedure

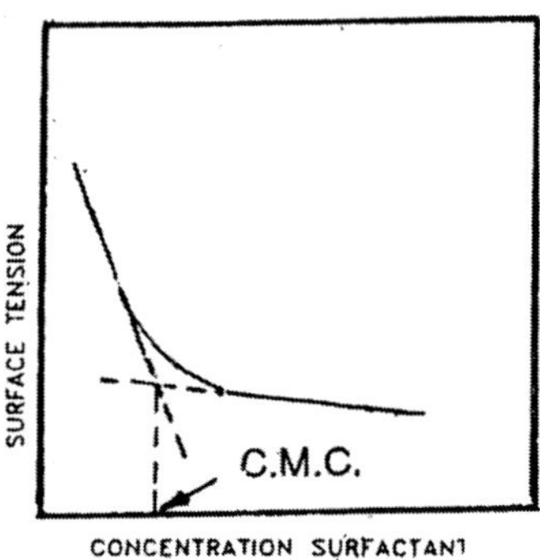

Fig. 58.

Prepare a series of 0.001%, 0.002%, 0.005%, 0.01%, 0.02%, 0.05%, 0.1%, 0.2% and 0.5% w/v concentrations of solutions of sodium lauryl sulphate from a 1% w/v solution of sodium lauryl sulphate by dilution.

Determine the surface tensions of each of the different concentrated solution of sodium lauryl sulphate by using Stalagamometer as described in the above experiment. From the data obtained, prepare a graph by plotting concentration on x axis against the surface tension of the corresponding concentration on y axis (Fig. 58). The concentration corresponding the break point in the curve yields critical micellar concentration of the sodium lauryl sulphate.

Report

The critical micellar concentration of the given surfactant ——— g/100 ml of the solution. The coventional expression of the critical micellar concentration is millimole/litre of solution (i.e. mM/litre)

Using colligative properties such as osmotic pressure and lowering of freezing point also, the critical micellar concentration of a surfactant can be found out. The association of monomeric ions or molecules into micelles at critical micellar concentration causes a marked change in the colligative

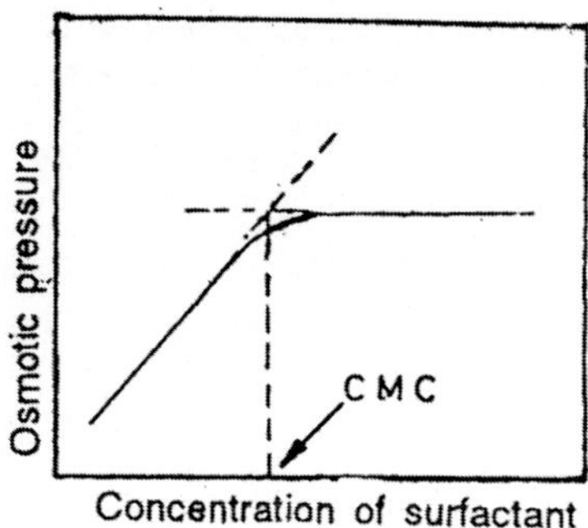

Fig. 59.

properties of the solutions of association colloid. For example, the concentrations of surfactants on X axis plotted against their corresponding osmotic pressures on Y axis may yield a curve as shown in Fig. 59.

In this, the osmotic pressure (depends upon the number of particles) increases with concentration of surfactant gradually and at critical micellar concentration at which aggregation of surfactant molecules into micelles occurs leads to a sharp change in the colligative property (i.e. it levels off) because the number of effective particles decreases drastically and there is a sudden change in osmotic pressure.

5. *Determination of Hydrophile-Lipophile balance (HLB) value of a polyhydric alcohol fatty acid ester surfactant*

Principle

Hydrophile-lipophile balance (HLB) value indicates the balance between the hydrophilic and lipophilic nature within a surfactant molecule. The determination is based on the following equation

$$HLB = 20\left(1 - \frac{S}{A}\right)$$

where S = saponification number of the ester

A = acid number of the fatty acid forming the ester

This equation can be used for determining HLB values of polyhydric fatty acid esters such as glyceryl monostearate, sorbitan mono-oleate (span 80), sorbitan monolaurate (span 20), triethanolamine oleate, polyoxy ethylenesorbitan mono-oleate (tween 80), polyoxy ethylene sorbitan monolaurate (Tween 20) etc.

Procedure

(a) *Determination of saponification number*

Weigh 2 grams of the surfactant and transfer into a round bottom flask. Add 25 ml of alcoholic potassium hydroxide (2.82 grams in 100 ml of alcohol). Reflux for 30 minutes. Cool the reaction mixture and titrate with 0.5 N HCl using phenolphthalein as indicator. Let this value be A. Perform a blank titration and let this value be 'B' then,

Saponification number

$$= \frac{(B - A) \times 0.02805 \times \text{normality of HCl}}{\text{Weight of sample} \times 0.5}$$

(b) *Determination of acid number*

Render the above saponified mixture acidic by adding excess hydrochloric acid. Extract the mixture with solvent ether (successive extration using 20 ml of ether). Take the combined extracts in a beaker and evaporate the ether over a water - bath to get a residue. Weigh about 500 mg of the residue and treat with 10 ml of alcohol and 10 ml of ether. Titrate against 0.1 N potassium hydroxide using phenolphthalein as indicator.

The acid number is obtained by using the formula

Acid number

$$= \frac{\text{Titration value} \times 0.00561 \times \text{normality of KOH}}{\text{Weight of sample} \times 0.1} \times 1000$$

Substitute the values in the equation given and find out the HLB value.

For Tween 20, $S = 45.5$, $A = 276$, and HLB = 16.7

Report

The HLB value of the given surfactant is ——

6. *Effect of concentration on adsorption*

Principle

Adsorption of gas molecules increases with increase in pressure. In the same way, adsorption of solute molecules from its solution on the adsorbent increases with increase in the concentration of the solute in the solution. The adsorption of solute molecules from its solution can be obtained from the Langmuir's equation and is given by

$$\frac{c}{y} = \frac{1}{by_m} + \frac{c}{y_m}$$

Where c = equilibrium concentration of solute per 100 ml of solution.

y = amount of solute (x) adsorbed per gram of adsorbent i.e. $y = x/m$ where m is the mass of adsorbent used.

b = a constant

y_m = a constant and is the amount of solute to form a monomolecular layer for a particular solute.

A plot of c/y versus c yields a straight line. b and y_m are obtained from the intercept and slope respectively.

Procedure

Prepare 200 ml of 0.5 N oxalic acid by dissolving 6.303 grams of oxalic acid in water and making up the solution to 200 ml. Prepare from this solution 4 or 5 different dilutions (for example 0.25 N, 0.1 N, 0.05 N, and 0.005 N etc). Add 1 gram of charcoal to 50 ml of different dilutions and agitate frequently and allow to stand for the equilibrium to attain. Filter the solution separately and titrate against standard N/10 NaOH solution using phenolphthalein as indicator. Find out the amount of oxalic acid adsorbed per gram of the charcoal (x/m). From the data obtained, plot x/m versus c and also $\log \frac{x}{m}$ against $\log c$.

7. ***Determination of surface area occupied per surfactant molecule (cross sectional area of a surfactant molecule) using surface excess Γ (gamma) - by Gibbs adsorption equation.***

We know that

$$\Gamma = -\frac{C}{RT} \cdot \frac{d\gamma}{dc} \text{ (Refer the text)}$$

In terms of activity of surfactant, the above equation is given by

$$\Gamma = -\frac{a}{RT} \cdot \frac{d\gamma}{da}$$

$$= -\frac{1}{RT} \cdot \frac{d\gamma}{dlna} \left(\because \frac{a}{da} = \frac{1}{dlna} \right)$$

The above equation can be written in terms of concentration of surfactant if the solution is dilute

$$\Gamma = -\frac{1}{RT} \cdot \frac{d\gamma}{dlnc}$$

Procedure: Prepare a series of 0.001%, 0.002%, 0.005%, 0.01%, 0.02%, 0.05%, 0.1%, 0.2% and 0.5% w/v concentrations of solutions of sodium lauryl sulphate from a 1% w/v solution of the surfactant by dilution

Determine the surface tensions of each of the above solution by using Stalagmometer. From the data obtained plot surface tension (r) on y axis and log of the concentration of surfactant on x axis. The plot will take the shape as shown below

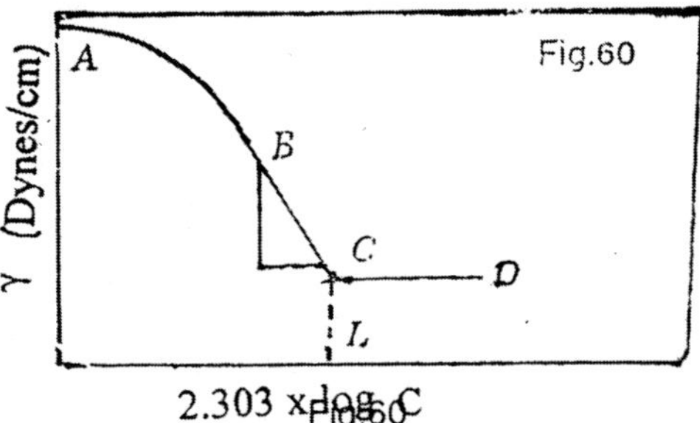

Fig.60

Portion of the curve $A - B$ is curved, $B - C$ is linear with a sharp decline in surface tension, and $C - D$ is horizontal indicating that further addition of surfactant does not alter the surface tension of the liquid. The point L corresponds to CMC. The point B indicates that saturation of surface with surfactant molecules has been reached, that is surface excess, Γ, does not increase further as the concentration in the bulk increases. However surface tension decreases greatly until the point 'C' is reached. The slope of the line is given by, $\frac{d\gamma}{2.303 \log C}$. The value of slope multiplied by $1/RT$ gives the value of Γ at a particular value of C. The unit is mole/cm^2

Number of molecules occupying 1 square centimeter

$$= \Gamma \times \text{Avogadros number}$$

$$= \Gamma \text{ mole/cm}^2 \times 6.023 \times 10^{23} \text{ mole}^{-1}$$

Reciprocal of this will give area occupied by one molecule and is given by

$$= \frac{1}{\Gamma \text{ mole/cm}^2 \times 6.023 \times 10^{23} \text{ mole}^{-1}}$$

V. RHEOLOGY

The term rheology was derived from two Greek words namely *rheo* (to flow) and *logos* (science). Rheology is the science that deals with the deformation of matter under the influence of stresses. The stresses may be

(a) *Tensile stress:* a stress applied perpendicularly to the surface of a body

(b) *Shearing stress:* a stress applied tangentially to the surface of a body.

(c) Stress applied at any other angle to the surface of a body.

The deformation are of two types.

Elastic deformation	Plastic deformation
It is spontaneous and reversible. The work spent for the deformation is recoverable when the body returns to the original position.	It is permanent and irreversible. The work spent for the deformation is dissipated as heat.

The flow properties or viscous behaviour of various pharmaceutical products ranging from simple liquids to semisolids such as ointments, gels, creams and pastes are very important for pharmacists in the following areas as detailed below.

1. ***For fluids***
   - Mixing of liquids
   - Particle size reduction of disperse system with shear.
   - Passage through orifices, including pouring, packaging in bottles, and passage through hypodermic needles.
   - Fluid transfer, including pumping and flow through pipes
   - Physical stability of disperse systems.
2. ***For semisolids***
   - Acceptable consistency and smoothness
   - Spreading and adherence on to the skin
   - Removal from jars or extrusion from tubes
   - Capacity of solids to mix with miscible liquids.
   - Release of the drug from the base
   - Mixing and packing into containers.
   - Physical stability and patient acceptability
   - Biological availability from skin and gastro-intestinal tract
3. ***For solids***
   - Flow of powders from hopper and into die cavities in tabletting and flow of powder into capsules during encapsulation.
   - Packageability of powdered or granular solids.

4. ***Processing***

- Production capacity of equipment
- Processing efficiency
- Correct choice of production equipment.

2. Viscosity

Viscosity is qualitatively defined as the resistance of a liquid to flow due to internal friction between different layers of liquid when it flows.

It may be treated mathematically as follows.

When the liquid flows (eg. liquid passing through a pipe) due to a shearing stress a plastic deformation occurs.

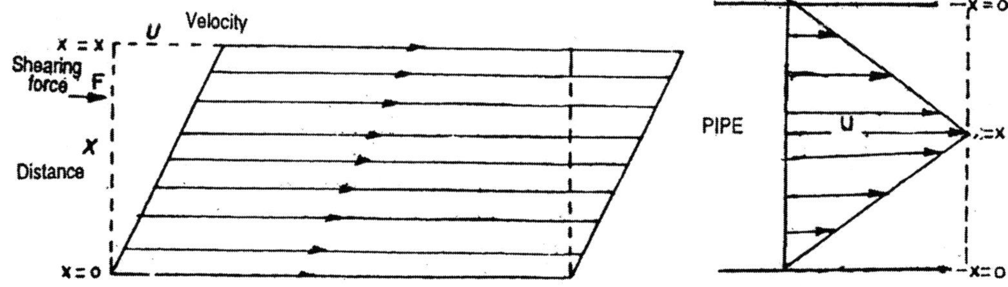

Fig. 61. Fig. 62.
Representation of movement of a liquid in a planar laminae and through a pipe

Due to this, there is a change of velocity between different layers of the liquid. That is, the velocity changes from zero (liquid at the periphery of the pipe) where the distance $x = 0$ from the base to a maximum value u at the topmost layer (In the case of liquid flowing through a pipe, the velocity will be maximum at the center of the pipe Fig. 62).

Let us consider the liquid is made up of infinitely thin parallel layers (laminae) each of area A on a horizontal base as shown in (Fig. 61).

The infinitesimal difference of velocity du between two layers of liquid separated by an infinitesimal distance dx is the velocity gradient and the change in velocity with distance is the rate of shear and is given by du/dx. The force per unit area required to produce a certain rate of shear is called the shearing stress S, i.e. $S = F/A$.

Shearing stress and shear rate are related by $S \propto \frac{du}{dx}$.

Introducing proportionality constant

$$S = \eta \frac{du}{dx} \quad \text{... (1)}$$

$$\text{or } \eta = \frac{\text{shearing stress}}{\text{rate of shear}} = \frac{S}{du/dx}$$

where η = coefficient of viscosity

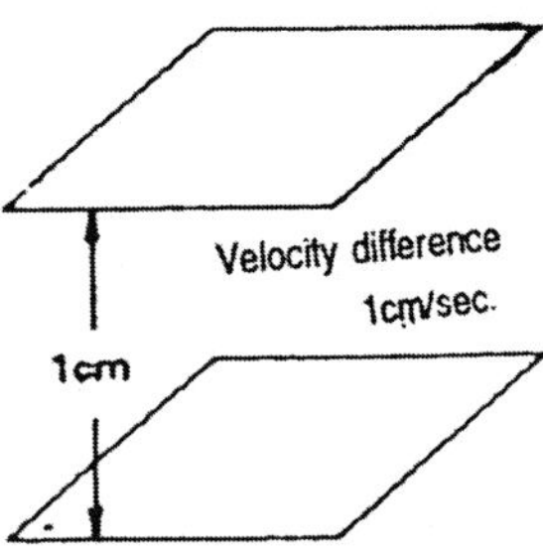

Fig. 63.

It may also be defined as the force (in dyne/square centimeter) required to maintain a velocity difference of 1cm/sec between two parallel layers of liquid of each one square centimeter separated by a distance of 1 centimeter (Fig. 63). If the force required is 1 dyne/square centimeter, the coefficient of viscosity (η) is said to be one poise (*P*)

The unit may be obtained by dimensional analysis

$$1 \text{ poise} = 0.1 \text{ Nsm}^{-2}$$

$$\eta = \frac{F}{A} \cdot \frac{dx}{dn} = \frac{\text{dyne} \times \text{cm}}{\text{cm}^2 \times \text{cm/sec}} = \frac{\text{dyne sec}}{\text{cm}^2}$$

(i.e. 0.1. Newton second per square meter)

Newton second is the SI unit for poise.

Liquids showing high coefficient of viscosity is said to be viscous and the liquid showing less coefficient of viscosity is said to be less viscous or mobile. For mobile liquids, the convenient unit is *centipoise* which is one hundredth of 1 *poise.* The reciprocal of viscosity is called fluidity (ϕ). (The unit is Poise^{-1})

$$\phi = \frac{1}{\eta} \qquad \text{... (2)}$$

2.1. Kinematic viscosity

Kinematic viscosity is the absolute viscosity (η) divided by the density of the liquid. The units are *stoke* and *centistoke.*

2.2. Viscosity of liquids

Poisuille was the first scientist who designed an equipment to find out viscosity of liquids. The equipment consists of a tall cylinder attached with a capillary flow tube at its lowest side at right angle to it (Fig. 64).

The liquid is filled upto the height '*h*' in the cylinder and a specified volume of liquid is collected into a reservoir through the capillary tube of length *l* and radius '*r*'. Then, the volume of liquid collected is given by

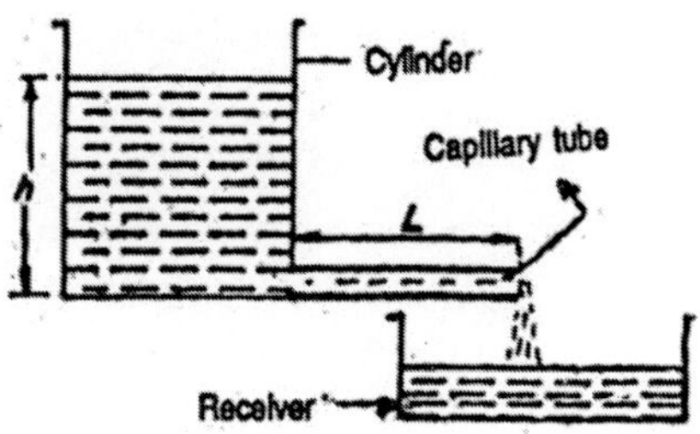

Fig. 64. Equipment to find out viscosity

$$V = \frac{\pi p r^4 t}{8\eta_l} \qquad \text{... (3)}$$

where *V* = volume of liquid collected

p = pressure head due to the liquid and is equal to '*hdg*', i.e. height × density × acceleration due to gravity.

r = radius of the capillary tube.

t = time upto which the liquid was collected.

η = coefficient of viscosity of the liquid.

l = length of the capillary tube.

Rearranging the formula for η (viscosity),

$$\eta = \frac{\pi}{8} \frac{pr^4 t}{Vl} \qquad \text{... (4)}$$

in which all the parameters are measurable and η can be calculated easily.

2.3. Effect of temperature on viscosity

It is fact that as the temperature of a system is increased. viscosity decreases. Approximately for one degree centigrade rise, the viscosity falls by 1 to 10%. It is mathematically given as

$$\eta = Ae^{E_a/RT} \qquad \text{... (5)}$$

$$\text{or } \ln \eta = \frac{E_a}{RT} + \ln A \qquad \text{... (6)}$$

where A = a constant

R = gas constant

T = thermodynamic temperature

E_a = energy of activation to move one molecule past another

However, there are some exceptions. For example, viscosity of methyl cellulose solution increases as the temperature increases.

Hence the viscosity is affected by temperature, it is necessary to report the viscosity of a system at a given temperature and in the determination of viscosity of substances, the temperature should be maintained constant throughout the experiment.

3. Types of Rheological Systems

It is broadly classified into two types

I. Newtonian systems

II. Non-Newtonian systems.

3.1. Newtonian systems

Rheological properties of a system are usually expressed in the form of a graph wherein shearing stress (on the x axis) is plotted against rate of shear (on the y axis) and this is called a *rheogram*.

If a system shows same values of 'η' (i.e. coefficient of viscosity) at different shearing rates at a given temperature, it is said to be a Newtonian system.

S. No.	Shearing stress	Shear rate	$\eta = \frac{\text{Shearing stress}}{\text{shear rate}}$
1	x_1	y_1	$x_1/y_1 = \eta$
2	x_2	y_2	$x_2/y_2 = \eta$
3	x_3	y_3	$x_3/y_3 = \eta$
.	.	.	.
.	.	.	.
.	.	.	.
n	x_n	y_n	$x_n/y_n = \eta$

The linear curve passes through the origin indicating that even a mild force can induce a flow. The curve also indicates that the values of η are constant at different shear rates (Fig. 65).

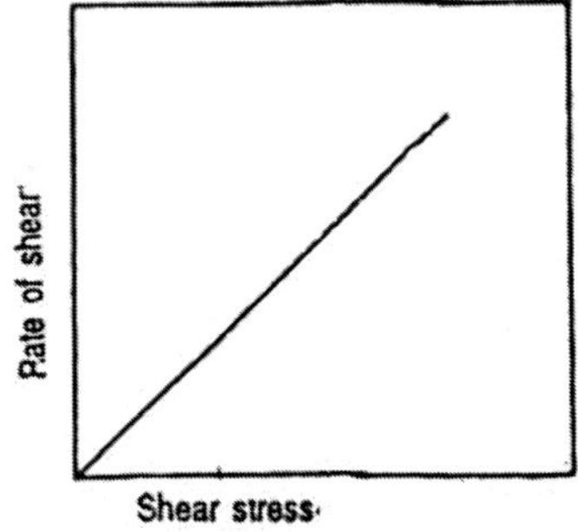

Fig. 65. Newtonian flow

Examples of some Newtonian liquids are water, simple organic liquids, true solutions, dilute suspensions and emulsions.

3.2. Non-Newtonian systems

A system is said to be non-Newtonian when it shows different η values at different shearing rates at a given temperature. Therefore the viscosity is often called *apparent* viscosity.

S. No.	Shearing stress	Shear rate	$\eta = \frac{\text{Shearing stress}}{\text{shear rate}}$
1	x_1	y_1	$x_1/y_1 = \eta_1$
2	x_2	y_2	$x_2/y_2 = \eta_2$
3	x_3	y_3	$x_3/y_3 = \eta_3$
.	.	.	.
.	.	.	.
.	.	.	.
n	x_n	y_n	$x_n/y_n = \eta_n$

There are three types of non-Newtonian systems. They are

1. Plastic systems
2. Pseudoplastic systems
3. Dilatant systems

3.2.1. Plastic systems

The rheogram of this system is shown in (Fig. 66).

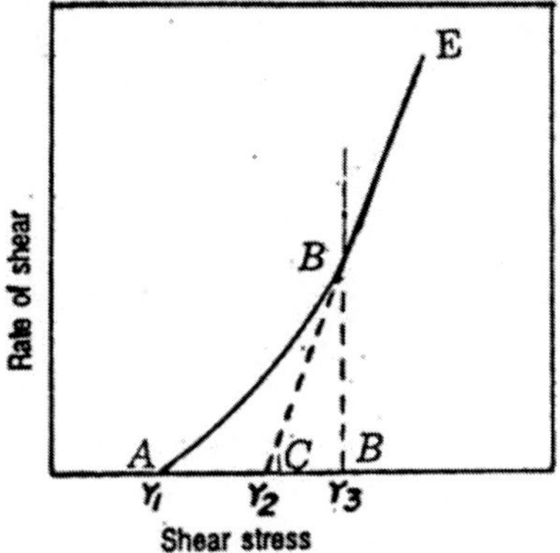

Fig. 66. Simple plastic flow

These systems were studied extensively by Bingham and hence, they are called as *Bingham bodies*. In this, the curve is not passing through the origin. It indicates that mild forces cannot induce a flow. The flow is possible only at a shearing stress of A or more. The minimum shearing stress 'A' which induces a flow is called *'yield value'*. The system behaves like a solid for stresses below the yield value. The curve obtained from shear stress A to shear stress B is not linear (i.e. the curve AD) The slope of the curve gradually increases until the point B and it indicates a gradual decrease in the viscosity of the system upto the point B (Slope of the curve is fluidity; reciprocal of the slope of the curve is viscosity). Therefore, the system which shows a gradual decrease in viscosity on increasing the shear stress is called *'shear thinning system'*. In this case, the *apparent plastic viscosity* (U or η_{pl}) is given by

$$\eta_{pl} \text{ or } U = \frac{S - \text{yield value}}{du/dx} \quad \dots (7)$$

It may be observed in the rheogram that there are three yield values. The stress at A is the low yield value. (y_1). The stress at B is the high yield value (y_3) and at C, occurs intermediate yield value (y_2). η_{pl} may be calculated by substituting either y_1 or y_2 or y_3 in the above equation.

The curve beyond B becomes linear (i.e. from D to E) and the system behaves just like Newtonian system thereafterwards.

Examples of plastic systems are *ointments, pastes and creams*

3.2.2. Pseudoplastic systems

The rheogram for pseudoplastic system is given in (Fig. 67).

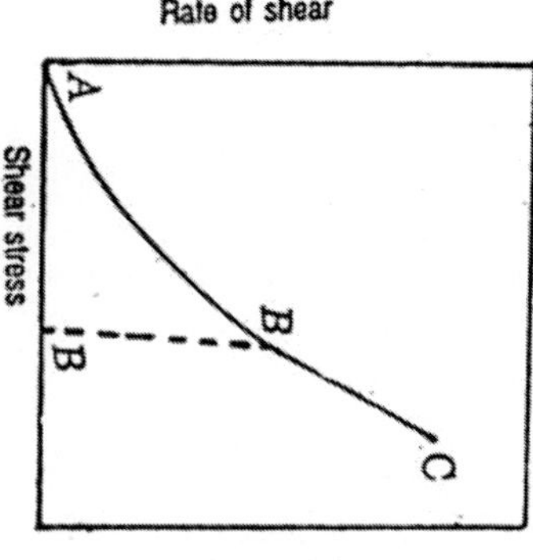

Fig. 67.

The curve passes through the origin which indicates that mild forces can induce a flow. There is no yield value for this system. The curve obtained from shear stress A to shear stress B is similar to plastic system (i.e. from A to C). Since the system is having both the characters of Newtonian and plastic, it is called pseudoplastic system. This is also a *'shear thinning system'*. In this case, the viscosity is given by the empirical power law

$$\eta = \frac{S^N}{du/dx}. \quad \dots (8)$$

where the value of N is greater than 1 (For Newtonian system, the value of N is 1). The values of N varies for different pseudoplastic systems. The greater the value of 'N' the more pseudoplastic is the system. The equation (8) can be rearranged and written in logarithmic form as

$$\log \frac{du}{dx} = N \log S - \log \eta.$$

Plotting the log of shearing stress (log S) versus the log of rate of shear, $\left(\log \frac{du}{dx}\right)$ a straight line is obtained with a slope of N (Fig. 68). However some pseudoplastic suspending agents do not conform to equation (8)

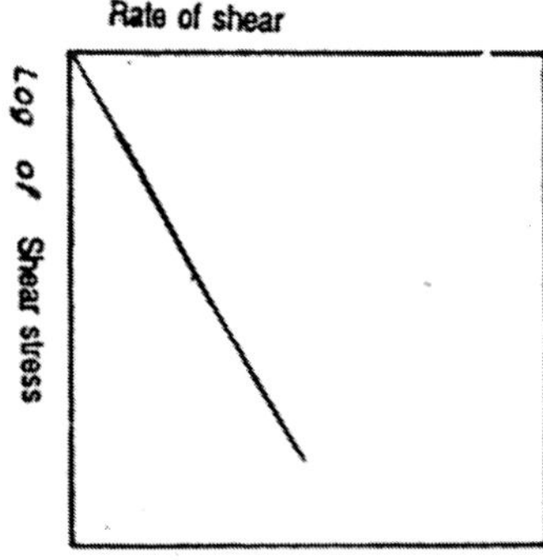

Fig. 68. Pseudo-Plastic flow

The curve beyond the point B becomes linear (i.e. from C to D) and the system behaves like Newtonian system thereafterwards.

To distinguish between plastic and pseudoplastic systems, it is necessary to obtain the flow behaviour at low shear rates.

Examples of pseudoplastic system are ***liquid dispersions of tragacanth, sodium alginate and sodium carboxymethyl cellulose.***

3.2.3. Dilatant systems

The rheogram for dilatant system is given in (Fig. 69).

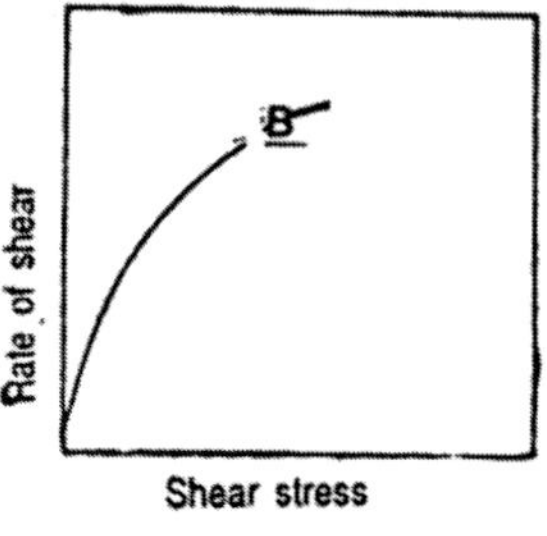

Fig. 69.

The curve passes through the origin and it indicates that mild forces can induce a flow. The slope of the curve gradually decreases until the point B. In this case, the viscosity of the system gradually increases and hence this system is called '*Shear thickening system*'.

The *apparent* viscosity of a dilatant system is given by the empirical power law.

$$\eta = \frac{S^N}{du/dx} \quad \text{... (9)}$$

where the value of N is less than 1.

Both the plastic and pseudoplastic systems show '*shear thinning*' and the dilatant systems show '*shear thickening*'.

Examples of dilatant system are concentrated deflocculated suspension. (about 50% or more) and suspensions of starch in water

3.3. Mechanism of shear thinning

Under the influence of shear in plastic and pseudoplastic systems having aggregates of dispersed particles (asymmetric network), there is progressive structural breakdown resulting in decrease in viscosity. Greater amount of breakdown occurs at higher shear rates. Consequently there is gradual decrease in viscosity. Once the structural breakdown is complete, the apparent viscosity becomes constant. i.e. the flow becomes Newtonian.

3.4. Mechanism of shear thickening

Shear thickening is expressed in **dilatant systems**. At rest, the particles **are closely** packed and so a minimum **void space is** present. The amount of vehicle **is sufficient** to fill the expanded void space and the particles can move relative to one another at low rates of shear. At rest the system is reasonably fluid. As the shear rate is increased, the bulk of the system expands, particles become open packed and the void space increases. The vehicle is now insufficient to fill the expanded void space. As one particle moves with respect to another, there is lot of structural build up which results in increased viscosity. Greater structural build up occurs at higher shear rates. Eventually the fluid system becomes a firm paste. Hence processing of dilatant systems in a mixer such as colloid mill leads to overloading and damaging the processing equipment especially at high shear rates

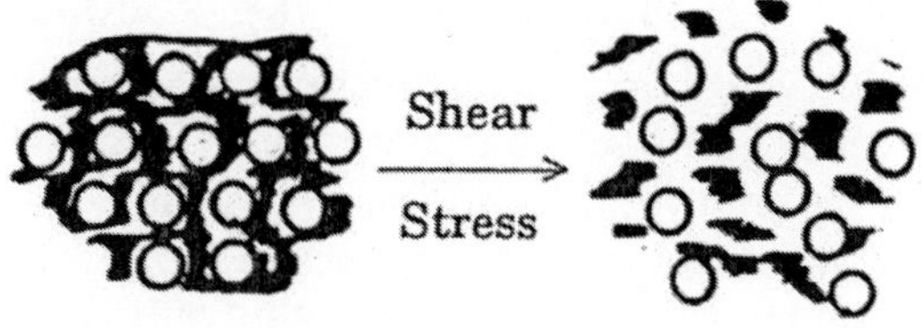

Dilatant system *at rest*	*Dilatant system at high shear rate*
Particles closely packed	Particles open packed
Less void space	More void space
Vehicle sufficient to fill the void space	Vehicle not sufficient to fill the void space
Less viscous and pourable	More viscous and non-pourable

3.5. Thixotropy

The plastic, pseudoplastic and dilatant systems at a given temperature, change their viscosities at varying shearing stresses. The behaviour of such systems are time dependent. It may be explained as follows.

(i) By gradually increasing the shearing stress on plastic or pseudoplastic systems, the apparent viscosity gradually decreases as a resxult of progressive breakdown of structure in the liquid medium at a given temperature. After removing the shearing stress, the viscosity is regained due to slow rebuilding of structure by Brownian motion. but not immediately but after some time lag. Consider the conversion of gel to sol and then sol to gel after removing the stress applied.

$$\text{Gel} \underset{\text{removing shear stress}}{\overset{\text{applying shear stress}}{\rightleftharpoons}} \text{Sol}$$

The conversion of sol to gel is not instantaneous but requires some time lag.

(ii) By increasing the shearing stress on dilatant system, the apparent viscosity gradually increases at a given temperature. After removing the shearing stress, the viscosity is decreased but not immediately but after some time. Consider the following conversion of sol to gel.

$$\text{Sol} \underset{\text{removing shear stress}}{\overset{\text{applying shear stress}}{\rightleftharpoons}} \text{Gel}$$

The conversion of gel to sol is not immediate but requires some time lag.

All the three systems, i.e. plastic, pseudoplastic and dilatant systems will change their viscosities gradually with respect to time even if a constant shearing stress is applied. Such a time dependant effect is called thixotropy which means *'change by touch'*. It is ***defined*** as ***a reversible isothermal transition from gel to sol in the case of shear thinning systems like plastic and pseudoplastic systems and from a sol to gel in the case of shear thickening systems like dilatant system, and the transition is time-dependent*** The thixotropy exhibited by plastic and pseudoplastic systems is called *positive thixotropy* and that of dilatant system is called *negative thixotropy* or *anti-thixotropy*.

A rheogram is obtained for a shear thinning system by plotting the rate of shear at various shear stresses. The curve is called 'up curve'. By reducing the shearing stress gradually on the above system, a 'down-curve' is obtained. Both the 'up curve' and 'down curve' are not super-imposable. The down curve is shifted to left side. This means the flow property of the system is not the same before and after the initial determination. Hence the viscosity of the sample depends upon its previous history. Therefore, the viscosities of the 'down curve' are lower than the viscosities of the 'up curve'. As a result, the 'down curve' is shifted to the left side of the 'up curve' in the rheogram (Fig. 70).

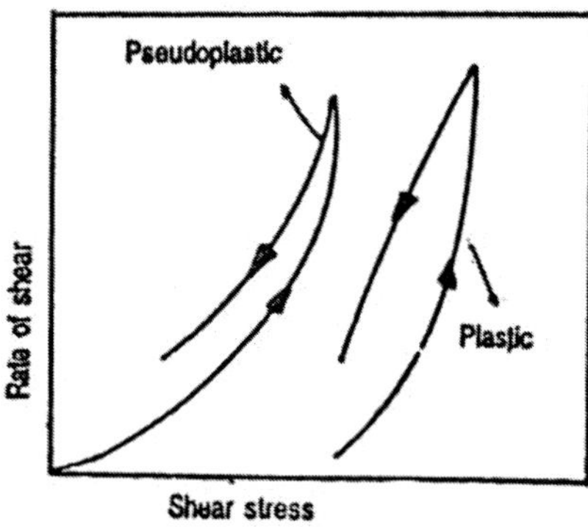

Fig. 70. Thixotropy in plastic and pseudoplastic system

The loop between the 'up curve' and the 'down curve' is called *'hysteresis loop'*. The area of the loop indicates the extent of structural breakdown.

An example of the system showing thixotropy is bentonite gel. It is made up of random network of hydrated elongated particles. On applying shearing stress, the net work is broken down and the elongated particles are aligned with their long axis parallel to the direction of flow and the interparticular links are broken and as a result the viscosity is reduced.

The antithixotropic rheogram for a dilatant system is as shown in (Fig. 71).

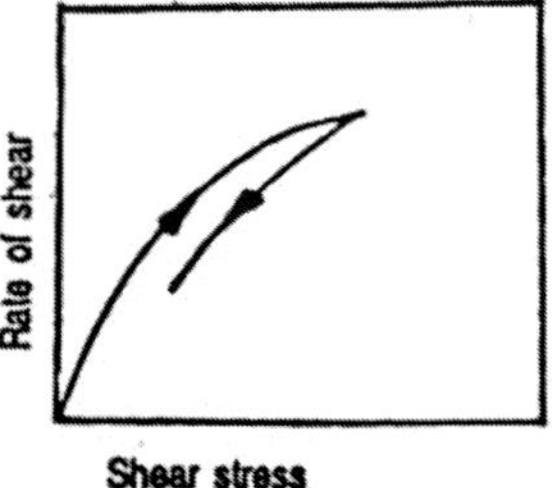

Fig. 71. Thixotropy in dilatant system

Examples of systems showing antithixotropic behaviour are magnesium magma and clay. The isothermal transition from gel to sol or sol to gel takes some time. It may range from a short period to very long period may be months. Any thixotropic system which takes undue time is considered practically irreversible. The time period to regain its original viscosity may be reduced by applying a gentle rolling or rocking motion (tumbling) to the system in a container. This is called *'rheopexy'* and it helps in bringing the particles to the original state. The rheopexy with the shear thinning system is called *positive rheopexy* and with the shear thickening system, it is called *negative rheopexy*.

4. Determination of Flow Properties

For Newtonian systems, the shear rate is directly proportional to the shearing stress and hence it is enough to find a single rate of shear for a shearing stress (i.e. one point determination.) The point obtained for this value in the graph may be extrapolated to the origin i.e. a line passing through the point and origin may be drawn. The line gives a complete rheogram. For non-Newtonian systems, one point determination determination is useless and hence a multipoint determinations should be undertaken. i.e. a number of rates of shear must be obtained at different shearing stresses to obtain a complete rheogram for plastic, pseudoplastic and dilatant systems.

The different instruments used for the determination of flow properties are

1. Ostwalds Viscometer
2. Ubbelohde Suspended Level Viscometer
3. Falling Sphere Viscometer
4. Cup and Bob Viscometer
5. Cone and Plate Viscometer.

Of these five viscometers, the first three viscometers are used for the determination of Newtonian flow and the last two are used for the determination of both Newtonian and non-Newtonian flows.

4.1. Ostwald's Viscometer

It is also called capillary viscometer. The apparatus Fig. 72 consists of a '*U*' tube the left arm of the tube has a 'bulging' at its lower part and there is a marking '*A*' above this bulb. The right arm of the tube also has a 'bulging' at the upper part and just below this bulb is a capillary tube as shown in the figure. There are two markings *B* and *C* above and below the bulb of the right arm.

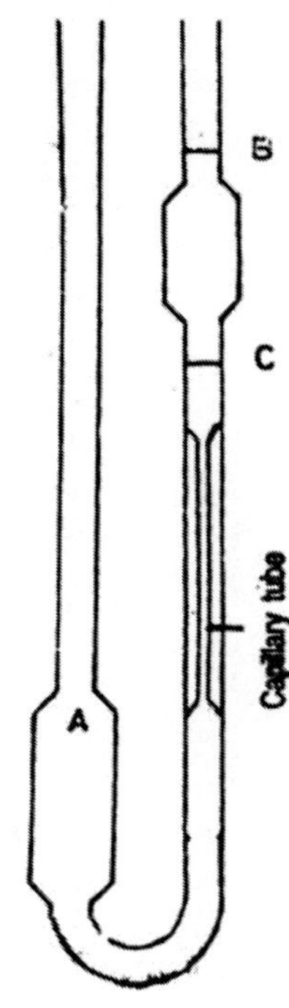

Fig. 72. Ostwald's Viscometer

The liquid is poured into the apparatus through the left arm upto the mark *A*. The liquid is sucked into the right arm slightly above the point *B* and the left arm is closed with the thumb to keep the liquid without dropping down. The apparatus is clamped vertically and the thumb is removed so as to allow the liquid to fall through the capillary under gravity. The time 't' taken for the liquid level to drop down from the point *B* to *C* is noted. The room temperature is also noted. As per Poisuille's equation.

$$\eta = \frac{\pi}{8}\frac{pr^4t}{Vl} = \frac{\pi}{8}\frac{hdgr^4t}{Vl}. \quad \ldots (10)$$

$$\eta = ctd$$

where c is instrument constant and is equal to

$$= \frac{\pi}{8}\frac{hgr^4}{Vl}. \quad \ldots (11)$$

The instrument constant is usually supplied along with the instrument by the manufacturer. By knowing the value of t and the density of the liquid d, the absolute viscosity of the liquid can be found out.

The relative viscosity of the liquid with respect to water can be found out as follows.

The experiment is undertaken for water as described above with the instrument. After cleaning and drying the instrument, the experiment is carried out with the liquid whose relative viscosity is to be found out.

$$\frac{\eta_l}{\eta_w} = \frac{ct_l d_l}{ct_w d_w} = \frac{t_l d_l}{t_w d_w} \quad \dots (12)$$

where subscript l =liquid and w =water

The viscosity of water η_w at a given temperature (may be room temperature) is found out. Then t_l, d_l, t_w, and d_w are determined. From these values, the relative viscosity of the liquid with respect to water can be found out. The relative viscosity of the liquid may be converted to absolute viscosity by multiplying the relative viscosity with the absolute viscosity of water. The viscosities of the liquid can be found out at different temperatures by keeping the instrument in a thermostat.

Sometimes the viscosity of the liquid is expressed as *kinematic* viscosity

$$\upsilon = \frac{\eta}{\rho} = \frac{\text{absolute viscosity}}{\text{density of the liquid}} \quad \dots (13)$$

Experimental precautions

1. Streamline flow must occur in the capillary
2. Unnecessary long flow time should be avoided.
3. There should not be any air bubble.
4. The instrument should be thoroughly cleaned and dried for each liquid.
5. Adequate temperature control should be ensured.
6. Correction may be made for surface tension which tends to raise or lower the meniscus of the liquid in the tube.

The disadvantage with the Ostwald's viscometer is that for relative viscosity determination, volume of liquid put into the apparatus should be constant so as to get correct reproducible result.

To avoid the above difficulties, Ubbelohde viscometer is used.

4.2. Ubbelhode viscomenter

It is a modified Ostwald's viscometer and in this another vertical tube (third arm) is attached to the bulb below the capillary part of the right arm parallel to '*U*' tube as shown in (Fig. 73).

A volume of liquid just sufficient to fill the bulb in the left arm is poured. By closing the left arm and the third arm with the thumbs, the liquid is sucked into the right arm (i.e. central tube) upto a level just above the point *B*. The central arm is now closed with the thumb after removing the thumbs from the other two arms and that keeps the level of the liquid just above the mark *B*. As the liquid below the capillary tube is ventilated down by the third arm, the volume of liquid in the right arm (central tube) remains constant. The rest of the experiment is similar to as described under Ostwald's viscometer.

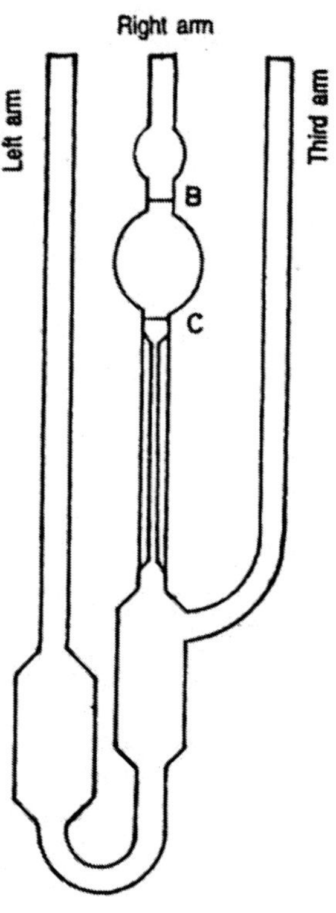

Fig. 73. Ubbelohde suspended level viscometer

1.3. Falling sphere viscometer (Hoeppler falling ball viscometer)

As per Stoke's law, a body falling through a viscous medium experiences a resistance or viscous drag that opposes the motion of the body. when the body falls through a liquid under the influence of gravity during which acceleration of the motion occurs at the initial period but when the gravitational force (acceleration) is balanced by the viscous drag, the body falls down at a uniform terminal velocity which can be determined in the falling sphere viscometer.

Viscous drag on the sphere = force responsible for downward motion due to gravity.

$$3\pi\, \eta d u = \frac{\pi}{6} d^3 g(\rho_s - \rho_l) \quad \text{... (14)}$$

where η = coefficient of viscosity
d = diameter of the sphere
g = acceleration due to gravity
u = terminal velocity
ρ_s = density of the sphere
ρ_l = density of the liquid

Rearranging the above equation

$$\eta = \frac{d^2 g(\rho_s - \rho_l)}{18u}. \quad \text{... (15)}$$

The diameter of the sphere may be obtained by using vernier caliper. ρ_l (density of the liquid) is determined using specific gravity bottle and the terminal velocity (u) by using the falling sphere viscometer and from these values the viscosity of the liquid may be calculated.

The apparatus (Fig. 74) consists of a tube having two markings A and B marked on the outer surface of the tube. The tube is filled with the liquid whose viscosity is to be determined. The tube is clamped vertically inside a constant temperature bath. Sufficient time is allowed to get all the air bubbles removed and the whole set up to attain the equilibrium temperature. A steel sphere (ball) is cleaned and allowed to reach the same temperature as that of the experiment by keeping in a thermostat. There is a guide tube on the fall tube through which the ball is allowed to fall and a hole in the guide tube prevents any airlock. The time 't' taken for the sphere to fall from A to B is noted. The terminal velocity is the ratio between the distance between the two markings A and B and the time 't'. By substituting all the values in the equation, the coefficient of the viscosity of the liquid is calculated.

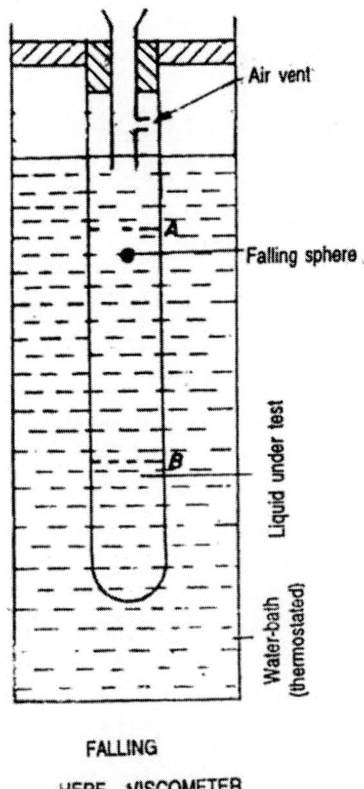

Fig. 74.

The equation is given assuming that the sphere is falling through a medium of infinite dimension. But in the experiment the liquid is contained in a cylinder. A correction factor (F) is introduced to nullify the effect of wall on the fall of the sphere.

$$F = 1 - 2.104d/D + 2.09d^3/D^3 \quad \ldots (16)$$

where d = diameter of the sphere

D = diameter of the tube

and the corrected viscosity $= \eta \times F$

The instrument can be used over a range of 0.5 to 200,000 poise. For best results, the ball (density) should be such that it takes not less than 30 seconds to fall from mark A to B.

(Red Wood Viscometer: It consists of a cylinder having an outlet at its bottom with a valve. Two sizes are available called No.1 and No.2. The specifications are detailed in British Pharmacopoeia. The liquid is filled upto the mark made in the cylinder. The valve is fully opened and the time taken for the liquid to drain out fully is reported as Redwood seconds. Thus, it is an empirical instrument.)

4.4. Rotational viscometer

In rotational viscometers a solid rotating body is immersed or suspended in a liquid/semi solid (whose viscosity is to be measured) and is subjected to a retarding force due to the viscous drag which is proportional to the viscosity of the liquid. The advantages of rotational viscometers are:

(a) it is possible to vary the shear rate over a wide range of values and

(b) measurements can be made continuously for extended periods at a given shear rate or shear stress.

Therefore, the rotational viscometer, with accurate temperature control, are useful for measuring the time dependency as well as shear dependency of the viscosities of non-Newtonian systems. The rotational viscometer are

1. Concentric cylinder viscometer (or co-axial cylinder viscometer or cup and bob viscometers)
2. cone and plate viscometers.

4.4.1. Cup and Bob viscometer

The cup and bob viscometer Fig. 75 consists of an outer cylinder A, (cup) which acts as a container for the liquid, and can be rotated at different speeds (different shearing stresses). An inner cylinder B (bob) is suspended freely by a torsion wire. Rotation of the outer cylinder A produces movements within the liquid in the gap separating the two cylinders and as a result the torque (indicating rate of shear) produced is transmitted to the inner cylinder B. This torque is measured in

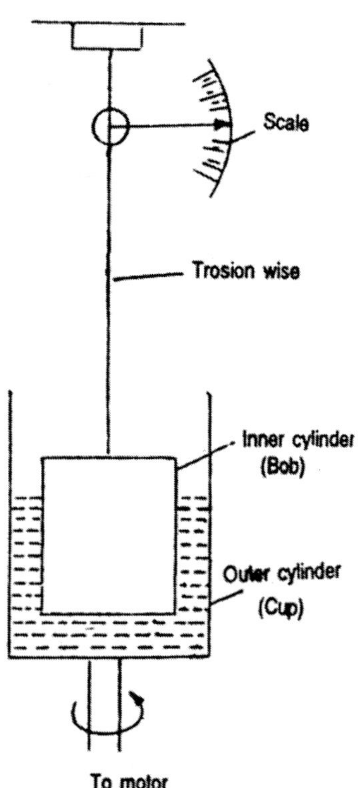

Fig. 75. Concentric cylinder viscometer. (coutte type)

terms of angular deflection θ of a pointer which moves on a scale.

If a steady laminar flow occurs within the liquid, the viscosity is calculated as follows:

$$\eta = \frac{C\theta\left(\frac{1}{r_1^2} - \frac{1}{r_2^2}\right)}{4\pi h\omega} \quad \text{... (17)}$$

where C = torsional constant of the wire

θ = angular deflection

r_1 and r_2 = radii of the inner and outer cylinders

h = height of the inner cylinder surrounded by the liquid.

ω = angular velocity of the outer cylinder

There are two types of viscometer

(a) *Couette type viscometer:* The cup is revolved. The viscous drag on the bob produced by the liquid results in a torque which is proportional to viscosity eg: *Mac Machael viscometer.*

(b) *Searle type viscometer:* It involves the principle of rotating the bob instead of the cup. eg: ***Stromer viscometer*** Fig. 76. For systems of viscosity more than 20 centipoise, it may be used. In this the cup is placed in a thermostat (constant temperature bath) on a stand and the bob is suspended into it. Both the cup and bob are allowed to reach the equilibrium temperature. The bob can be rotated by placing weight on a hanger through a winding pool which is attached to a hanger through a pulley. The number of revolutions of the bob can be counted with the help of a revolution counter. The data are converted to rpm. The weight is increased and the whole procedure is similar to the above.

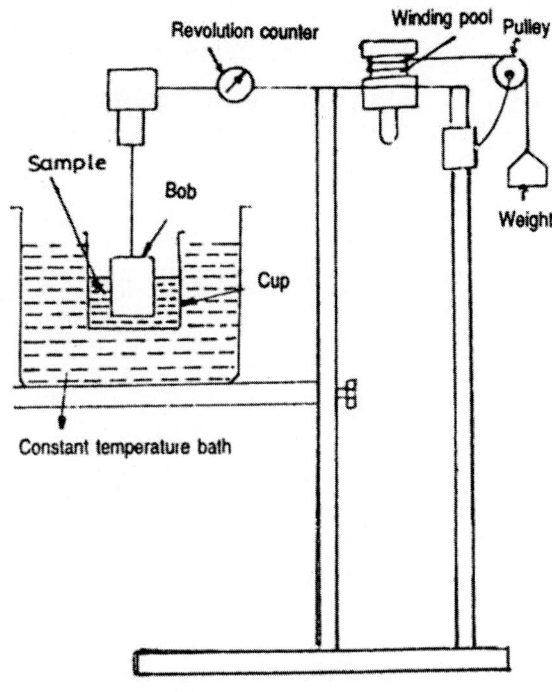

Fig. 76. Stromer viscometer (Searle type)

A rheogram can be obtained by plotting rpm versus the weight added. Making use of appropriate constants, rpm values are converted to actual shear rates (sec^{-1}) and the weights added into the units of shear (dynes cm^{-2}) In this case, the viscosity is calculated as follows

$$\eta = K_v \frac{w}{v} \quad \text{... (18)}$$

where w = weight in grams

V = rpm generated due to w.

K_v = instrument constant which can be determined by analysing an oil of known viscosity using the instrument.

The plastic viscosity may be calculated using the formula

$$U = K_v = \frac{W - W_f}{V} \quad \dots (19)$$

where W_f = yield value.

The yield value of a Bingham body (plastic system) is given by the expression.

$$f = K_f \times W_f \quad \dots (20)$$

where $K_f = K_v \times \frac{2\pi}{60} \times \frac{1}{2.303 \log (R_2/R_1)} \quad \dots (21)$

where R_2 = radius of the cup

R_1 = radius of the bob

Disadvantages of cup and bob viscometer

1. If the gap between the cup and bob is larger, there will be no uniform rate of shear.
2. Frictional heating may develop at higher rates of shear and hence a constant temperature bath is used to offset the temperature effect on viscosity of the liquid.
3. Filling and cleaning are often difficult.
4. The instrument requires more sample.
5. *Plug flow development:* In the cup and bob viscometer there is a variable shear stress within the sample across the gap between the cup and bob. This variation is mainly dependent upon the gap. In searle type viscometer, the bob is rotated and the cup is stationary. For the bob to be rotated, the shearing stress should necessarily be higher than the yield value. It may happen so, for a certain shearing stress of the bob, **Though** it is sufficiently high to exceed the yield value the shearing stress developed at the inner surface of the cup may be less than the yield value. In such a situation, the material at the inner surface of the cup remains as a solid plug without any flow. This phenomenon is plug flow. Chances of plug flow can be minimised by reducing the gap between the cup and bob. For that a bob as large as possible may be used. Laminar flow (rather than plug flow) of the system can be expected only when the shear stress at the wall of the cup exceeds the yield value).

Plug flow may be important when pastes and concentrated suspensions flow out of the container through an orifice. For example, in the case of tooth paste obtained from its container, the paste experiences a higher shear stress when pressed at the circumference of the tube aperture. As a result the consistency drops at the points of stress and this facilitates extrusion of the paste in the core as a plug. However this phenomenon is not desirable in obtaining rheograms of plastic systems with cup and bob viscometer.

4.4.2. Cone and plate viscometer

In cone and plate viscometer, all the disadvantages mentioned under cup and bob viscometer are overcome.

The cone and plate viscometer Fig. 77 essentially consists of a smooth

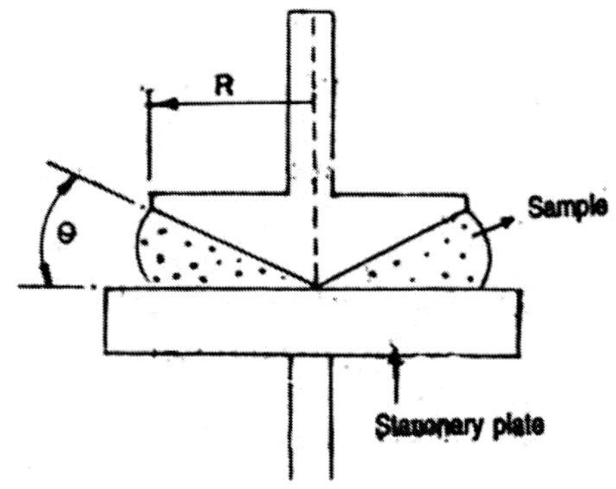

Fig. 77. Cone and plate viscometer

plate and a cone. During operation, the sample is placed at the centre of the plate, which is then slowly raised so that the tip of the cone comes in contact with the sample. At this position, the cone to plate angle is ordinarily less than 1°C. The sample is sheared in the narrow gap between the plate and the cone when the plate is driven by a variable speed motor. The torque transmitted through the sample to the cone is measured. The viscosity is given by

$$\eta = \frac{3A/2\pi R^3}{B/Q} \quad \dots (22)$$

where A = torque on the cone

R = radius of the cone

B = radial velocity of the plate

Q = angle between the cone and the plate and is less than $\pi/360$ radians

Advantages:

1. Rate of shear is constant throughout the sample and hence no chance for plug flow.
2. Cleaning is easy and requires less time
3. Temperature stabilization is also good.
4. It needs vary little sample for the study. That is a sample volume of 0.1 to 0.2 ml will do.
5. Rates of shear can be increased or decreased in a predetermined and reproducible manner.
6. This serves as a valuable aid for the determination of hysteresis loop obtained in thixotropic systems and also in determining thixotropic coefficient.

5. Commercial Viscometers

1. Ferrante – Portable viscometer
2. Brookfield synchrolectric viscometer
3. Ferrante – Shirley cone and plate viscometer
4. Extrusion viscometer

5.1. Ferranti – Portable viscometer (for bulk liquids)

In this the rotating outer cylinder is inverted and immersed in the liquid. The inner cylinder is attached to a pointer on a scale through a torque spring which is beryllium copper spring. (Fig. 78) There is a guard ring shown in Fig. 78.

The outer cylinder is driven by a synchronous motor with a three to five speed gear box. The gear box can provide a range of 1 rev/min upto 300 rev/min. The mean shear rates vary from 930 to 0.15 sec^{-1}. Amount of sample required is usually about 100 ml. For a given rpm (rate of shear) and the angle of deflection (shearing stress),

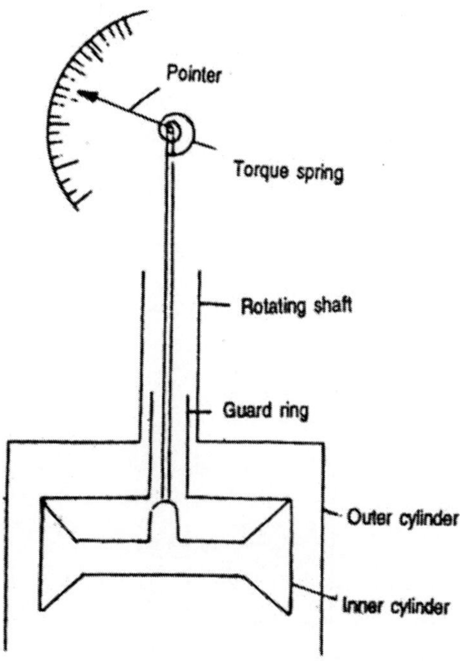

Fig. 78. Ferranti portable viscometer

the viscosity may be read directly from the literature table supplied by the manufacturer.

5.2. Brookfield synchrolectric viscometer

It is used as a comparative instrument (Fig. 79) since it does not provide results in terms of absolute shear. A bob is immersed in the sample liquid. The bob carries a rotating spindle which is driven through a calibrated beryllium copper spring which in turn is mounted on a motor shaft. The spindle is also attached to a pointer which gives the displacement of the spindle due to viscous drag of the sample. Since both the pointer and the scale revolve, the readings are complicated. However it is possible to clamp the pointer. In this viscosity changes cannot be followed while increasing the shearing stress and hence it is used for comparing the apparent viscosities of non-Newtonian systems.

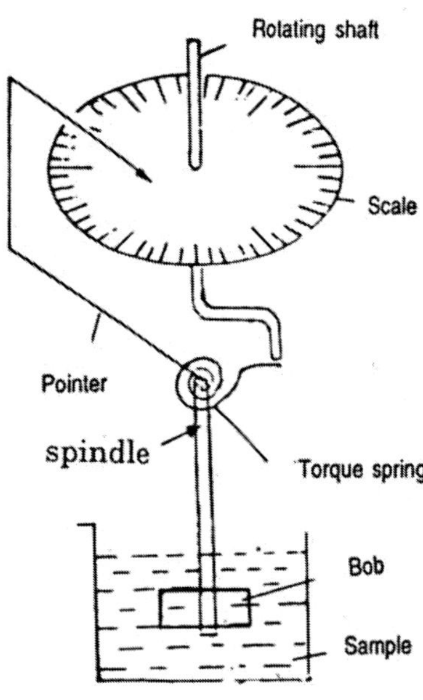

Fig. 79. Brookfield Viscometer

5.3. Ferranti – Shirley cone and plate viscometer

It is very popularly used to study the change of flow properties of a rheological system continuously by varying the shear rates and to study thixotropy.

This viscometer Fig. 80 consists of a stationary flat plate and a rotating cone. The usual plate to cone angles are about 0.3° so that only small samples (0.5 to 1 ml) are required. The plate is maintained at a constant temperature.

The rate of shear for small angles is constant and is given by

$$\frac{A}{B} \qquad \ldots (23)$$

where A = rotation (rad/sec)

B = cone angle (rad)

The cone is driven by a variable speed motor and the rate of shear is capable of being varied over a wide range from 0 to 18000 sec^{-1}. A torsion spring is interposed between the cone (i.e. the driving shaft of the cone) and the driving shaft in order to measure the shearing stress on a galvanometer connected to a potentiometer circuit.

It is possible to obtain recording of shear rates and shearing stresses simultaneously. This enables to obtain flow curves automatically on an $x-y$ recorder.

A rheological system is taken in between the cone and the plate. The rate of shear is varied continuously and the corresponding shearing stresses are recorded simultaneously on $x-y$ recorder. From the rheograms obtained, one can make out whether the system is Newtonian, plastic, pseudoplastic or dilatant.

For thixotropic studies, a sample is placed in between the cone and plate in the instrument. The rate of shear is

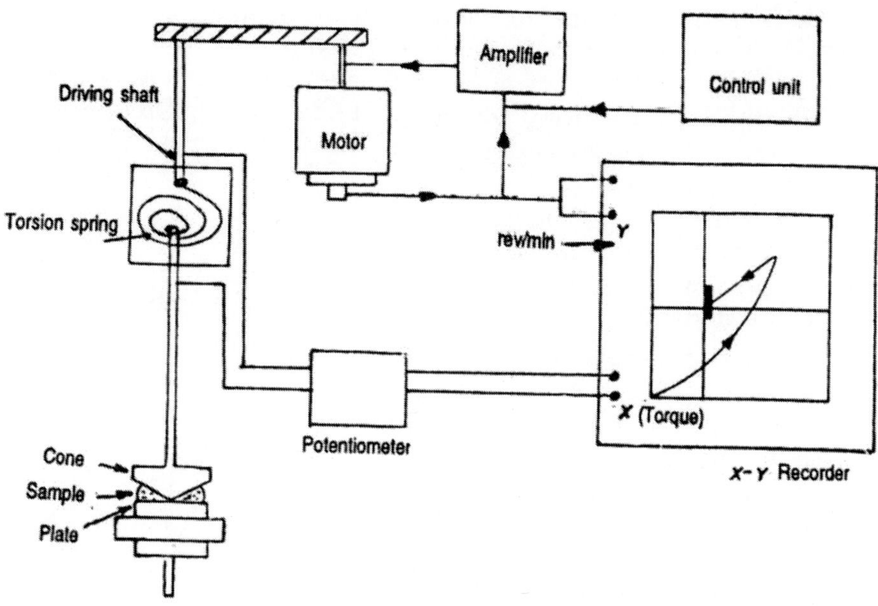

Fig. 80. Ferranti-shirely cone and plate viscometer

gradually increased and the corresponding shear stresses are recorded simultaneously on the $x-y$ recorder to get the 'up-curve'. Then the rate of shear is gradually decreased in the sample and the corresponding shearing stresses are recorded simultaneously on the $x-y$ recorder to obtain the 'down curve'. Thus it is possible to demonstrate the time-dependent effect of stresses on rheological systems as well as how the previous history of the sample alters its physical properties.

5.4. Extrusion viscometer

It is suitable for butter and semi-solid preparations. It consists of a simple cylinder 4 cm long and 1.25 cm in diameter with a circular orifice. Inside the cylinder is a plunger which could be moved at a uniform speed.

A sample of any ointment or paste or cream which has got consumer acceptability is kept in the cylinder. The thrust just required to extrude the material is recorded. Whether the sample of ointment or paste or cream is having the same thrust for the subsequent batches are tested. Any inhomogeneity due to substandard material, agglomerate of particles or air bubble will be indicated by the fluctuation in the recorded thrust.

6. Viscoelasticity

Materials which exhibit viscous properties of liquids and elastic properties of solids are called ***viscoelastic materials.*** Pharmaceutical systems which belong to this class are creams, ointments, suppositories, suspensions and emulsifying and suspending agents. Biologic materials such as blood, sputum and cervical fluid also show viscoelastic properties.

Rheograms obtained by plotting shear stress against shear rate can provide information which can be used to characterise pharmaceutical products. For this purpose, we mainly employ rotational viscometers. In these, the continuous shear produces deformation and alteration of material during measurement. Whereas in the measurement of viscoelastic properties of the materials, the structure is not destroyed and hence the measurements provide information on intermolecular and interparticular forces in the materials.

Viscoelastic behaviour comprises both viscous flow and elasticity. Hence, two basic elements of mechanical models are used to represent their behaviour. One is the *helical spring* which gives the elastic behaviour and other is a *dashpot* which is nothing but a cylindrical container with a loosely fitting piston filled with a Newtonian liquid which gives the viscous flow. Thus, the viscoelastic behaviour of a semisolid can be described by the combination of the dashpot and spring. The mechanical models are of two types - the Maxwell element and Voigt-Kelvin element. Maxwell element (Fig. 81) is obtained by connecting a spring and dashpot in *series* and when they are connected in *parallel*, they form Voigt-Kelvin element. (Fig.82)

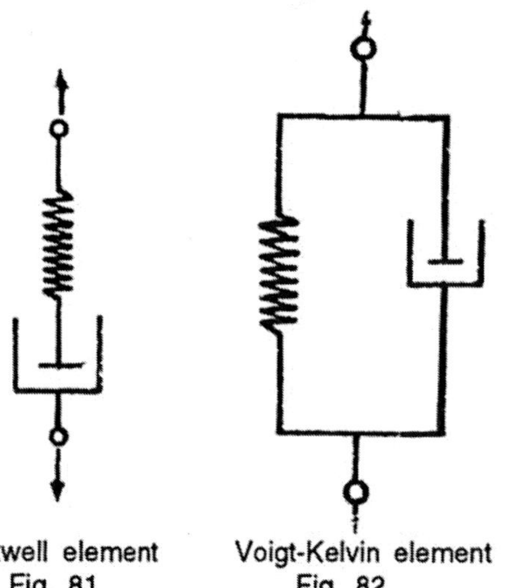

Maxwell element
Fig. 81

Voigt-Kelvin element
Fig. 82

Most materials need more than one Maxwell or Voigt-Kelvin element to characterise their rheological behaviour and to describe their deformation curves under stress. One simple model is the **Burgers** model. (Fig.83)

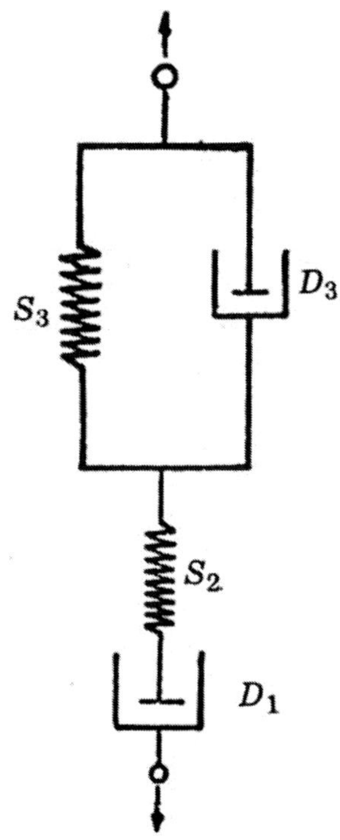

Fig. 83 Burger's model

A creep-deformation -time curve of Burgers' body is shown in Fig. 84

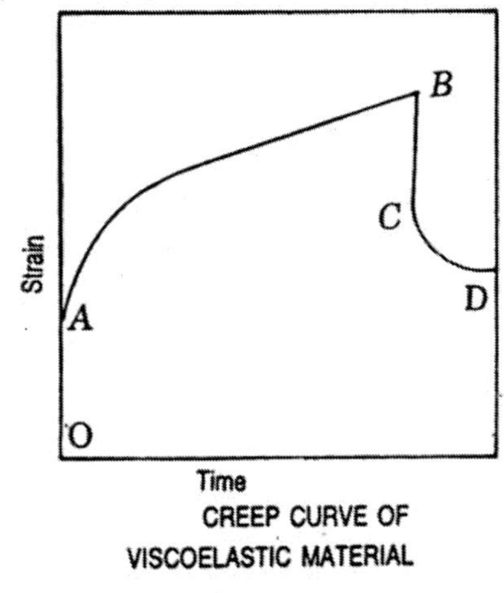

CREEP CURVE OF VISCOELASTIC MATERIAL

Fig. 84

The curve *OAB* represents period of time when the model is under a constant stress. It consists of two segments. The first segment *OA* represents the instant stretching of spring 2 (S_2) under applied stress and as a result, the material is elongated from *O* to *A*. This corresponds to elastic stretching of bonds between primary structural units. If the stress is removed at *A*, the material would recover and regain the original structure completely. The second segment *AB* represents the combination of the recoverable deformation of spring 3 (S_3) which is retarded by dashpot 3 (D_3) (both connected in parallel) and the non recoverable creep of dashpot 1 (D_1). The initial strongly curved region which represents recoverable deformation corresponds to breaking and reformation of interparticle bonds. The straight line region of the curve corresponds to the creep of dashpot 1 (D_1) and this in turn represents that some of the bonds break so slowly that they reform within the test period. The rupture of interparticle bonds that occur in the initial strongly curved region releases some structural units and as a result they flow past one another to produce the permanent deformation.

When the stress is removed at time *T*, recovery occurs. The recovery is represented by *BCD*. On the removal of stress, spring 2 (S_2) retracts instantly and the meterial contracts along *BC* which is equal to *OA*. The retraction of spring (S_3) is retarded by dashpot 3 (D_3) along *CD*.

Viscoelastic materials exhibit a range of relaxation or retardation. If the mean relaxation time is very long as compared to the time of measurement, the material behaves as an elastic solid. If it is very short as compared to the time of measurement the material behaves as a viscous liquid. When both (i.e. mean relaxation time and time of measurement) are comparable in magnitude, the material is viso-elastic.

6.1. Measurement of Viscoelasticity

Creep (permanent or non-recoverable deformation) and stress relaxation (*recoverable strain or elongation; stress/unit strain is called compliance which is reciprocal of modulus*) can be measured with coaxial-cylinder viscometer provided with sensing devices. It consists of an inner cylindrical bob and an outer concentric cylindrical cup (Fig 85). The material is taken in the annular gap between the two cylinders (i.e. cup and bob). The material is subjected to oscillations with small amplitudes or strains. This is accomplished by causing the outer cylindrical cup to rotate sinusoidally through small angles. The stress given to the outer cylinder is transmitted to the inner cylindrical bob by the material in the gap. As a result the inner cylindrical bob will also rotate sinusoidally. Dynamic viscosities and various moduli are measured through sensing devices as a function of frequency and temperature.

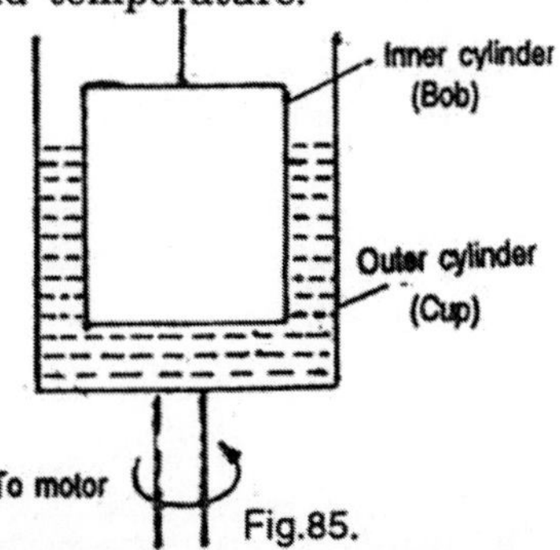

Fig.85.

7. Determination of Thixotropic Coefficient

Thixotropic properties of plastic and pseudoplastic systems can be quantified by the following methods.

7.1. Measurement of structural break down with time at constant rate of shear

A typical rheogram is shown in Fig. 86

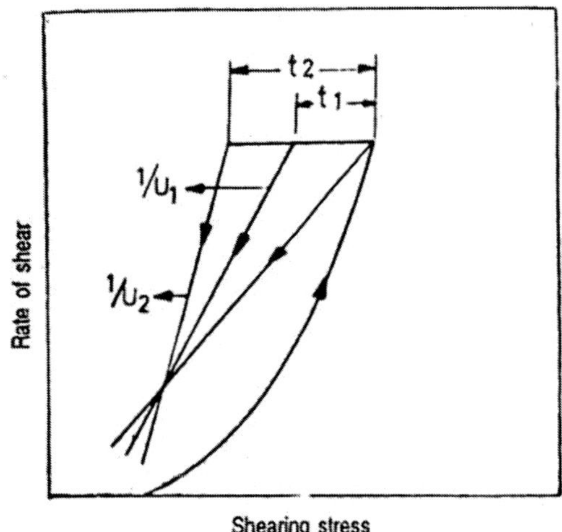

Fig.86. Structural Breakdown in Plastic system with time at constant rate of shear

The study of this can be undertaken using cone-plate Ferranti-Shirley type viscometer. An 'up-curve' and a 'down curve' are obtained after subjecting the sample upto a particular rate of shear 'B' and then removing the stress gradually. This rheogram is plotted on $x-y$ recorder.

Another sample from the same material is taken and kept between the cone and plate in the viscometer. The rate of shear is increased upto the point B (i.e. up curve) and is subjected to a constant rate of shear for a period of t_1 seconds and a 'down curve' is obtained on the same rheogram as shown in the figure.

A third sample from the same material is subjected to the same experiment as above but this time the sample is kept at constant rate of shear at B for t_2 seconds. A down curve is again drawn on the same rheogram which is shown in the figure. The thixotropic coefficient (B) is given by

$$\beta = \frac{U_1 - U_2}{\ln \frac{t_2}{t_1}} \quad \text{... (24)}$$

where U_1 and U_2 = plastic viscosities of the latter two down curves after subjecting it to a constant shear rate for t_1 and t_2 seconds respectively. The choice of the shear rate is arbitrary. Slopes of the down curves give reciprocal of plastic viscosities.

7.2. Measurement of structural breakdown due to increasing rate of shear

The rheogram obtained is shown in Fig. 87. Using cone and plate viscometer, the 'up-curve' and 'down curve' for a material are obtained as described in the first experiment. For first sample of the material, the rate of shear is increased gradually to V_1, and the down curve is obtained. The second sample of the same material is subjected to a shear rate V_2 and then a down curve is obtained. All the curves are shown in the figure. The thixotropic coefficient is

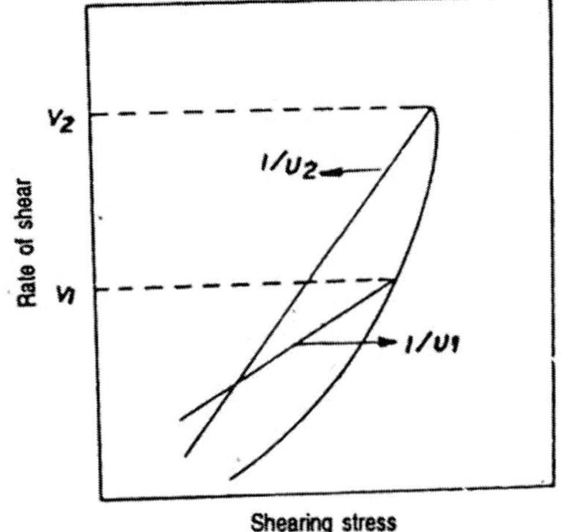

Fig. 87. Structural Breakdown in a plastic system under increasing rate of shear

$$M = \frac{U_1 - U_2}{\ln\left(\frac{V_2}{V_1}\right)} \quad \ldots (25)$$

M indicates the fall in shear stress per unit increase in the rate of shear. The unit is degrees sec/cm^2. U_1 and U_2 are the plastic viscosities of the two down curves exposed to a maximum shear rates V_1 and V_2 respectively. The value of M depends on the values of V_1 and V_2 chosen. Slopes of the down curves give reciprocal of plastic viscosities.

Thixotropic coefficient is calculated for every batch of ointments, pastes or creams to ascertain that the flow property and thixotropic properties of every batch remains the same with the flow and thixotropic properties of a standard preparation of an ointment, paste or cream which had good stability during storage period with good consumer acceptability (psychorheology). Thus the determination serves as one of the quality control measures for semi-solid forms.

8. Rheology of Suspensions

The flow properties of suspensions depend upon their rheological characters. The presence of dispersed particles in the liquid continuous medium (especially in suspensions containing more percentage of dispersed phase) causes streamlines of liquid around the particles to be distorted and as a result the viscosity of the system is increased (due to insufficient liquid which can act as lubricant).

The apparent viscosity of a flocculated suspension is greater than that of a similar suspension having deflocculated particles and hence more stable. The floccules in the suspension produce streamline flow which can withstand mild stresses. Hence flocculated suspension has an yield value and behaves like a plastic or pseudoplastic system (If all the liquid medium is entrapped within the floccules it acts as plastic material. If some amount of liquid medium is left over it acts as pseudoplastic system).

It also exhibits thixotropy. The rheological property of suspensions decides the pourability, ease of injectability, sedimentation, its redispersibility and the elegancy of the appearance. A suspension may be formulated as follows.

(a) Deflocculated particles in Newtonian vehicles

(b) Deflocuulated particles in non-Newtonian vehicles

(c) Flocculated particles in Newtonian vehicles

(d) Flocculated particles in non-Newtonian vehicles.

Of the four, the fourth type is more stable and has lot of advantages. Highly concentrated suspensions exhibit dilatant flow.

9. Rheology in emulsions

Dilute emulsions show Newtonian type flow. Highly concentrated emulsions and creams show plastic flow and has excellent thixotropic properties. The important property influencing viscosity of emulsions are

1. Phase volume ratio
2. Viscosity of the continuous phase
3. Aggregation of globules
4. Nature and proportion of emulsifying agent
5. Globule size and size distribution.

10. Rheology of ointments and creams

Ointments and creams show plastic and thixotropic behaviour. Determination of rheological behaviour and thixotropic coefficients of a standard preparation and comparison of this property with subsequent batches of preparations serve as a guide for quality control measures, for stability, spreadability, performance and elegance of the preparation [Earlier practice of judgement during manufacture by an expert about the products "feel" and "body" is no longer acceptable since it is subjective and not scientific].

Thixotropic pharmaceutical preparations have high consistency in the container under storage and hence more physical stability. Yet they are easily pourable and spreadable at the time of use. They are easily injectable. The injected thixotropic preparation sets as a gel at the site of administration (intra-muscular) from where the drug is released slowly and show sustained or prolonged action. An example is concentrated parenteral suspension containing 40 to 70% w/v of procaine penicillin *G* in water (a depot action preparation) which is having inherent thixotropy and shear thinning properties.

Suggestions for Practicals

1. Determination of viscosity of a liquid

Principle

Refer the text

Procedure

Using Ostwalds viscometer, find out the time for the liquid and water separately to flow from the mark B to C. From the values obtained calculate viscosity, fluidity and Kinematic viscosity.

(a) Absolute viscosity of the liquid is = Ctd (Poise)

where C = instrument constant.

t = time taken by the liquid to flow from B to C.

d = density of the liquid.

(b) Kinematic viscosity of the liquid $= ct$ stokes

(c) Relative viscosity of the liquid (η_l) with respect to water (η_w) is

$$\eta_{rel} = \frac{\eta_l}{\eta_w} = \frac{t_l\, d_l}{t_w\, d_u}$$

(There is no unit for relative viscosities)

Substituting the η_w at a given temperature, the experimental values of t_l, t_w, d_l and d_w, the relative viscosity of the liquid can be found out. The multiplication of the relative viscosity of the liquid and the viscosity of the water gives the absolute viscosity of the liquid in poise.

(d) The instrument constant of the Ostwald's viscometer can be found out by using the equation $C = \frac{\eta}{td}$

2. Effect of concentration on the viscosity of a liquid

Prepare 5%, 10%, 15% and 20%. v/v solution of glycerin in water. Find out the relative viscosities of these solutions with respect to water using Ostwald's viscometer. Prepare a graph by plotting the different concentrations on x-axis against the corresponding relative viscosities on y axis. Observe the graph and report the effect of concentrations on viscosity.

3. Rheological properties of non-Newtonian system and determination of thixotropic coefficient of such systems

(Refer the text)

VI. SOLUTION AND DISTRIBUTION LAW

A solution is defined as a mixture of two or more components whose relative amounts may vary within some limits. A *solution* is physically and chemically homogeneous and it consists of one or more substances called *solutes* dissolved and evenly distributed in a medium called the solvent. The particles of the solute and the *solvent* are in chaotic thermal motion and are uniformly distributed throughout the entire volume of the solution.

Solutions may be gas in gas, liquid in gas, solid in gas, gas in liquid, liquid in liquid, solid in liquid, gas in liquid, liquid in solid and solid in solid. The term solution is frequently applied to a homogeneous system that is liquid. In pharmacy, solutions of solids in liquids, liquids in liquids and gases in liquids are of primary concern.

Solutions of solids in liquids may be put into two types – *solutions of non-electrolytes and solutions of electrolytes.* When sugar (non-electrolyte) is dissolved in water, it produces a solution – a molecular dispersion i.e. the solute sugar is dispersed in the form of molecules in water. When sodium chloride (electrolyte) is dissolved in water to obtain a solution, it yields an ionic dispersion i.e. the solute sodium chloride is dispersed as ions (Na^+ and Cl^-) into water.

1. Expression of concentration

The concentration of a solution may be given either as a quantity of solute in a definite volume of solution or as a quantity of solute in a definite mass of solvent or solution.

1.1. The various expressions are

Percent by mass (c): It is the number of mass units (in grams) contained in 100 mass units (in 100 grams) of solution.

Molarity (c): It is the number of moles (or gram molecular weight) of solute dissolved in 1 litre of solution.

Molality (m): It is the number of moles of solute dissolved in 1000 g of solvent.

Normality (N): It is the number of gram equivalents of solute dissolved in 1 litre of solution.

Mole fraction (x): The mole fraction of a constituent is the fraction of total number of moles present in the solution or it is the ratio of the number of moles of one constituent (solute) of a solution to the total number of moles of all the constituents (solutes and solvent)

$$x = \frac{\text{number of moles of solute}}{\text{number of moles of solute (or solutes)} + \text{number of moles of solvent}} \quad \dots (1)$$

Number of moles

$$= \frac{\text{weight of a substance}}{\text{molecular weight of the substance}}$$

1.2. *Molar ratio*

For a binary system (i.e. one solute and one solvent), it is the ratio of the number of moles of the solute to the number of moles of the solvent (Mole percent may be obtained by multiplying mole fraction by 100)

In pharmacy, three concentration terms are often used. They are:

1. ***Percent by weight*** (%w/w): It is the number of grams of solute in 100 grams of solution.
2. ***Percent by volume*** (% v/v): It is the number of ml of solute in 100 ml of solution
3. ***Percent weight by volume*** (% w/v): It is the number of grams of solute in 100 ml of solution.

2. Solubility

When a substance (solute) dissolves in water, a solution results. The ability of a substance to dissolve in a solvent is quantified as its solubility. The solubility of a solute in a particular solvent is measured by its concentration in a saturated solution. A solution is said to be saturated when it contains the maximum amount of solute that a solvent can dissolve at a particular temperature. As temperature influences solubility, temperature must be specified whenever the solubility of a component (or solute) is expressed. A saturated solution of a solute at a particular temperature will be in equilibrium with the solute undissolved.

Under certain conditions, a supersaturated solution can be obtained. It is the solution that contains more solute than the solvent can dissolve at a definite temperature. This may be obtained simply by cooling a saturated solution carefully to a lower temperature (without any precipitation). However, this supersaturated solution is metastable and the excess solute may be precipitated by shaking, by scratching the sides of the container or by introducing a small crystal of the solute.

2.1. Determination of solubility

Determination of solubility of solids in solvent is usually undertaken in two steps.

1. Preparation of a saturated solution at a particular temperature desired.
2. Analysis of the saturated solution.

To obtain a saturated solution at the required temperature, an excess of powdered solute is added to a solvent in a vessel and then stirred for several hours keeping the vessel in a constant temperature bath until equilibrium has been achieved.

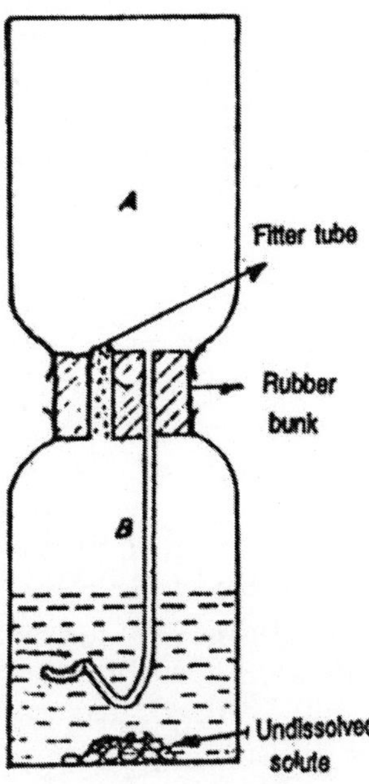

Fig. 88. Solubility determination apparatus

A sample of the saturated solution is separated from the undissolved solid by filtration. Enough care should be taken to ensure that filtration is carried out at the temperature desired for the solubility determination and that no loss of volatile component (solvent) occurs. The solution is, then analysed.

In order to obtain very accurate results, the following apparatus shown in Fig. 88 may be used. This apparatus consists of two bottles '*A*' and '*B*' attached with a rubber bunk. There are two holes within the rubber bunk one carrying a capillary tube bent at one end and the other carrying a filter tube packed with glass wool.

The solute and solvent are added to the lower bottle '*B*' and agitated in a thermostat until a saturated solution is achieved. It may take 24 hours or more. The apparatus, after the saturated solution is complete, is inverted in the thermostat so that the solution can filter through the filter tube into the other empty bottle '*A*'. The bend present in the capillary tube prevents the transference of undissolved solid into the empty bottle '*B*'. The apparatus is removed from the thermostat and the solution is analysed.

Analysis of the filtered solution may be undertaken by any suitable chemical analysis or by gravimetric analysis if the solute is non-volatile and undecomposed at the temperature of evaporation of the solvent. Physical measurements such as electrical conductivity (for sparingly soluble electrolytes) optical rotation (for optically active compounds), specific gravity or refractive index may be used. The technique of isotope dilution analysis may also be applied. Method of analysis depends on the physico-chemical properties of the solute.

Once the amount of solute in a sample of solution has been determined, the concentration in 100 ml of solution can easily be arrived at by calculation.

Another method involves the preparation of a saturated solution at a higher temperature and allowing the solution to cool to room temperature. In this method, a known amount of solute is taken with a known quantity of solvent in a stoppered vessel. The mixture is slowly heated on a water bath with agitation and the temperature at which all the solute just disappears is noted. The vessel is cooled and the temperature at which the first crystal of the solute reappears is noted. The two temperatures should differ very little, if no supersaturated solution has been produced. The solubility at the mean of these two temperatures can, then, be obtained by analysis.

Solubility of a substance in a solvent depends on the nature of the solute and the solvent, and the interactions involved. A quantitative prediction of solubility of a solute in a solvent can be made and that too after considering polarity, dielectric constant, acid-base reactions and other factors.

In general, polar solvents dissolve polar solutes and non-polar solvents dissolve non-polar solutes. Semipolar solvents such as acetone and alcohol act as intermediate solvents.

Crystalline solids have low solubility. The insoluble nature is due to the stable crystalline arrangement and low intermolecular forces between solvent and solute. Melting point can be considered as a measure of intermolecular forces among solute molecules. Higher the melting point of a solute, the less soluble is the solute in a liquid.

Electrolytes have appreciable solubility and their solubility is largely governed by electrostatic forces of attraction and repulsion. They are easily soluble in a solvent with high dielectric constant. For example water has high dielectric constant and is a good solvent for polar substances (electrolytes).

It may be said that solubility of a solute in a solvent may be predicted by the solute-solute, solvent-solvent, and solute-solvent attractions. When the adhesive forces (attraction between unlike molecules i.e. solute-solvent molecules) are more than the cohesive forces (attraction between like molecules i.e. solute-solute or solvent-solvent molecules), the solubility of a solute in a solvent or the miscibility of a liquid in some other liquid is generally enhanced.

3. Solubility of Gases in Liquids

Solutions of gases in liquids include liquid ammonia and hydrochloric acid (hydrogen chloride gas in water). Effervescent preparations (when added to water) and aerosols may be considered as solutions of gases in liquids. Most of the soft drinks are solutions of gases.

Solubility of a gas in a liquid represents the concentration of dissolved gas in equilibrium with the gas above the solution.

3.1. Factors affecting solubility of gases in liquids

Solubility of a gas in a solvent depends on temperature, pressure, presence of salts, and chemical reaction if any, between the gas and the solvent.

(a) *Effect of pressure*

The effect of pressure on the solubility of a gas in a solvent is given by *Henry's law* which states that in a dilute solution, the mass of a gas which dissolves in a given volume of a liquid at a constant temperature is directly proportional to the partial pressure of the gas. The Henry's law is

$$c = \sigma p \qquad \dots (3)$$

where c = concentration of the dissolved gas in grams per litre of solvent

p = partial pressure in mm of Hg of the undissolved gas above the solution. It is obtained by subtracting the vapour pressure of the solvent from the total pressure of the solution.

σ = proportionality constant and is referred to as the solubility coefficient.

In short, the solubility of gases increases with increase in pressure and on the release of pressure, the solubility decreases and the gas escapes.

Sparingly soluble gases such as oxygen and nitrogen obey Henry's law and gases which are slightly soluble such as carbon-dioxide and chlorine react partially with water and show considerable deviation from Henry's law. Very soluble gases such as hydrogen chloride and ammonia do not obey Henry's law.

Solubility of gases can be expressed by *Bunsen absorption coefficient*. It is the volume of a gas in litres reduced to NTP, dissolved by one litre of a liquid at a fixed temperature and at one atmospheric pressure of the gas.

In a mixture of gases, the solubility of each gas is considered separately and the pressure appearing in the Henry's law is the partial pressure of the gas under consideration. The partial pressure is the pressure of the gas that would be exerted if it occupied the same volume as the mixture of gases.

Total pressure is the sum of partial pressures of each gas.

(b) *Effect of temperature*

The dissolution of a gas in water is normally attended by the liberation of heat (exothermic) and hence the solubility of most gases decreases with rise in temperature. One must be careful when opening the containers containing gaseous solutions under elevated temperatures. It is advisable to reduce the temperature either by immersing in ice or ice-cooled water before opening such containers.

(c) *Effect of electrolytes and non-electrolytes*

Solubility of a gas in a solvent is reduced by the addition of electrolytes such as sodium chloride or non-electrolytes such as sugar. This is referred as *salting out*. This is due to more affinity between the solvent and the electrolytes or non-electrolytes than between the solvent and the gas.

(d) *Effect of chemical reaction*

Chemical reaction if any, between a gas and a solvent will greatly increase the solubility of the gas in the solvent. For example hydrogen chloride gas reacts with water by hydrogen bonding when it dissolves in water. This increases the solubility of hydrogen chloride gas in water. This is about 10,000 times more than the solubility of oxygen in water.

4. Solubility of Liquids in Liquids

Hydroalcoholic solutions (mixture of water and alcohol), aromatic waters (*Peppermint water, Dill water and Chloroform water*), spirits (*Chloroform spirit*), and elixirs (*Piperacine Citrate Elixir*) are some of the examples for liquid in liquid solutions. Lotions, sprays, and medicated oils may contain two or more miscible oils.

4.1. Ideal and Real solutions

The volume of an ideal solution at a given temperature and pressure is equal to the sum of the volumes of its pure components at the same temperature and pressure.

In general, the molecules in ideal solutions assume similar molecular sizes, equal attractive and repulsive forces between like and unlike molecules and there will be no chemical interactions.

Ideal solutions obey *Raoult's law* over the whole range of composition at all temperatures. According to this law at a definite temperature, the partial pressure (P_A) of a component (A) in a liquid mixture is equal to the vapour pressure in the pure state (P_A°) multiplied by the mole fraction of the component (X_A) in the solution. It is expressed as

$$P_A = P_A^\circ X_A \qquad \dots (4)$$

Mixtures of nearly adjacent compounds in a homologous series (eg. benzene-toluene, methanol-ethanol, hexane-heptane etc) at low temperatures behave as ideal solutions.

There may be deviations from Raoult's law. The liquid-liquid mixtures showing deviations are called real (or non-ideal) solutions. The deviations may be negative leading to increased solubility. This may be due to hydrogen bonding between polar components. If the deviation is positive, it leads to decreased solubility and it may result from the association of the molecules of one of the components to form dimers (association of two molecules of the same substance) or polymers of high order. It has been suggested that positive deviation in most cases is due to the difference in the cohesive forces or internal pressures of the molecules of each constituent.

The internal pressure (P_i) in cal/cm^3 is given by

$$P_i = \frac{\Delta H_v - RT}{V} \quad \dots (5)$$

where ΔH_v = heat of vaporisation

R = Gas constant and

V = molar volume of the liquid at temperature T.

4.2. Solutions of liquids in liquids

The solutions of liquids in liquids are of three classes.

1. Liquids that are completely miscible
   e.g. alcohol-water
2. Liquids that are partially miscible
   e.g. phenol-water; ether-water
3. Liquids that are practically immiscible
   e.g. Benzene-water.

4.3. Solubility of completely miscible liquids

These liquids are miscible with each other. e.g. alcohol water, methanol-water etc. The separation of this type of solution is effected by *fractional distillation*. There are three types of solutions in completely miscible liquids.

1. Azeotropic solution with maximum boiling point e.g. Hydrogen chloride-water
2. Azeotropic solution with minimum boiling point e.g. Ethyl alcohol-water
3. Zeotropic solution e.g. Methyl alcohol-water

Azeotropic mixtures (solution): a complete separation (of two miscible liquids) is not possible by fractional distillation.

Zeotropic mixture (solution) - a complete separation (of two miscible liquids) is possible by fractional distillation.

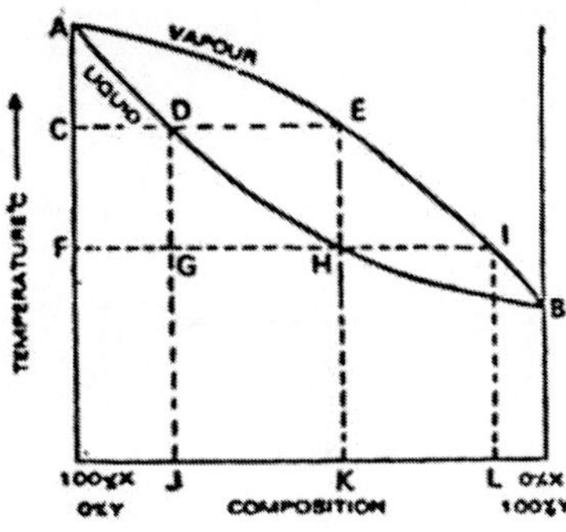

Fig. 89

4.4. Theory of fractional distillation

The curves *AEB* and *ADB* are the temperature composition curves for the vapour and liquid respectively for the completely miscible liquids x and y. (Fig.89) (x with high boiling point and y with low boiling point).

At the boiling temperature 'c' the composition of liquid mixture is represented by J. This liquid mixture forms a vapour in equilibrium with it. The composition of the vapour is given by K. The vapour when condensed will yield the liquid corresponding to point H and this liquid will be richer in more volatile liquid Y. If this liquid is subjected to distillation, it will boil at F. The vapour formed will correspond to the composition at point I which on condensation will yield liquid corresponding to the composition to the point L. In this way by repeating the process of fractional distillation, it is obvious that we can get almost pure Y. This is the principle involved in fractional distillation.

4.5. Phenol-Water system (Solubility of partially miscible liquids)

The above curve represents the miscibility of phenol and water. The left

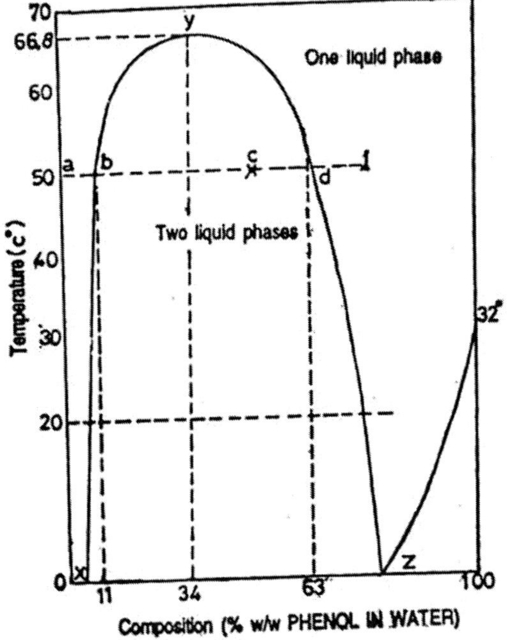

Fig. 90

hand side of the parabolic curve represents one of the two conjugate solutions which represents the percentage of phenol in water. The right hand side of the curve represents the other conjugate solution that gives the % of water in phenol. The two solution curves meet at the maxima on the temperature-composition curve of the system. This point represents a temperature of 66.8° and a composition of 34% phenol in water (*w/v*). Therefore, the temperature at which the two conjugate solutions or layers merge into one another forming a single layer is called critical solution temperature (CST) or upper consolate temperature. Thus at any temperature above the critical solution temperature and outside the curve the phenol-water system exists as single layer. Within the parabolic curve, the phenol-water system exists in two liquid phases (i.e. two conjugate solutions) - one is phenol in water and the other is water in phenol. For example, at 50°C, a mixture of equal proportion of phenol and water will form two layers whose compositions are given by *b* and *d*. The line joining the points *abcd* (at 50°) is called 'tie line'. (The relative amounts of two layers at the point '*c*' is given by *cd/bc*).

The determination if initial solution temperature can be used for testing the purity of phenol and other such substances.

4.5.1. Some examples other than phenol-water system

1. Methanol - Cyclohexane system
2. Hexane - Aniline system
3. Carbon disulphide - Methanol system

4.5.2. Systems showing lower critical solution temperatures

1. Trimethylamine - water system
2. Diethylamine - water system
3. 1 - methyl piperidine - water system

4.5.3. Systems showing both upper and lower critical solution temperature

1. Nicotine - water system
2. glycerin - m. toluidine system
3. β-picoline-water system

4.6. Ternary Systems

Addition of a third liquid to a pair (two components) of partially miscible liquids produce a ternary system. (Fig. 91)

In the Fig. 91 each corner of the triangle represents a 100% of a component *A*, *B* or *C*. The sides of the triangle *AB*, *BC* and *CA* represent a binary mixture (i.e. mixture of two liquids) of *A* and *B* along *AB*, *B* and *C* along *BC*

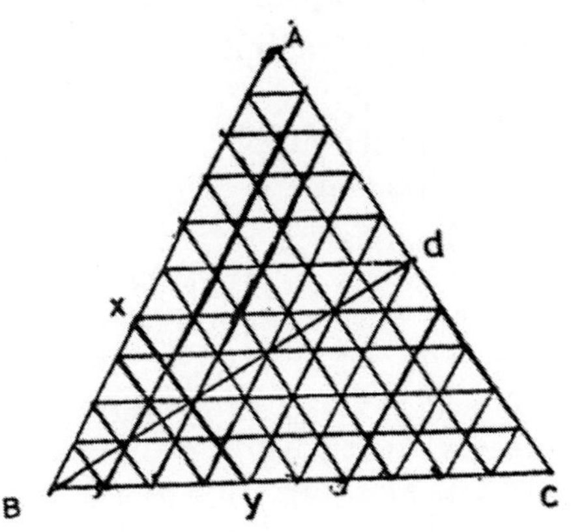

Fig. 91 Ternary System

and C and A along CA. The area within the triangle represents all the possible combinations of A, B and C (a three component system)

Any line drawn from the corner to a point on the opposite side represents a constant ratio of two components and increasing concentration of the other (i.e. the third) component if one moves towards the corner on the line. For example in the figure on the line Bd, A and C will be in a constant ratio and as one proceeds from d to B on the line, the amount of B will be increasing and at B it is 100% of B.

If a line is drawn parallel to one side of the triangle, the proportion of one component will be constant on the line and there will be varying concentrations of the other two components. For example, in the figure, the line xy is parallel to the side AC. Along xy, the proportion of B will be constant and as one moves on the line xy, (from x to y or y to x) there will be varying concentrations of A and C (for more details, refer under phase Equilibria)

In a ternary system, there may exist three possibilities

1 A three component system one pair of which is partially miscible

2. A three component system two pairs of which are partially miscible

3. A three component system, each pair of which is partially miscible i.e. with three pairs of partially miscible liquids.

If the miscibility of the third liquid added to the other two liquids (partially miscible) differs greatly, the mutual miscibility of the partially miscible liquids will be decreased. On the other hand, the mutual miscibility (or solubility) of the other two liquids will be increased if the third added has some solubility (or miscibility) with both the liquids.

Applications

Triangular diagrams are useful in the study and in formulations of solutions containing two immiscible liquids and a mutually soluble liquid. They are also useful in the study of emulsions, solubilised products, in the preparation of microencapsulated products using phase coacervation technique and in cosmetic formulations involving three liquid phases.

5. Solubility of Non Electrolytes in Liquids

It is possible to predict the solubility of a solute forming an ideal solution since it is dependent on temperature, melting point of the solid and molar heat of fusion (ΔH_f). It is difficult to predict the solubility of solids forming non-ideal (real) solutions because of the complicating factors involved.

5.1. Ideal Solution

When the heat of solution is equal to the heat of fusion (i.e. when ΔH is zero), the solution formed is termed as an *ideal solution.* There is no volume change and the solute-solute, solvent-

solvent and solute-solvent interactions are about the same. For such an ideal solution, the solubility can be predicted from its heat of fusion. The equation derived from thermodynamic considerations is

$$-\log X_2^i = \frac{\Delta H_f}{2.303\,R}\left(\frac{T_0 - T}{T_o\,T}\right) \quad \ldots (6)$$

where X_2^i = ideal solubility of the solute expressed in mole fraction (the superscript i indicates ideal)

T_0 = melting point in absolute temperature of the solid solute

T = absolute temperature of the solution.

ΔH_f = molar heat of fusion of the solid state and can be determined using *differential scanning calorimeter*

The equation does not apply when $T > T_0$ and at temperatures considerably below the melting point.

5.2. Non-ideal solution

When the heat of solution has a positive or negative value, the solution is termed as *non-ideal*. This non-ideality is due to various attractive forces involved between solute, solvent and solute-solvent molecules.

The solute-solute interaction may be ion-ion interaction, dipole-dipole interaction or induced dipole-induced dipole interaction.

The attractive forces present in solvents may be dipole-dipole or induced dipole-induced dipole.

The solute-solvent interaction may be any one of the four

1. ion-dipole interaction
2. dipole-dipole interaction
3. dipole induced – dipole interaction or
4. induced dipole – induced dipole interaction.

In dealing with non-ideal solutions, activity of a solute must be considered. The conventional concentration terms do not indicate the physical or chemical activity of the species (i.e. solute molecules). But activity takes into account any intermolecular attraction or repulsion, interaction between solute-solvent in solution, association, and ionisation. It measures the net effectiveness of a chemical species. Thus activity may be considered as a *corrected concentration.*

Activity a_2 is the concentration X_2 multiplied by the *activity coefficient* γ_2. When concentration is expressed in terms of mole fraction, the activity is

$$a_2 = X_2\,\gamma_2 \quad \ldots (7)$$

Converting to logarithms

$$\log a_2 = \log X_2 + \log \gamma_2 \quad \ldots (8)$$

Multiplying by (minus),

$$-\log a_2 = -\log X_2 - \log \gamma_2$$

$$-\log a_2 + \log \gamma_2 = -\log X_2$$

$$-\log X_2 = -\log a_2 + \log \gamma_2 \quad \ldots (9)$$

In an ideal solution $a_2 = X_2^i$ since $\gamma_2 = 1$

Expressing ideal solubility in terms of activity

$$-\log a_2 = -\log X_2^i = \frac{\Delta H_f}{2.303\,R}\left(\frac{T_o - T}{T_o T}\right) \quad \ldots (10)$$

Combining the last two equations, (9) and (10)

$$-\log X_2 = \frac{\Delta H_f}{2.303\,R}\left(\frac{T_o - T}{T_o T}\right) + \log \gamma_2 \quad \ldots (11)$$

The activity coefficient depends on the nature of both the solute and the solvent as well as on the temperature of the solution. All the factors must be considered before the solubility can be predicted for non-ideal solution.

The $\log \gamma_2$ appearing in the equation is obtained from the consideration of intermolecular forces of attraction involved in the solution process or the work done in the process of solution.

The process of solution may be considered to occur in three steps.

1. removal of a molecule from the solute
2. creation of a hole in the solvent to accommodate solute molecule
3. placing of the solute molecule in the hole created in the solvent.

Consider the subscripts $_{22}$, $_{11}$ and $_{12}$ appearing in W_{22}, W_{11} and W_{12} as the energy of interaction between solute-solute molecules, solvent-solvent molecules, and solvent-solute molecules respectively. The work required to free a molecule from two adjacent molecules from the solute is $2W_{22}$. The hole created in this process closes and the work gained is - W_{22}. The net work for the first step becomes $2W_{22} - W_{22} = W_{22}$. (The free molecule is considered to be in vapour state). The work required to create a hole in the solvent to accommodate the solute molecule (second step) is W_{11}. The freed molecule from the solute is now placed in the hole created in the solvent and for this the work gained is $-W_{12}$ and because of this the hole is closed and for this the work gained is $-W_{12}$. Hence, the total work gained for the third step is $(-W_{12}) + (-W_{12}) = -2W_{12}$

The overall work involved in all the three steps is $(W_{22} + W_{11} - 2W_{12})$. The activity coefficient term $\ln \gamma_2$ of solubility appearing in the equation for non-ideal solution is proportional to the total work involved in the three steps and also to the volume of solute (considered as supercooled liquid) and the fraction of total volume occupied by the solvent. (Scatchard and Hildebrand solubility approach) Then, the $\ln \gamma_2$ is given as

$$\ln \gamma_2 = (W_{22} + W_{11} - 2W_{12}) \frac{V_2 \phi_1^2}{RT} \quad \text{... (12)}$$

where V_2 = molar volume of solute (considered as supercooled liquid)

ϕ_1 = volume fraction of the solvent

The term W_{12} can be regarded as approximately equal to the geometric mean of W_{11} and W_{22} since *van der Waals* forces of attraction between molecules follow a geometric mean rule (the term '*W*' actually represents attractive forces) In other words, the interaction between different molecules (i.e. W_{12}) is equal to the square root product of the interaction among similar molecules (i.e. W_{11} and W_{22}),

$$\text{or } W_{12} = \sqrt{W_{11} W_{22}} \quad \text{... (13)}$$

Substituting this in the above equation, we obtain

$$\ln \gamma_2 = (W_{11} - 2\sqrt{W_{11} W_{22}} + W_{22}) \frac{V_2 \phi_1^2}{RT}$$

Since

$(W_{11} - 2\sqrt{W_{11} W_{22}} + W_{22}) = (\sqrt{W_{11}} - \sqrt{W_{22}})^2$, the equation is written as

$$\ln \gamma_2 = (\sqrt{W_{11}} - \sqrt{W_{22}})^2 \frac{V_2 \phi_1^2}{RT} \quad \text{... (14)}$$

where the terms $\sqrt{W_{11}}$ and $\sqrt{W_{22}}$ are known as *solubility parameters*. Replacing $\sqrt{W_{11}}$ and $\sqrt{W_{22}}$ by δ_1 and δ_2 for the solvent and solute respectively and writing the equation in terms of common logarithm, we get

$$\log \gamma_2 = (\delta_1 - \delta_2)^2\ 2.303\ \frac{V_2\,\phi_1^2}{RT} \quad \text{... (15)}$$

Substituting this value for $\log \gamma_2$ in the equation,

$$-\log X_2 = \frac{\Delta H_f}{2.303\,R}\left(\frac{T_0 - T}{T_0 T}\right) + \log \gamma_2 \quad \text{... (16)}$$

we get

$$-\log X_2 = \frac{\Delta H_f}{2.303\,R}\left(\frac{T_0 - T}{T_0\,T}\right) + (\delta_1 - \delta_2)^2 \frac{V_2\,\phi_1^2}{2.303\,RT} \quad \text{... (17)}$$

This gives the mole fraction solubility for non-polar and moderately polar solutes.

The terms δ_1 and δ_2 which represent cohesion between like molecules, may be obtained from heats of vapourisation, internal pressure, surface tension or other properties.

When heat of vapourisation and molar volume for the solute (or solvent) are available, δ value can be obtained. It is the square root of internal pressure. For solvent or solute,

$$\delta = \left(\frac{\Delta H_v - RT}{V_l}\right)^{1/2} \quad \text{... (18)}$$

where ΔH_v = heat of vapourisation with respect to molar volume of the solvent or solute

V_l = molar volume of the liquid compound at the required temperature.

In the case of solid solute, the solute is melted and the liquid volume is obtained and extrapolated to the temperature under consideration.

5.3. Extended Hildebrand solubility approach (EHS approach)

This method is used to calculate the solubility of polar and non-polar solutes in solvents ranging from non-polar hydrocarbons to highly polar solvents such as alcohols, glycols and water. It is applicable to solid in liquid, liquid in liquid and gas in liquid solutions

The equation for solubility of non-ideal solution is

$$-\log X_2 = \frac{\Delta H_f}{2.303R}\left(\frac{T_0 - T}{T_0 T}\right) + \log \gamma_2 \quad \text{... (19)}$$

$$\text{or, } -\log X_2 = -\log X_2^i + \log \gamma_2 \quad \text{... (20)}$$

$$\text{where } -\log X_2^i = \frac{\Delta H_f}{2.303R}\left(\frac{T_0 - T}{T_0 T}\right) \quad \text{... (21)}$$

X_2^i = ideal solubility of the solute expressed in mole fraction

$$\text{i.e. } -\log X_2 = -\log X_2^i + (W_{22} + W_{11} - 2W_{12}) \frac{V_2 \phi_1^2}{RT} \quad \text{... (22)}$$

(refer eqn:)

The solubility equation for EHS approach is

$$-\log X_2 = -\log X_2^i + A(W_{11} + W_{22} - 2W) \quad \text{... (23)}$$

$$\text{where } A = \frac{V_2 \phi_1^2}{2.303RT} \text{ and } W = W_{12} \quad \text{... (24)}$$

In the EHS approach, the term $\log \gamma_2$ is partitioned into two terms γ_v (it represents physical or Van der waals forces) and γ_r (it represents residual forces)

$$\log \gamma_2 = \log \gamma_v + \log \gamma_r \quad \text{... (25)}$$

$$\log \gamma_v = A(\delta_1 - \delta_2)^2 \quad \text{... (26)}$$

$$\log \gamma_r = A(2\delta_1\delta_2 - 2W) \quad ... (27)$$

$$\log \gamma_2 = A(\delta_1^2 + \delta_2^2 - 2\delta_1\delta_2) + A(2\delta_1\delta_2 - 2W)$$

$$= A(\delta_1^2 + \delta_2^2 - 2\delta_1\delta_2 + 2\delta_1\delta_2 - 2W)$$

$$= A(\delta_1^2 + \delta_2^2 - 2W) \quad ... (28)$$

Substituting the value of $\log \gamma_2$ in equation (20) we obtain,

$$-\log X_2^i = -\log X_2^i + A(\delta_1^2 + \delta_2^2 - 2W) \cdots (29)$$

$-\log X_2^i$ may be obtained from a knowledge of ΔH_f, T_0 and T. *Log* γ_2 is btained from a knowledge of drugs leal solubility, X_2^i and its mole fraction solubility, X_2 in a particular solvent sysem.

$$W = \frac{1}{2}\left[\delta_1^2 + \delta_2^2 - \log\left(X_2^i / X_2\right) / A\right]$$

This equation has been applied to polar and non-polar solutes in individual solvents as well as in mixed solvents and it provides an accurate prediction of the mole fraction solubility of a polar drug in binary solvent system.

5.4. Mechanism of solution process

The readers are to refer first in chapter 1 of this book regarding intermolecular forces. A solvent may function in one or more of several ways.

When an ionic salt is dissolved in water, solution process takes place and it involves separation of cations and anions of the salt with orientation of molecules of the solvent around the ions. Such orientation of solvent molecules about the ions of the solute is called solvation (hydration if the solvent is water). It is possible only when the solvent is highly polar, that is dipoles of the solvent are attracted and held by the ions of the solute. The solvent also must possess the ability to solvate the ions of the solute and keep the ions apart with minimal energy and this is due to the dielectric constant of the solvent.

A polar liquid like water may exhibit solvent action also by its ability to break a covalent bond in the solute and bring about ionisation of the latter. For e.g., hydrogen chloride dissolves in water and functions as an acid as a result of the following dissociation

$$\left[HCl + H_2O \rightleftarrows H_3^+O + Cl^- \right]$$

The ions thus formed are maintained in solution by the same mechanism as ionic salts.

The third mechanism of solvent action of polar solvent is by coupling of solvent and solute molecules through hydrogen bond formation. For example, lower molecular weight alcohols are soluble in water due to water-alcohol association complex through hydrogen bonding.

```
  H           R           H       R
  |           |           |       |
H-O - - - H - O - - - H - O - H - O
```

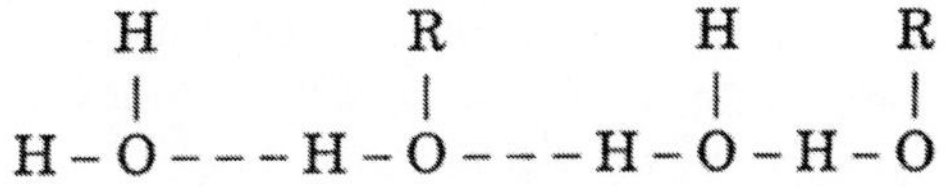

As the molecular weight of the alcohol increases, it becomes progressively less polar and less able to compete with water molecules for a place in the lattice arrangement of water formed through hydrogen bonding

```
[    H           H           H           H ]
[    |           |           |           | ]
[  H-O - - - H - O - - - H - O - - - H - O ]
```

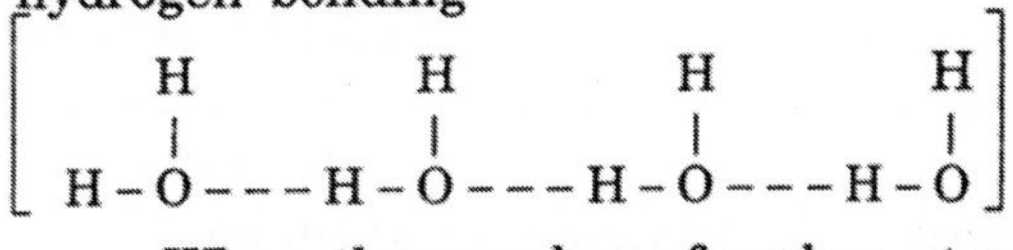

When the number of carbon atom in alcohol reaches five, its solubility in water is reduced materially. When the number of hydroxyl groups in the alcohol is increased, its solubility in water is increased for the above reason that alcohols can get into lattice arrangement of water. eg. sugars, many glycosides and polyethylene glycols are very soluble in water.

Solubility of ethers, aldehydes, ketones, acids, and acid anhydrides in water and in other polar solvents also is due to the formation of an association complex between solute and solvent by means of the hydrogen bonds. These compounds contain a strongly electronegative oxygen atom which is capable of association with water through hydrogen bond formation eg. Acetone dissolves in water freely because of following association

$$(H_3C)_2CO + H_2O \rightarrow (H_3C)_2CO \ldots H-\underset{|}{O}\!-\!H$$

When the number of carbon atom reaches five in these molecules, their solubility in water is reduced materially. In amines, nitrogen is less electro negative (than oxygen) and forms a weaker hydrogen bond and thus amines are as soluble as alcohols containing an equivalent chain length

Solvent action of non-polar liquids involves a different mechanism. They only can dissolve other non-polar substances in which the bonds between molecules are weak. The forces usually involved are of the induced dipole-induced dipole type, eg. Fixed oil or a fat or a hydrocarbon like wax is dissolved in petroleum ether. There are exceptions also. Polar substance like alcohol dissolves in a non-polar liquid like benzene. In this the alcohol molecule induces a temporary dipole in the benzene molecule which forms an association complex with the solvent molecules. This binding force is called a permanent dipole-induced dipole force. Some generalisations may be summarised.

1. The greater the structural similarity between solute and solvent, the greater the solubility eg. Phenol is insoluble in petroleum ether but soluble in glycerin.
2. Organic compounds containing polar groups ($-OH$, $-CHO$, $=CO$, $-CHOH$, $-CH_2OH$, $-COOH$, NO_2, $-NH_2$, and $-SO_3H$) are capable of forming hydrogen bonds with water are soluble in water provided that the molecular weight of the compound is not too great. Non-polar or very weak polar groups such as hydrocarbon radicals reduce the solubility of compounds in water. Similarly the greater the number of carbon atoms in the radical, the greater is the decrease in solubility.
3. Introduction of halogen into an organic compound decreases solubility because of increased molecular weight without a proportional increase in polarity.
4. Between molecules, if the number of carbon atoms are same and the number of polar groups are more, the molecule with more polar groups show more solubility. eg. Pyrogallol is more soluble in water than phenol.
5. Relative position of the polar groups influence solubility in water eg. Resorcinol (*m*-dihydroxy benzene) is more soluble than catechol (*o*-dihydroxy benzene) and the latter is more soluble than hydroquinone (*p*-dihydroxy benzene).
6. Polymers and compounds of high molecular weight which could not form hydrogen bonding with water are generally insoluble.
7. High melting points are indicative of low solubility for organic compounds since cohesive forces between molecules are very high.
8. The *cis* form of an isomer is more soluble than the *trans* form.

9. Solvation, a strong attractive force between solute and solvent enhances the solubility of the solute.
10. Acids, especially strong acids, usually produce water soluble salts when reacted with nitrogen containing organic bases.

6. Thermodynamics of the Solution Process

When a solid (A) dissolves in a solvent, two steps may be involved. The solid absorbs energy (heat) to become liquid and then the liquid dissolves (or mixes) in the solvent.

$$A_{(solid)} \rightleftarrows A_{(liquid)} \rightleftarrows A_{(solution)}$$

Disregarding the first step (i.e. energy needed for melting is disregarded) and assuming the solid as a liquid (a supercooled liquid) going into solution, the process is given as

$$A_{(liquid)} \rightleftarrows A_{(solution)}$$

For the dissolution process to be spontaneous at constant temperature and pressure, the net free energy change should be negative i.e. ΔG should be negative in the equation given

$$\Delta G = \Delta H' - T\Delta S \qquad \text{... (30)}$$

($\Delta H'$ refers to heat involved for the liquid solute to go into solution)

$\Delta H'$ and ΔS determine the free energy change. That is, if ΔG is negative, the reaction is spontaneous and as a result dissolution is favoured.

If heat is the source of energy in effecting solution, a heat-releasing effect and a heat absorbing effect should be considered beyond that required for melting the solid. In the process of solution, it has been already discussed that there are three steps involved in terms of solute-solute molecules, solvent-solvent molecules and solvent-solute molecules interactions. In the absence of solute-solvent interaction, there is only an absorption of heat (heat absorbing effect) to separate solute and solvent molecules to effect solution. If there is significant interaction between solute and solvent molecules (generally exothermic) the quantity of heat in excess of that needed to overcome the solute-solute and solvent-solvent molecular forces is liberated. When these opposing heat effects (i.e. heat releasing effect of solute-solvent interaction and heat-absorbing effect of solvent-solvent interaction and solute-solute interaction) are equal, there will be no change of temperature. That is, when ΔH is zero and there is no change in volume in the solution process, an ideal solution results. (Equation relating ideal solubility has already been discussed).

If $\Delta H'$ (heat of solution) is positive or negative, the solution is a non-ideal one. Solubility is favoured with negative heat of solution while, with a positive heat of solution, it is opposed.

The other term that determines the free energy change (and therefore, spontaneity of a reaction) is ΔS, the entropy change which is a measure of disorderliness or randomness. A physical change or a chemical change (reaction) is favoured if ΔS increases. Though $\Delta H'$ is zero, the entropy change (ΔS) is not zero for an ideal solution.

In a non-ideal solution, $\Delta H'$ is not zero and ΔS can be equal to, greater than, or less than the entropy of mixing found for an ideal solution. A non-ideal solution in which $\Delta H'$ is not zero and the entropy of mixing is equal to that of an ideal solution is termed ***'regular solution'***. Regular solutions are encountered usually with non-polar and weakly polar solutes and solvents.

When there is association among solvent or solute molecules in a non-ideal solution (i.e. $\Delta H'$ is not zero), the entropy change is usually greater than that for an ideal solution. The enthalpy change ($\Delta H'$) in such a solution is positive. Such non-ideal solutions, in general, show more solubility with unsymmetrical molecules than with symmetrical molecules.

The third type of non-ideal solutions shows entropy change that is less than that for an ideal solution. This type of non-ideal solutions can occur with polar solutes and solvents. The enthalpy change is negative favouring dissolution. This dissolution may be opposed by unfavourable entropy change (i.e. less entropy change).

7. Factors affecting Solubility

7.1. *Temperature*

In general temperature increases the solubility of a solid that dissolves with absorption of heat ***(endothermic process).*** The system removes the constraint of higher temperature by increasing its solubility. This tendency is an example of *Le Chatelier's principle.* Most of the solids show this type of solution. Temperature rise decreases the solubility of a solid that dissolves with evolution of heat (exothermic process).

Effect of temperature on the solubility of salts can be shown with the use of solubility curves. (Fig. 92) It may be observed for $Na_2SO_4 \cdot 10H_2O$ (hydrated). The dissolution is endothermic upto a temperature of 32°C and hence there is increase in solubility and thereafterwards (i.e. after transition from hydrated form to unhydrated form - indicated by the break in the curve) the dissolution is exothermic resulting in decrease in solubility with increase in temperature.

There is continuous increase in solubility of potassium nitrate as the temperature is increased (endothermic process) and with calcium acetate there

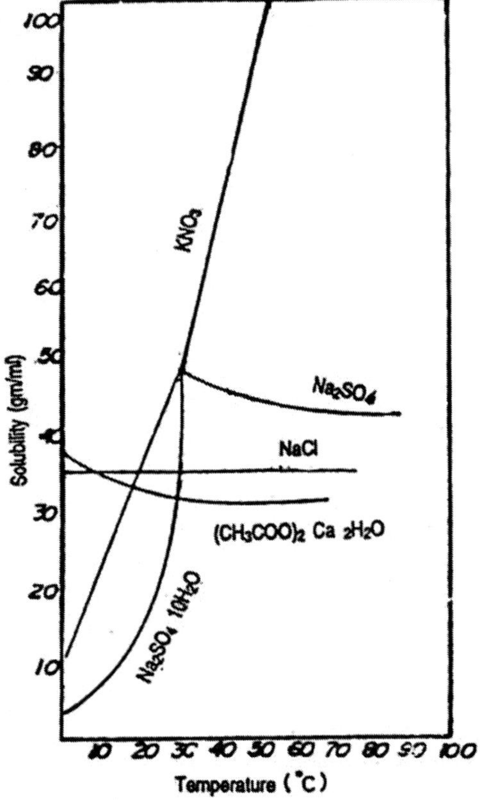

Fig. 92. Effect of heat on solubility

is opposite effect i.e. the solubility decreases (though not appreciably) with increase in temperature *(exothermic process).*

In the case of sodium chloride there is no appreciable amount of heat evolved or absorbed during the dissolution indicating heat of solution is approximately zero.

The equation that relates the solubility, temperature and heat of solution for a solid that goes into solution may be given as

$$A_{(\text{solid})} \rightleftarrows A_{(\text{solution})}$$

$$\log K_s = \frac{-\Delta H}{2.303\,RT} + J \quad \text{... (31)}$$

where J is a constant.

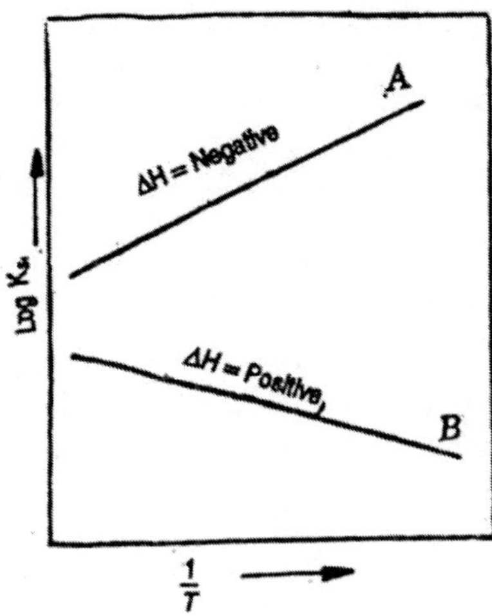

Fig. 93

When heat is absorbed in the solution process, the relation between log of saturation solubility ($\log K_s$) and the reciprocal of the absolute temperature is shown in the Fig. 93 as (*A*). In this case, as the temperature increases $\left(\frac{1}{T}\text{ decreases}\right)$ and the solubility increases (eg. KNO_3) (Fig. 93).

When heat is released (heat of solution is negative) in the solution process, the relation between log K_S and $\frac{1}{T}$ is shown in Fig. 93 as (*B*). In this case a rise in temperature decreases the solubility (eg. calcium acetate).

When heat is neither absorbed nor evolved, solubility remains unchanged with variation in temperature. A close example of this is sodium chloride.

7.2. *Particle size*

The size as well as the surface affects the solubility of solids. Generally solubility increases with decrease in particle size which results in excess surface free energy due to increase in surface area.

The equation relating the size and the solubility is given approximately as

$$\log \frac{S}{S_0} = \frac{2\gamma M}{2.303\, RT\rho r} \quad \text{... (32)}$$

where S = solubility of fine particles

S_0 = solubility of relatively larger particles

γ = surface tension of the particles. (difficult to obtain)

r = radius of the fine particles

M = molecular weight of the solid

ρ = density of the solid

R = gas constant

$= 8.314 \times 10^7$ erg mole^{-1} deg^{-1}

T = absolute temperature

M/ρ may be replaced by V, the molar volume i.e. the volume per mole of particles and the equation becomes

$$\log \frac{S}{S_0} = \frac{2\gamma V}{2.303\, RTr} \quad \text{... (33)}$$

This equation may be used for solid or liquid particles such as those in suspensions or emulsions.

The increase in solubility with decrease in particle size ceases when the particles have a very small radius, and any further decrease in size causes a decrease in solubility. It is due to electrical charges on the particles which become important as the size of the particles decreases.

Also the configuration of a molecule and the kind of arrangement in the crystal has some influence on solubility. Symmetric particles may be less soluble than unsymmetric particles. The molecules of amino acid alpha alanine which pack compactly in the crystal with high lattice energy, show low solubility than the molecules of alpha amino-*n*-butyric acid which pack less efficiently in the crystal with reduced crystal energy.

7.3. *Solvent*

The solubility of a solid depends on the nature of the solvent. There is variation in solubility of a solid in different solvents. In general polar solutes dissolve in polar solvents and non-polar solutes dissolve in non polar solvents (like dissolves like).

Solubility of a solid in a solvent may be affected by the addition of some other solvent which may bring about changes in the properties of the first solvent. Frequently, to increase the solubility of weak electrolyte as well as non-electrolytes a mixture of solvents is used.

The phenomenon of increasing solubility of poorly soluble substances by the use of more than one solvent is known as co-solvency. The co-solvency technique is used in the preparation of elixirs wherein poorly soluble drugs are dissolved in a mixture of water and alcohol.

7.4. *Solubility of weak electrolytes (pH effect)*

Most of the drugs are either weak acids or weak bases which in general are less soluble in water. Their solubility is influenced by pH. They react with bases or acids to form the respective salts which are soluble in water.

Carboxylic acids with more than five carbon atoms are insoluble in water. They form soluble salts with dilute solution of hydroxides, carbonates and bicarbonates. Hydroxy acids such as tartaric acid and citric acid are quite soluble in water. But their alkali metal salts are more soluble. Aromatic acid such as benzoic acid reacts with sodium hydroxide to form the salt, sodium benzoate, which is water soluble.

Many organic compounds such as alkaloids, antihistamines, local anaesthetics, etc. contain basic nitrogen atoms. They form soluble salts with acids. Barbiturates and sulphonamides are weak acids and they form soluble salts with metallic alkali sodium hydroxide.

Adjustment of pH to an optimum value may be necessary to obtain a clear homogeneous solution of drug substances with maximum therapeutic effectiveness.

The salt of a weak acid (weak electrolyte) such as sodium sulphacetamide or sodium phenobarbitone may precipitate from aqueous solution below a certain pH. The pH below which precipitation occurs may be obtained as follows.

Consider the free acid form of a drug as HD and the soluble ionised form as D^-. The equation representing the saturated solution of this slightly soluble weak acid is

$$HD_{(solid)} \rightleftarrows HD_{(solution)}$$

$$HD_{(solution)} + H_2O \rightleftarrows H_3O^+ + D^-$$

The equilibrium constant for the solution equilibrium is given as follows since the concentration of the un-ionized form in solution $[HD]_{solution}$ remains almost constant.

$$K_a = \frac{\left[H_3O^+\right]\left[D^-\right]}{[HD]} \quad \text{... (34)}$$

$$\text{or } [D^-] = K_a \frac{[HD]}{[H_3O^+]} \quad \text{... (35)}$$

The total solubility S of the drug may be given as

$$S = [H\,D] + [D^-] \quad \text{... (36)}$$

(i.e. the solubility of unionized and ionized drug)

Representing the solubility of unionized drug [HD] by S_o. The expression becomes

$$S = S_o + K_a \frac{S_o}{[H_3O^+]} \quad \text{... (37)}$$

$$\text{or } S - S_o = K_a \frac{S_o}{[H_3O^+]} \quad \text{... (38)}$$

Writing in logarithmic form

$$\log (S - S_o) = \log Ka + \log S_o - \log [H_3O^+] \quad \text{... (39)}$$

$$\text{or } \log (S - S_o) - \log Ka - \log S_o = - \log [H_3O^+] \quad \text{... (40)}$$

$$pH_D = pK_a + \log \frac{S - S_o}{S_o}$$

where $- \log [H_3O^+] = pH_D$

$- \log K_a = pK_a$

where pH_D is the pH below which the drug precipitates from solution as the undissociated acid.

7.5. *Combined effect of Solvent and pH*

The combined effect of solvent and pH can be studied by determining the solubility of a weak electrolyte in a buffered solution. The addition of a solvent such as alcohol (co-solvent effect) to a buffered aqueous solution may affect the solubility of weak electrolytes in two ways

1. may increase the solubility of the unionized molecule of the weak electrolyte by adjusting the polarity of the solvent to a more favourable value or
2. may decrease the dissociation of the weak electrolyte (i.e. pK_a increases) reducing the solubility.

7.6. *Solubility of slightly soluble electrolyte*

For a saturated solution of sparingly soluble electrolyte AB in contact with the undissolved electrolyte, the equilibrium may be represented as follows

$$\underset{\text{undissolved solid}}{AB_{(s)}} \rightleftarrows \underset{\text{dissolved undissociated (molecules)}}{AB} \rightleftarrows \underset{\text{dissolved dissociated (ions)}}{A^+ + B^-}$$

Species in solution

The overall equilibrium is

$$AB_{(solution)} \rightleftarrows A^+ + B^-$$

According to Law of Mass action, the equilibrium constant in terms of concentration is

$$K = \frac{[A^+]\,[B^-]}{[AB]}$$

where $[AB]$ indicates $[AB]_{(solution)}$

Since $[AB]_{(solution)}$ remains constant, the equation may be written as

$$K_{sp} = [A^+]\,[B^-]$$

where K_{sp} = ***solubility product*** of the compound AB

(a) *Effect of common-ion*

If a compound that carries a common ion. (for example B^-) is added to the above system, there is a momentary increase in the ionic product as shown

$$[A^+]\,[B^-] > K_{SP}$$

In order to reestablish the equilibrium $[A^+]\,[B^-] = K_{SP}$ some of AB will precipitate out. The same will be the effect if a compound containing the ion $[A^+]$ is added. Thus, the addition of a compound bearing a common ion reduces the solubility of sparingly soluble salt.

Therefore, the solubility of a sparingly soluble salt is decreased by the addition of a second salt that carries a similar ion to that of the first. This is known as ***common-ion effect***.

(b) *Effect of indifferent electrolyte*

An opposite effect to that of common-ion will be produced if salts carrying no common-ion (*indifferent electrolytes*) is added to a solution of slightly soluble electrolyte. Such indifferent electrolytes even increase the solubility at moderate concentrations as they tend to lower the activity coefficient.

The solubility product of a sparingly soluble salt (*AB*) in terms of the concentration of ions produced at equilibrium is

$$K_{sp} = [A^+]\,[B^-]$$

It is only an approximation and from the more exact thermodynamic relationship

$$K_{sp} = a_{A^+} \cdot a_B \qquad \text{... (41)}$$

where a_{A^+} and a_{B^-} are the activities of the respective ions A^+ and B^-

Replacing the activity by the product of concentration and activity coefficients (γ)

$$K_{sp} = [A^+]\,[B^-]\,\gamma_A \cdot \gamma_{B^-} \qquad \text{... (42)}$$

$$= [A^+]\,[B^-]\,\gamma_\pm^2$$

$$\text{or } \frac{K_{sp}}{\gamma_\pm^2} = [A^+]\,[B^-]$$

$$\text{Solubility} = [A^+] = [B^-] = \frac{\sqrt{K_{sp}}}{\gamma_\pm} \qquad \text{... (43)}$$

The solubility of slightly (or sparingly) soluble salts can be increased by preventing the precipitation and it can be carried out by tying up or by reducing the concentration of one of the ions by adding indifferent electrolytes. For example, solubility of iron compounds can be increased by citrates or with similar compounds (In this case, complex is formed with one of the ions and not with the compound).

In accordance with solubility product principle, addition of soluble iodide (KI) should decrease the solubility of mercuric iodide (HgI). Instead the solubility is increased due to the formation of more soluble complex salt K_2HgI_4. In this case iodide ion (I^-) does not function as a common-ion.

7.7. *Effect of non-electrolytes on the solubility of electrolytes*

Electrolytes dissolve in water because of dissociation of the dissolved molecules. This dissociation is influenced by the dielectric constant of the solvent (i.e. polar solutes dissolve in polar solvents).

The solubility of sparingly soluble salt in water is decreased if a water soluble non-electrolyte such as alcohol is added to the aqueous solution. This effect is due to the lowering of dielectric constant and this in turn reduces the dissociation of the dissolved salt. Though there is lowering of dielectric constant, the effect is more due to competition for water molecules. This competition depends on the affinity. Alcohol has more affinity than the sparingly soluble salt and hence it dislodges the sparingly soluble salt resulting in precipitation.

7.8. *Effect of electrolytes on the solubility of non-electrolytes*

The solubility of non-electrolytes depends on the weak intermolecular bonds (hydrogen bonds) formed with water molecules. Any attempt that reduces this intermolecular forces will decrease the solubility of non-electrolytes. Thus, when an electrolyte (which is having more affinity towards water) is added to a solution of non-electrolyte in water, the solubility of non-electrolyte is decreased. This effect is taken advantage of in the precipitation of proteins.

7.9. *Effect of complex forming substances*

The apparent solubility of some solutes in a liquid may be increased or decreased by the addition of a substance that forms a complex which is more or less soluble.

Iodine is very slightly soluble in water (0.03%). But iodine is more soluble in a concentrated solution of potassium iodide because iodine forms a complex with potassium iodide (i.e. polyiodide)

The apparent water solubility of 3-amino-benzoic acid has been shown to increase by the addition of dicarboxylic acids due to the formation of complexes between them. Caffeine forms complexes with organic acids and the complex is more soluble than the caffeine itself. This technique of enhancing the solubility of drugs is not popular especially when intended for internal use.

It is also possible that a drug may form an insoluble complex with other ingredients. For example, gentisic acid forms a complex with caffeine that is less soluble than caffeine alone. Tetracycline forms an insoluble complex with calcium ions present in milk or any preparation containing calcium salts.

Liquid pharmaceutical preparations which are multicomponent systems consist of more than a single drug in solution. These several drugs together with pharmaceutical adjuncts may interact in solution and form complexes which may be less soluble than the simple solubility of drug/adjuncts alone in a solvent. Hence simple solubility profiles of individual drugs/adjuncts cannot be used to predict solubilities of ingredients. Hence each multicomponent system must be separately studied for the complicating effects drugs/adjuncts interactions.

7.10. *Effect of surfactants*

Solubility of weak acidic and basic drugs may be enhanced by the technique *micellar solubilisation*. Solubilising action of surfactants involves this micellar solubilisation. These surfactants (normally non-ionic surfactants) form micelles above their CMC and bring about solubilisation.

Effect of surfactants on the solubility of drugs can be considered in quantitative terms. When a weakly acidic drug is dissolved in aqueous solution of a non-ionic surfactant, the total solubility (D_T) may be given as

$$D_T = D_S + D_S^- + D_M + D_M^-$$

where D_S and D_S^- represent concentrations of the unionized and the ionized forms of the drug in the aqueous solution outside the micelles and D_M and D_M^- represent concentrations of the unionized and ionized drug within the micelles.

Taking into account the partitioning of the drug in the ionised and unionised forms in between the interior of the micelle and the aqueous solution outside the micelle quantitatively and also the total amount of drug present in the ionised and unionised forms in the aqueous solution in the absence of surfactant *Rippie et al.* obtained the following expression

$$\frac{D_T}{D_{T*}} = 1 + (M)\left[\frac{[H^+]\,K' + K_a K''}{K_a + [H^+]}\right] \quad \dots (44)$$

where D_T = total solubility of the drug as given by $D_S + D_S^- + D_M + D_M^-$

(M) = volume fraction of surfactant as micelles in solution

$[H^+]$ = hydrogen ion concentration at a definite pH

K' = partition coefficient for the unionised drug between the aqueous solution and the micelle

K'' = partition coefficient for the ionised drug between the aqueous solution and the interior of the micelle

K_a = dissociation constant of the drug

D_{T^*} = total drug solubility in the solution in the absence of surfactant at a definite pH.

Similarly for a weaker base (such as procaine)

$$\frac{D_T}{D_{T^*}} = 1 + (M)\left[\frac{K_a K' + [H^+]\,K''}{K_a + [H^+]}\right] \quad \text{... (45)}$$

where K_a is the dissociation constant of the D^+ which is the cationic acid of the drug.

The above equations 1 and 2 may be used to calculate the total drug solubility in a solution of definite pH and having a volume fraction (M) of surfactant (such as polysorbate 20) present in the form of micelles for a weakly acidic drug such as phenobarbitone and a weakly basic drug such as procaine respectively.

[***Note:*** Solubilisation, in general, may be defined as the spontaneous passage of poorly soluble molecules into an aqueous solution promoted by a suitable technique other than temperature and the solution is thermodynamically stable.]

The solubilisation of poorly soluble drugs may be brought about by

(a) using micelles of a surfactant (*micellar solubilisation*)

(b) using a complexing agent of the solute (eg. solubilisation of iodine in water by using the complexing agent KI.)

(c) using a cosolvent of water like alcohol, glycerin etc. (*cosolvency*) Eg. Elixirs.

(d) using a chemical modification of drugs to form water-soluble derivatives, eg. Phenobarbitone to phenobarbitone sodium, atropine to atropine sulphate, etc.

(e) using larger amounts of additives. It is called *hydrotropy*, eg. using large concentrations of sodium benzoate on the solubility of caffeine. The mechanism is complicated and it may involve complexation, cosolvency, oriented clusters of hydrotrophic agent, etc.

Thus *solubilisation* involves not only the solute and the solvent but also some other additive or agent whereas the *solution* involves only the solute and the solvent.

8. Buffer solutions

A buffer solution is one which resist a change of pH on addition of an acid or alkali or, on dilution with a solvent. The pH of pure water is 7 and the water has no buffer action. Hence, when it is exposed to atmosphere, the water may absorb or dissolve carbon-dioxide present in air and get equilibrated with the carbon dioxide in air. As a result, there is a sharp change in pH of the water from 7 to 5.7. Solutions of neutral salts also lack ability to resist pH change on the addition of small amounts of acid or alkali.

A buffer solution contains a weak acid and its salt (e.g. acetic acid and sodium acetate) or a weak base and its salt (e.g. ammonium hydroxide and ammonium chloride). Apart from this two general types of buffers, a third type comprises two salts. (e.g. monobasic potassium phosphate and dibasic potassium phosphate)

8.1. Buffer action

Buffer solutions undergo only small changes of pH on the addition of small amounts of acid or basé. For example, if 1 ml of 0.01 M hydrochloric acid is added to 1 litre of pure water, the pH is reduced to 5.0 from 7.0. On the other hand, if the acid is added to 0.01 M buffer solution containing equal quantities of acetic acid and sodium acetate in water the pH change is only by 0.09 units. From this, it is clear that a buffer solution resists change of pH upon the addition of small quantities of acid or alkali.

8.2. Mechanism of buffer action

If a small quantity of 0.1N HCl is added to the buffer solution, the base ties up the hydrogen ions released by HCl.

$$(HCl + H_2O \rightleftharpoons H_3O^+ + Cl^-)$$

$$CH_3COO^- + H_3O^+ \rightleftharpoons CH_3COOH + H_2O$$

If an alkali (NaOH) is added to the buffer solution, the free acid of the buffer solution neutralises the base added

$$CH_3COOH + NaOH \rightarrow CH_3COONa + H_2O$$

Thus, the change in pH is resisted by the addition of small quantities of strong acid.

The buffer action of a weak base and its conjugate acid (ammonia - ammonium chloride pair) may be explained as follows.

If an acid is added, the ammonia combines with the hydronium ion produced by the reaction of HCl with H_2O.

$$\text{i.e. } HCl + H_2O \rightleftharpoons H_3O^+ + Cl_-$$

$$NH_3 + H_3O^+ \longrightarrow NH_4^+ + H_2O$$

If an alkali (NaOH) is added, it combines with the NH_4^+ ion produced by the dissociation of NH_4Cl (i.e. $NH_4Cl \rightarrow NH_4^+ + Cl^-$). The ammonium ion being an acid combines with the alkali which dissociates into Na^+ and OH^-

$$NH_4^+ + OH^- \longrightarrow NH_3 + H_2O.$$

Thus the change in pH is resisted.

In addition to these general types, a third type comprises two salts such as monobasic potassium phosphate KH_2PO_4 and dibasic potassium phosphate K_2HPO_4. This is actually a weak-acid-conjugate- base buffer. In this $H_2PO^{4^-}$ serves as the weak acid and HPO_4^{-2} as its conjugate base.

When hydroxyl ion (an alkali) is added H_2PO_4 reacts with OH^- ion

$$H_2PO_4^- + OH^- \longrightarrow HPO_4^{2-} + H_2O.$$

When a hydronium ion (an acid) is added HPO_4^{2-} reacts with H_3O^+

$$HPO_4^{2-} + H_3O^+ \longrightarrow H_2PO_4^- + H_2O.$$

Thus, the mechanism of buffer action is just the same as for acetic acid and sodium acetate.

8.3. Buffer equation

Buffer equation may be obtained by considering the effect of sodium acetate on the ionisation of acetic acid (the salt and the acid have an ion common with them i.e. acetate ion, CH_3COO^-)

The dissociation constant for the acid is given as

$$CH_3COOH \rightleftharpoons CH_3COO^- + H_3O^+$$

$$Ka = \frac{[CH_3COO^-]\,[H_3O^+]}{[CH_3COOH]} = 1.75 \times 10^{-5} \quad [0.0000175]$$

If sodium acetate is added to the acetic acid solution, it ionises to produce acetate ions ($CH_3COONa \rightleftharpoons CH_3COO^- + Na^+$) and it results in the increase in the concentration of CH_3COO^- momentarily. To re-establish the constant $Ka = 1.75 \times 10^{-5}$, the hydrogen ion term in the numerator is instantaneously decreased. This results in the increase of concentration of CH_3COOH in the denominator i.e. the reaction $H_3O^+ + CH_3COO^- \rightarrow CH_3COOH + H_2O$ is favoured. Thus the constant K_a remains unaltered.

The pH of the final solution (i.e. the buffer solution) is obtained from the above equation.

By rearrangement

$$[H_3O^+] = K_a \frac{[CH_3COOH]}{[CH_3COO^-]}$$

Since CH_3COOH ionises only slightly (i.e. to an extent of 0.0000175 mole / liter), the concentration of CH_3COOH may be considered to represent the total concentration of acid in the solution and can be replaced by [acid]. The acetate ion (CH_3COO^-) is contributed entirely by sodium acetate as the contribution by the acid is negligible, Therefore $[CH_3COO^-]$ may be replaced by [salt]

$$\text{Therefore } [H_3O^+] = K_a \frac{[\text{acid}]}{[\text{salt}]}$$

Expressing in logarithmic form,

$$\log [H_3O^+] = \log K_a + \log [\text{acid}] - \log [\text{salt}]$$

Reversing the sign

$$-\log [H_3O^+] = -\log K_a - \log [\text{acid}] + \log [\text{salt}]$$

$$\text{or } pH = pK_a + \log \frac{[\text{salt}]}{[\text{acid}]}$$

This is known as **Henderson-Hasselbalch** equation for a weak acid and its salt.

Buffer equation for a weak base and its salt may be obtained as follows

$$[OH^-] = K_b \frac{[\text{base}]}{[\text{salt}]}$$

$$\text{or } \frac{K_w}{[H_3O^+]} = K_b \frac{[\text{base}]}{[\text{salt}]}$$

$$\left(\text{Since } K_w = H_3O^+ \times OH^- \text{ or, } OH^- = \frac{K_w}{H_3O^+}\right)$$

where K_w = ionic product of water

Expressing in logarithmic terms,

$$\log K_w - \log [H_3O^+] = \log K_b + \log [\text{base}] - \log [\text{salt}]$$

$$\text{or, } -\log [H_3O^+] = -\log K_w + \log K_b + \log [\text{base}] - \log [\text{salt}]$$

$$= pH - pK_w - pK_b + \log \frac{[\text{base}]}{[\text{salts}]}$$

In fact, there will be some difference in the pH of the solutions, since the *activity coefficient* of the components varies with concentrations. Taking into account the *activity coefficients*, the Henderson-Hasselbalch equation for a weak acid and its conjugate base may be give as

$$\text{pH} = pK_a + \log \frac{[\text{salt}]}{[\text{acid}]} + \log \gamma_{Ac^-}$$

Where γ_{Ac^-} indicates the activity coefficient of the acetate (CH_3COO^-) ion.

However, for most practical purposes Henderson-Hasselbalch equation is satisfactory.

Example:

What is the pH of a buffer solution prepared by mixing 10 ml of N/100 acetic acid $pK_a = 4.76$ with 20 ml of N/10 sodium acetate?

Total volume

$= 30$ ml (i.e. $10 + 20$)

The salt concentration [salt]

$$= \frac{20}{30} \times \frac{1}{10} \text{ g equiv/litre}$$

$$= \frac{2}{30} \text{ g equiv/litre}$$

The acid concentration [acid]

$$= \frac{10}{30} \times \frac{1}{100} \text{ g equiv/litre}$$

$$= \frac{1}{300} \text{ g equiv/litre}$$

$$\text{pH} = pK_a + \log \frac{[\text{salt}]}{[\text{acid}]}$$

$$= 4.76 + \log \frac{2/30}{1/300}$$

$$= 4.76 + \log \frac{600}{30}$$

$$= 4.76 + \log 20$$

$$= 4.76 + 1.30$$

$$= \mathbf{6.06}$$

What is the molar ratio [salt]/[acid] required to prepare an acetate buffer of pH 5.5. Express the concentration in mole percent ($pK_a = 4.76$)?

$$\text{pH} = pK_a + \log \frac{[\text{salt}]}{[\text{acid}]}$$

$$\text{i.e. } 5.5 = 4.76 + \log \frac{[\text{salt}]}{[\text{acid}]}$$

$$\text{or, } \log \frac{[\text{salt}]}{[\text{acid}]} = 5.5 - 4.76 = 0.74$$

$$\frac{[\text{salt}]}{[\text{acid}]} = \text{anti log of } 0.74$$

$$= 5.494 \text{ or } 5.5$$

The mole ratio of salt to acid is $\frac{5.5}{1} = 5.5$

Mole percent = mole fraction × 100

Mole fraction of salt

$$= \frac{5.5}{1 + 5.5} = \frac{5.5}{6.5} = 0.846 \text{ or } 0.85$$

Mole fraction of acid

$$= \frac{1}{1 + 5.5} = \frac{1}{6.5} = 0.15$$

$$\text{Mole \% of salt} = \frac{5.5}{6.5} \times 100 = 85\%$$

$$\text{Mole \% of acid} = \frac{1}{6.5} \times 100 = 15\%$$

Thus the Henderson - Hasselbalch equation can be used for calculating the ratio of molar concentrations of acid and its salt in a buffer solution to produce a solution of required pH after rearranging the equation to

$$\log \frac{[\text{base}]}{[\text{salt}]} = pH - pK_a$$

Different proportion of salt to acid (weak acid) will have different pH. However, if the proportion is maintained the pH remains the same irrespective of concentrations of acid and salt used. Consider the following sodium acetate and acetic acid buffer system in different concentrations but with same proportion.

Sodium acetate : Acetic acid (in moles/litre)	pH
0.575 : 1.0	4.5
0.0575 : 0.1	4.5
0.00575 : 0.01	4.5

It may be understood that the same proportion of salt to acid has the same pH. However increase in concentration has a greater buffer capacity. Thus, the actual concentration needed to maintain a certain pH in a pharmaceutical liquid preparation would depend chiefly on the desired buffer capacity which is discussed later in this chapter.

8.4. Factors influencing the pH of buffer solutions

pH of buffer solutions may be affected by

1. alteration of ionic strength by the addition of neutral salts.
2. dilution with moderate amounts of water.
3. with rise in temperature, the pH of acetate buffers rises whereas that of borate buffers decreases. The temperature effect is more with basic buffers due to K_w than with acidic buffers.

8.5. Determination of pH

pH determination may conveniently be carried out with a pH meter. This may also be undertaken with the use of pH indicators. Indicator method is only an approximate one. A pH indicator may be considered as a weak acid or weak base that acts like buffers. It exhibits different colours at different pH value. Colour change is exhibited when the degree of dissociation of an indicator varies.

Universal indicator is a mixture of several indicators to cover a wide range of pH. For example a mixture of methyl red, methyl yellow, bromothymol blue, thymol blue and phenolphthalein covers the range pH 1 to 11.

8.6. Pharmaceutical significance of pH

pH has an important role in the preparation of pharmaceutical products and also in ensuring the action of certain drugs with respect to solubility, stability, activity and absorption.

(a) Solubility

For drugs which are weak acids or bases, the solubility depends on pH. When a salt of weak acid such as the sodium salt of the weak acid is dissolved in water, it will dissociate into free acid ion and sodium ion. If the pH of the solution is lowered it will begin to precipitate from the solution when the conjugate acid formed exceeds its solubility in the solvent.

Consider the following reactions which occur when a salt of weak acidic drug (NaD) is dissolved in water

$$\text{Na}D \longrightarrow \text{Na}^+ + D^-$$

$$\text{D}^- + \text{H}_2\text{O} \longrightarrow \text{HD} + \text{OH}^-$$

HD = conjugate acid formed with water

Then, the pH below which precipitation of the acid (*HD*) occurs may be given as

$$\text{pH}_{(\text{p})} = \text{pK}_\text{a} + \log \frac{\text{C}_\text{S} - \text{S}_0}{\text{S}_0}$$

where $\text{pH}_{(\text{p})}$ = pH below which precipitation occurs

K_a = ionisation constant for the conjugate acid, *HD*

C_S = aqueous solubility of *HD* and D^- i.e. total amount of drug in solution (unionised + ionised)

S_0 = aqueous solubility of *HD* (i.e. of unionised drug)

The analogous equation for salts of weak bases and strong acids can be given as $\text{pH}_{(\text{p})} = pK_a + \log \dfrac{S_0}{C_S - S_0}$

Where pK_a = dissociation constant of the protonated form of weak base.

(b) *Drug stability*

Drug instability is due to the conversion of the drug into unwanted substances. This conversion of the drug into unwanted substance may be due to the catalytic effect of acids or bases i.e. due to hydrogen-ion concentration. Maintaining the pH within optimum range increases the solubility of certain pharmaceutical products. For example decomposition of morphine solution is negligible when exposed to a temperature of 100°C even for an hour if the pH is below 5.5. Whereas neutral and alkaline solutions decompose extensively. The stability of many disperse systems such as emulsions is often pH dependent.

(c) *Drug activity*

Some drugs need an optimum pH range for maximum activity. For example, benzoic or salicylic acid remain unionised in an acid environment. Thus unionised form has pronounced antibacterial activity whereas the ionised form at alkaline pH has practically no such activity. The activity of acridines and quaternary ammonium compounds is also affected by pH.

(d) *Drug absorption*

The rate of absorption of drugs from G.I. tract is affected by the degree of dissociation which is influenced by pH and lipid solubility. Drugs which are weak organic acids remain unionised in acidic pH of the stomach and are absorbed better. The degree of acidic or basic character and the pH of the physiological medium (G.I fluid – acidic pH; intestinal fluid – alkaline pH) influence the drug absorption. Usually the non-ionised form is soluble in lipids and is well absorbed through cellular membranes which are lipoidal in nature.

In general, weakly acidic drugs are better absorbed in stomach (acidic pH) and weakly basic drugs are better absorbed from intestine (alkaline pH).

8.7. Buffer capacity

Resistance to changes in pH on the addition of an acid or alkali is referred to as buffer action. The magnitude of the resistance of a buffer solution to pH change is called its *buffer capacity*. The buffer capacity may otherwise be called as *buffer coefficient*, *buffer index*, or *buffer value* and is given by

$$\beta = \frac{\Delta B}{\Delta pH}$$

where β = buffer capacity

ΔB = small increment in gram equivalent per liter of strong base added to the buffer solution, to produce a pH change (i.e. ΔpH)

Buffer capacity of a buffer solution is 1 when 1 g equivalent of strong base (or acid) is added to 1 liter of the buffer solution it brings in a change of 1 pH unit.

Van Slyke, the biochemist introduced a more exact equation for buffer capacity and is given by

$$\beta = 2.3C \frac{K_a\,[H_3O^+]}{(K_a + [H_3O^+])^2}$$

where C = total buffer concentration (i.e. sum of the molar concentrations of the acid and the salt)

This equation may be used to calculate the buffer capacity at any hydrogen ion concentration.

Buffer capacity is at maximum when there is equal concentration of acid and its salt. This is realised when $pH = pK_a$. Consider an acetate buffer containing 0.1 mole each of acetic acid and sodium acetate in 1 liter of solution. The pK_a value of this solution at 25°C is 4.76. From Henderson equation, the pH is

$$pH = pK_a + \log \frac{[salt]}{[acid]}$$

$$pH = 4.76 + \log \frac{[0.1]}{[0.1]} = 4.76.$$

Maximum buffer capacity may be derived from the buffer capacity formula of *Van Slyke* when $pH = pK_a$ i.e. when $H_3O^+ = K_a$. Substituting $[H_3O^+]$ for K_a the *Van Slyke* equation becomes

$$\beta_{max} = 2.3C \frac{[H_3O^+]^2}{([H_3O^+] + [H_3O^+])^2}$$

$$= 2.3C \frac{[H_3O^+]^2}{(2[H_3O])^2} = 2.3C \frac{[H_3O^+]^2}{4[H_3O^+]^2}$$

$$= 2.3C \cdot \frac{1}{4}$$

$$\beta_{max} = 0.576C.$$

where C = total buffer concentration (i.e. [salt] + [acid])

For example the maximum buffer capacity of an acetate buffer with a total concentration of 0.040 mole/1 litre is $0.576 \times 0.040 = 0.023$

Addition of a base to a buffer solution containing an acid and its salt produces a change in concentration of the salt and acid. This may be given by a modified equation:

$$pH = pK_a + \log \frac{[salt] + [base]}{[acid] - [base]}$$

Buffer capacity decreases with the addition of increased concentrations of a base. This may be understood by considering the following example.

Consider the acetate buffer containing 0.1 mole each of acetic acid and sodium acetate in 1 liter of solution. Before the addition of any base the pH is given (pK_a of acetic acid = 4.76) as

$$pH = pK_a + \log \frac{[salt] + [base]}{[acid] - [base]}$$

$$= 4.76 + \log \frac{(0.1 + 0)}{(0.1 - 0)} = 4.76$$

To the above system if 0.01 mole of sodium hydroxide is added, the pH of the buffer solution is given as,

$$pH = 4.76 + \log \frac{(0.1 + 0.01)}{(0.1 + 0.01)} = 4.85$$

Then the change in pH

$$= 4.85 - 4.76 = 0.09$$

Then the buffer capacity

$$= \frac{\Delta B}{\Delta pH} = \frac{0.01}{0.09} = 0.11$$

If 0.06 mole of sodium hydroxide is added, the pH of the buffer solution is given as

$$pH = 4.76 + \log \frac{(0.1 + 0.06)}{(0.1 - 0.06)} = 5.36$$

The change in pH (i.e. ΔpH) is $5.36 - 4.76 = 0.60$ units

$$\text{Then, } \beta = \frac{\Delta B}{\Delta pH} = \frac{0.06}{0.60} = 0.10$$

From the above consideration, it may be seen that with the addition of more sodium hydroxide, the buffer capacity decreases. This occurs because of reduction in acid reserve.

The buffer capacity increases with an increase in the total concentration of the buffer constituents. For example if 0.01 mole of base is added to the above acetate buffer system

$$pH = 4.76 + \log \frac{(0.1 + 0.01)}{(0.1 - 0.01)} = 4.85$$

If the same 0.01 mole of base is added to the buffer system after raising the concentration to 1.0 molar, the pH change is

$$pH = 4.76 + \log \frac{(1.0 + 0.01)}{(1.0 - 0.01)} = 4.77.$$

Thus if the concentration of buffer solution is 0.1 molar, the addition of 0.01 mole of the base produces a pH 4.85 whereas to a concentration of 1.0 molar, addition of 0.01 mole of the same base produces a pH 4.77. The decrease in pH from 4.85 to 4.77 indicates increase in buffer capacity.

The same may be understood by considering *Van Slyke* equation $\beta_{max} = 0.576C$) for maximum buffer capacity. When C is increased, buffer capacity increases and with a decrease in C, the buffer capacity decreases.

Relatively concentrated solution of strong acids and bases also have the ability to resist a change in pH on the addition of an acid or alkali.

The buffer capacity of solution of a strong acid is directly proportional to the hydrogen ion concentration

$$\beta = 2.303\ [H_3O^+]$$

The buffer capacity of a solution of a strong base is

$$\beta = 2.303\ [OH^-]$$

The total buffer capacity is the sum of the separate capacities

$$\beta = 2.303\ ([H_3O^+ + [OH^-])$$

8.8 Biologic Buffers

Blood pH is maintained at about 7.4 by the buffers present in plasma as well as by the buffers in the erythrocytes. The plasma contain carbonic acid / bicarbonate and acid / alkali sodium salts of phosphoric acid as buffers. In the erythrocytes, the buffers are haemoglobin / oxyhaemoglobin and acid / alkali potassium salts of phosphoric acid. The total buffer capacity is 0.028 gram equivalents per litre/pH unit. The physiological pH range of blood is 7.0 to 7.8. When the pH of the blood goes below 6.9 or above 7.8, the life is said to be in danger.

The pH of tear solution is about 7.4 with a range of 7.0 to 8.0.

8.9. Pharmaceutical buffers

Usually for the preparation of buffer solutions, weak bases and their salts are not used since many bases are volatile and their solutions have high temperature coefficients

Some pharmaceutical buffers are

1. HCl and KCl — pH 1.2 to 2.2
2. HCl and potassium hydrogen phthalate — pH 2.2 to 5.0
3. NaOH and potassium hydrogen phthalate — pH 4.2 to 5.8
4. NaOH and potassium dihydrogen phosphate — pH 5.8 to 8.0
5. Boric acid, NaOH and KCl — pH 8.0 to 10.0

KCl is a neutral salt and is added to adjust the ionic strength of the buffer system.

8.10. Buffer capacity and tissue irritation

If the pH of the externally applied liquids such as ophthalmic solutions or of parenteral liquids deviates considerably from the normal pH of the relevant body fluid, it may cause irritation. Of greater importance than the pH of the liquid are the buffer capacity and volume of solution used in relation to the volume of body fluid with which the solution will come in contact.

Tissue irritation will be minimal when there is

1. lower buffer capacity and volume for the solution to be used.
2. larger buffer capacity and volume for the physiologic fluid with which the solution comes in contact.

Most of the solutions used for the eye are buffered and parenteral solutions are usually not buffered and if buffered, the buffer has low buffer capacity

8.11 Stability and therapeutic action

Most of the ophthalmic drugs for ophthalmic use are weakly acidic or basic. At low pH, these drugs dissociate and go into solution and they remain stable. However, the therapeutic effect is lower as only the undissociated form is able to penetrate the lipoidal membrane. Hence there must be a compromise between the pH of optimum stability and the pH of maximum therapeutic effect. When the solution is instilled, the pH slowly changes to that of tear solution (pH 7.4) and the weak acid or base (i.e. the drug) gets into the undissociated form which provides for maximum therapeutic effect.

9. Isotonic solutions

Solutions having same osmotic pressures are termed isotonic solutions. ***Pharmaceutically an isotonic solution is one which is having same osmotic pressure as that of blood or lacrimal fluid (tear solution)***

Solution which are not isotonic are termed *paratonic* solutions. Paratonic solutions may be hypotonic or hypertonic. Isotonic solutions, when they come in contact with tissues such as eye, nasal tract or other body tissues or when introduced into blood by injection (intravenous), do not cause swelling or contraction of the tissues. But paratonic solutions produce unwanted effects.

The effect of paratonic solutions may be demonstrated. A solution having 0.9 g of sodium chloride in 100 ml of solution is an isotonic solution. A 2.5% solution of sodium chloride is hypertonic. If red blood cells are suspended in the 2.5% solution of sodium chloride the water within the cells passes out through the cell membrane to attain equilibrium with the salt solution surrounding. This passage of water out of the cells causes the cells to shrink and become crenated. When this occurs, the salt solution (2.5% NaCl solution) is said to *hypertonic* with respect to the blood cell contents. Alternatively, if the red blood cells are suspended in a solution containing 0.1% of sodium chloride, water from the surrounding solution enters into the blood cells through cell membrane. As a result the cells swell and finally burst open with the liberation of hemoglobin. This bursting of cells is called ***hemolysis***. In this instance, the salt solution (i.e. 0.1% NaCl solution) is said to be hypotonic with respect to the blood (i.e blood cells).

The red blood cell membrane may permit the entry of solute molecules such as urea, ammonium chloride, alcohol and boric acid and hence it does not act as a perfect cell membrane Isotonic definition given already refers to a solution which is isotonic only when the blood cells are impermeable to the solute molecules and permeable to the solvent molecules. Such a membrane which allows only solvent molecules to pass through may be considered as an ideal semipermeable membrane. *Mucous membrane* of the eye acts as a true semipermeable membrane.

It has been suggested that the term isotonic should be restricted to solutions having equal osmotic pressures with respect to a particular membrane separating the solutions. Hence a new term is defined on the basis of sodium chloride concentration. The new term is the *isotonicity value*. This is the concentration of aqueous sodium chloride solution having the same colligative properties as the solution in question. However it is to be born in mind that solutions having an isotonicity value of 0.9 g of sodium chloride in 100 ml of solution need not necessarily be isotonic with respect to living membranes concerned. Inspite of that, many of the solutions are roughly isotonic in this sense.

9.1. Measurement of Tonicity

The tonicity of solutions of drugs may be estimated by the methods based on

1. Hemolysis
2. Colligative properties.

Only the methods based on colligative properties of solutions will be discussed in this chapter.

9.2. Calculation of Tonicity using L_{iso} values

The student may be aware of colligative properties such as lowering of vapour pressure, elevation of boiling point, depression of freezing point and osmotic pressure of solutions. These colligative properties depend on number of particles and not on the nature of solute. The freezing point depression for solutions of electrolytes (both weak and strong) and non electrolytes may be given by the equation

$$\Delta T_f = K_f C \qquad \text{... (46)}$$

where

ΔT_f = freezing point depression

K_f = molal depression constant

c = molar concentration

But actual freezing point depression is always greater than the value obtained by using the above equation. This is, ofcourse, due to the deviation from ideal behaviour of solutions. To compensate for this deviation Vant Hoff '*i*' factor is introduced. The factor expresses the departure of real solutions of non-electrolytes from the laws of ideal solution (Raoult's law). In otherwords, the '*i*' represents the number of times greater that the colligative effect is for a real solution (of electrolytes or non electrolytes) than for an ideal solution.

$$\text{i.e. } T_f = iK_f C \qquad \text{... (47)}$$

In order to overcome the above difficulty a new factor L which is equal to iK_f is introduced. The equation now becomes

$$\Delta T_f = LC \qquad \text{... (48)}$$

$$\text{or } L = \frac{\Delta T_f}{C} \qquad \text{... (49)}$$

The L value can be obtained from the freezing point lowering of a solution of a compound that represents a given ionic type at a molar concentration C that is isotonic with body fluids such as blood and lacrimal fluid. The specific value for L is represented as L_{iso}. Thus L_{iso} is defined as the specific value of L which is equal to iK_f at a concentration of a drug which is isotonic with blood or lacrimal fluid.

The L_{iso} value for 0.9% of sodium chloride whose freezing point depression is 0.52°C and hence isotonic with blood or lacrimal fluid is

$$L_{iso} = \frac{\Delta T_f}{c} \qquad \text{... (50)}$$

$$L_{iso} = \frac{0.52}{0.154} = 3.4$$

0.154 appearing in the denominator represents the molar concentration of 0.9% W/V sodium chloride solution and can be obtained as follows:

molarity (c) = moles *per volume*

where

$$\text{moles} = \frac{\text{weight in gram of a solute}}{\text{molecular weight of the solute}}$$

$$\text{and volume in terms of liter} = \frac{\text{volume}}{1000 \text{ ml}}$$

(i.e. the volume of the solution is given terms of liter (i.e. in fractions of liters)

$$\frac{\text{moles}}{\text{volume}} = \frac{\text{weight in grams of the solute}}{\text{molecular weight of the solute}} \div \frac{\text{volume}}{1000}$$

$$\text{or } c = \frac{W}{M} \div \frac{V}{1000} \text{ or } \frac{W}{M} \times \frac{1000}{V} \quad \ldots (51)$$

(where V is the volume of solution)

For 0.9% w/v of sodium chloride, the molarity is given by

$$c = \frac{0.9}{58.45} \times \frac{1000}{100} = 0.154$$

(the volume of solution is 100 ml since 0.9% w/v indicates 0.9 gram of sodium chloride in 100 ml of solution).

Average L_{iso} Values for Various Ionic Types

Type	L_{iso}	Examples
Nonelectrolytes	1.9	Sucrose, glycerin, urea, camphor
Weak Electrolytes	2.0	Boric acid, cocaine, phenobarbital
Didivalent electrolytes	2.0	Magnesium sulfate, zinc sulfate
Uniunivalent electrolytes	3.4	Sodium chloirde, cocaine hydrochloride, sodium phenobarbital
Unidivalent electrolytes	4.3	sodium sulfate
Diunivalent electrolytes	4.8	Zinc chloride
Unitrivalent electrolytes	5.2	Sodium citrate
Triunivalent electrolytes	6.0	Aluminum chloride, ferric iodide
Tetraborate electrolytes	7.6	Sodium borate, potassium borate

Isotonic Values

Substance	M	E	$\Delta T_f^{1\%}$	L_{iso}
Alcohol, dehydrated	46.07	0.70	0.41	1.9
Aminophylline	456.46	0.17	0.10	4.6
Ammonium chloride	53.50	1.08	0.64	3.4
Amphetamine sulfate	368.49	0.22	0.13	4.8
Antipyrine	188.22	0.17	0.10	1.9
Antistine hydrochloride (Antazoline hydrochloride)	301.81	0.18	6.0	0.11
Apomorphine hydrochloride	312.79	0.14	0.08	2.6
Ascorbic acid	176.12	0.18	0.11	1.9
Atropine sulfate	694.82	0.13	0.07	5.3
Aureomycin hydrochloride	544	0.11	0.06	3.5
Barbital sodium	206.18	0.29	0.29	3.5

Substance	M	E	$\Delta T_f^{1\%}$	L_{iso}
Benadryl hydrochloride (Diphenhydraminehydrochloride)	291.81	0.20	0.34	3.4
Boric acid	61.84	0.50	0.29	1.8
Butacaine sulfate	710.95	0.20	0.12	8.4
Caffeine	194.19	0.08	0.05	0.9
Caffeine and sodium benzoate	-	0.25	0.28	-
Calcium chloride $2H_2O$	147.03	0.51	0.30	4.4
Calcium gluconate	448.39	0.16	0.09	4.2
Calcium lactate	308.30	0.23	0.14	4.2
Camphor	152.23	0.20	0.12	1.8
Chloramphenicol (Chloromycetin)	323.14	0.10	0.06	1.9
Chlorobutanol (Chloretone)	177.47	0.24	0.14	2.5
Cocaine hydrochloride	339.81	0.16	0.09	3.2
Cupric sulfate $5H_2O$	249.69	0.18	0.11	2.6
Dextrose H_2O	198.17	0.16	0.09	1.9
Dibucaine hydrochloride (Nupercaine hydrochloride)	379.92	0.13	0.08	2.9
Emetine hydrochloride	553.56	0.10	0.06	3.3
Ephedrine hydrochloride	201.69	0.30	0.18	3.6
Ephedrine sulfate	428.54	0.23	0.14	5.8
Epinephrine bitartrate	333.29	0.18	0.11	3.5
Epinephrine hydrochloride	219.66	0.29	0.17	3.7
Ethylhydrocupreine hydrochloride (Optochin)	376.92	0.17	0.10	3.8
Ethylmorphine hydrochloride (Dionin)	385.88	0.16	0.09	3.6
Eucatropine hydrochloride (Euphthalmine hydrochloride)	327.84	0.18	0.11	3.5
Fluorescein sodium	376.00	0.31	0.18	6.9
Glycerin	92.09	0.34	0.20	1.8
Homatropine hydrobromide	356.26	0.17	0.10	3.6
Lactose	360.31	0.07	0.04	1.7
Magnesium sulfate $7H_2O$	246.50	0.17	0.10	2.5
Menthol	156.26	0.20	0.12	1.8
Meperidine hydrochloride (Demerol hydrochloride)	283.79	0.22	0.12	3.7
Mercuric chloride (Mercury bichloride)	271.52	0.13	0.08	2.1
Mercuric cyanide	252.65	0.15	0.09	2.2
Mercuric succinimide	396.77	0.14	0.08	3.3
Methacholine chloride (Mecholyl chloride)	195.69	0.32	0.19	3.7
Methamphetamine hydrochloride (Desoxyephedrine hydrochloride)	185.69	0.37	12.3	0.22

Substance	M	E	$\Delta T_f^{1\%}$	L_{iso}
Metycaine hydrochloride	292.82	0.20	0.12	3.4
Mild silver protein	-	0.18	6.0	0.11
Morphine hydrochloride	375.84	0.15	0.09	3.3
Morphine sulfate	758.82	0.14	0.08	6.2
Naphazoline hydrochloride (Privine hydrochloride)	246.73	0.27	0.16	3.3
Neomycin sulfate	-	0.11	0.06	-
Neostigmine bromide (Prostigmine bromide)	303.20	0.22	0.11	3.2
Nicotinamide	122.13	0.26	0.15	1.9
Penicillin G potassium	372.47	0.18	0.11	3.9
Penicillion G Procaine	588.71	0.10	0.06	3.5
Penicillin G sodium	356.38	0.18	0.11	3.8
Phenacaine hydrochloride (Holocaine hydrochloride)	352.85	0.20	0.11	3.3
Phenobarbital sodium	254.22	0.24	0.14	3.6
Phenol	94.11	0.35	0.20	1.9
Phenylephrine hydrochloride (Neosynephrine hydrochloride)	203.67	0.32	0.18	3.5
Physostigmine salicylate	413.46	0.16	0.09	3.9
Physostigmine sulfate	648.45	0.13	0.08	5.0
Pilocarpine nitrate	271.27	0.23	0.14	3.7
Potassium acid phosphate (KH_2PO_4)	136.13	0.43	0.25	3.4
Potassium chloride	74.55	0.76	0.45	3.3
Potassium iodide	166.02	0.34	0.20	3.3
Procaine hydrochloride	272.77	0.21	0.12	3.4
Quinine hydrochloride	396.91	0.14	0.08	3.3
Quinine and urea hydrochloride	547.48	0.23	0.14	7.4
Scopolamine hydrobromide (Hyoscine hydrobromide)	438.32	0.12	0.07	3.1
Silver nitrate	169.89	0.33	0.19	3.3
Sodium acid phosphate ($NaH_2PO_4H_2O$)	138.00	0.40	0.24	3.2
Sodium benzoate	144.11	0.40	0.24	3.4
Sodium bicarbonate	84.00	0.65	0.38	3.2
Sodium bisulfite	104.07	0.61	0.36	3.7
Sodium borate $10H_2O$	381.43	0.42	0.25	9.4
Sodium chloride	58.45	1.00	0.58	3.4
Sodium iodide	149.92	0.39	0.23	3.4
Sodium nitrate	85.01	0.68	0.39	3.4
Sodium phosphate, anhydrous	141.98	0.53	0.31	4.4
Sodium phosphate $2H_2O$	178.05	0.42	0.25	4.4

Substance	M	E	$\Delta T_f^{1\%}$	L_{iso}
Sodium phosphate $7H_2O$	268.08	0.29	0.17	4.6
Sodium phosphate $12H_2O$	358.21	0.22	0.13	4.6
Sodium propionate	96.07	0.61	0.36	3.4
Sodium sulfite, exsiccated	126.06	0.65	0.38	4.8
Streptomycine sulfate	1457.44	0.07	0.04	6.0
Strong silver protein	-	0.08	0.05	-
Sucrose	342.30	0.08	0.05	1.6
Sulfacetamide sodium	254.25	0.23	0.14	3.4
Sulfadiazine sodium	272.27	0.24	0.14	3.8
Sulfamerazine sodium	286.29	0.23	0.14	3.9
Sulfanilamide	172.21	0.22	0.13	2.2
Sulfathiazole sodium	304.33	0.22	0.13	3.9
Tannic acid	-	0.03	0.02	
Tetracaine hydrochloride (Pontocaine hydrochloride)	300.82	0.18	0.11	3.2
Tetracycline hydrochloride	480.92	0.14	0.08	4.0
Tripelennamine hydrochloride (Pyribenzamine hydrochloride)	291.83	0.30	0.17	3.8
Urea	60.06	0.59	0.35	2.1
Zinc chloride	139.29	0.62	0.37	5.1
Zinc phenolsulfonate	555.84	0.18	0.11	5.9
Zinc sulfate $7H_2O$	287.56	0.15	0.09	2.5

where M = Molecular weight of the drug

E = Sodium chloride equivalent of drug

$\Delta T_f^{1\%}$ = freezing point depression value of a 1% solution of the drug

L_{iso} = molar freezing point depression of the drug at a concentration approximately isotonic with blood and lacrimal fluid

9.3. Adjustment of Tonicity of hypotonic solutions

In order to render a hypotonic solution isotonic, sodium chloride, dextrose or any other suitable substance may be added. The purpose of addition is to lower the freezing point to –0.52°C and to make it isotonic with body fluids (blood serum or lacrimal solution)

Two methods are available for calculating the percentage of sodium chloride or dextrose needed. They are the ***cryoscopic method*** (i.e. freezing point depression method) and ***sodium chloride equivalent method.***

9.4. Cryoscopic Method

The freezing point depression values of a number of 1% solutions of drug substances are listed in the table given under $\Delta T_f^{1\%}$. These values have been determined theoretically or experimentally. If the value is not found for a drug in the table, it may be arrived at from the molecular weight of the drug and the L_{iso} value of the ionic species.

The depression of the freezing point varies with dilution and is not absolutely proportional to the concentrations and this can be illustrated by considering procaine HCl. A 3% solution of procaine HCL has a freezing point depression of 0.33°C and therefore 1% solution of procaine chloride should have a value of 0.11°C(0.33/3). But the actual value is 0.12°C. Since adjustment need not be absolutely isotonic, as approximate adjustment will do. However, the adjustment made to be isotonic should be as exact as practicable.

The calculation involved for the amount of sodium chloride needed may best be illustrated with an example.

Let us find out the amount of sodium chloride needed to render 100 ml of 1% solution of procaine hydrochloride isotonic with blood serum. A 1% solution of procaine HCl has a freezing point depression of 0.12 as given in the table. In order to make this solution isotonic, a sufficient quantity of sodium chloride should be added to bring down the freezing point value to −0.52°C. The drug solution already has a freezing point depression of 0.12. The additional depression needed is 0.52°C − 0.12°C = 0.40°C. Therefore to produce this much of freezing point (i.e. 0.40°C) depression, sodium chloride must be added. A 0.9% sodium chloride has a freezing point depression value 0.52°C. By the method of proportion,

$$\frac{0.9}{x} = \frac{0.52}{0.40}$$

$$\text{i.e. } 0.52 \times x = 0.9 \times 0.40$$

$$x = \frac{0.9}{0.52} \times 0.40 = 0.69\% \frac{W}{V}$$

This may also be obtained by considering a 1% sodium chloride whose freezing point depression value is 0.58. Using the method of proportion

$$\frac{1}{x} = \frac{0.58}{0.40}$$

$$0.58x = 0.40 \times 1$$

$$x = \frac{1}{0.58} \times 0.40 = 0.69\% \frac{W}{V}$$

Where x is the amount of sodium chloride required for 100 ml of solution having 1% procaine hydrochloride to make it isotonic

The solution can be prepared by dissolving 1 g of procaine hydrochloride and 0.69 g of sodium chloride in sufficient water and then making up the solution to 100 ml with water.

Example

How much of sodium chloride is needed to render 150 ml of atropine sulphate solution containing 3 gram isotonic with lacrimal fluid. (The freezing point depression value of 1% atropine sulphate is 0.07°C).

The percentage of given atropine sulphate is given by

$$\frac{3}{150} \times 100 = 2\% \text{ solution}$$

1% solution has a freezing point depression value of 0.07°C. Then for 2% solution, $0.07 \times 2 = 0.14$°C. The freezing point depression value of the given solution is 0.14°C. To make this solution isotonic, a further depression in freezing point is needed. This is 0.38 (0.52 − 0.14). By the method of proportion.

$$\frac{1}{x} = \frac{0.58}{0.38}$$

$$= 0.58 \times x = 1 \times 0.38$$

$$\text{or } x = \frac{1}{0.58} \times 0.38 = 0.65 \frac{W}{V}$$

Thus for 100 ml 0.65 g of sodium chloride is needed and for 150 ml, the amount is

$$\frac{0.65}{100} \times 150 = \mathbf{0.975\ g}$$

The solution is prepared by dissolving 3 grams of atroprine sulphate and 0.975 g of sodium chloride in sufficent quantity of water and making up the solution to 150 ml with water.

Thus in order to arrive at the amount of sodium chloride required to render a hypotonic solution of a drug isotonic with blood or lacrimal fluid, two steps of calculation may be needed.

The first step involves finding the freezing point depression required to be depressed. This is easily obtained by subtracting the freezing point depression value of the given drug solution (let it be *a*) from the freezing point depression value of the blood or lacrimal fluid which is 0.52°C.

i.e. $(0.52 - a^\circ) = x^\circ$

The next step is to find out the percent of sodium chloride needed to produce x° of depression in freezing point and that may be given as

$$\frac{1\%}{\%\text{ of NaCl required}} = \frac{0.58^\circ}{x^\circ}$$

where 1% indicates the percentage of sodium chloride and for which the freezing point depression is 0.58°C.

Example

How much sodium chloride is required to render 100 ml of 1% solution of physostigmine sulphate isotonic with lacrimal secretion. The freezing point depression value of 1% physostigmine sulphate is 0.08°

Freezing point value of the drug is 0.08

Freezing point required to be depressed is $0.52 - 0.08 = 0.44°C$

The percent of sodium chloride needed to depress by 0.44° is $\frac{1\%}{x} = \frac{0.58}{0.44}$

$$x = \frac{0.44}{0.58} \times 1 = 0.76\%\ W/V$$

The solution is prepared by dissolving 1 g of physostigmine sulphate in a little amount of water and then 0.76 g of sodium chloride is added. To this sufficient water is added to produce 100 ml of solution.

Example

How much sodium chloride is required to render 200 ml of a solution containing 4 gram of procaine hydrochloride to render it isotonic with blood serum. The freezing point depression value of 1% procaine hydrochloride is 0.12°

The percent of given procaine HCl solution is 2% i.e. $\frac{4}{200} \times 100$

Freezing point value of this 2% solution is $0.12 \times 2 = 0.24°C$

Freezing point required to be depressed is $0.52 - 0.24 = 0.28°C$

The percent of sodium chloride required to produce a depression of 0.28° is

$$\frac{1\%}{x} = \frac{0.58}{0.28}$$

$$= \frac{0.28°}{0.58} \times 1$$

$$= 0.482 \text{ or } 0.48\%$$

i.e. 0.48% or 480 mg per 100 ml and for 200 ml, the sodium chloride needed is 960 mg.

9.5. Sodium chloride Equivalent Method

Sodium chloride equivalent (or tonicic equivalent) of a drug is the amount of sodium chloride equivalent to 1 gram of drug osmotically. It is designated as *E*. The *E* values for a number of drugs are given in the table.

This method involves simply multiplying the quantity of the given drug by the sodium chloride equivalent (*E* value) and subtracting this value from 0.9 g of sodium chloride which produces an isotonic solution with body fluids in 100 ml of solution.

The calculation may be illustrated with an example.

Example

What is the quantity of sodium chloride to make a solution of 1 g of procaine HCl in 100 ml of water to make it isotonic.

The quantity of the drug is 1 gram. Multiplying by its *E* value, 0.16, we get $1 \times 0.16 = 0.16$ g.

0.16 g is the quantity of sodium chloride osmotically equivalent to 1 gram of the drug. 0.9 g is required for every 100 ml of solution and hence the amount of sodium chloride needed in 0.9 – 0.16 = 0.74%

The solution is prepared by dissolving 1 gram of procaine hydrochloride and 0.74 g of sodium chloride in a sufficient quantity of water and than making up the solution to 100 ml with water.

We can make use of the method of proportion to obtain the amount of dextrose needed to adjust the tonicity. Since sodium chloride equivalent of dextrose is 0.16,

$$\frac{1 \text{ g of dextrose}}{0.16 \text{ gram of sodium chloride}} = \frac{x}{0.74}$$

$$\text{or or } x = \frac{1 \times 0.74}{0.16} = 4.62 \text{ gram}$$

9.6. White - Vincent Method

This method involves two steps. The first step is to find out the amount of water needed to prepare an isotonic solution with the given amount of drug. The second step is the simple addition of an isotonic or a buffered isotonic solution to make up to the final volume.

For example if one requires to prepare 20 ml of a 1% solution of ascorbic acid isotonic with body fluids, first the amount of the drug (in weight) is multiplied by the sodium chloride equivalent E. The amount of drug in 20 ml of 1% solution is 0.2 g.

$$0.2 \times 0.18 (0.18 \text{ is the } E \text{ value for ascorbic acid})$$

$$= 0.036$$

0.036 g is the quantity of sodium chloride that is osmotically equivalent to 0.2 g of ascorbic acid. By the method of proportion, the amount of water required to make this 0.2 g of ascorbic acid can be found out

$$\frac{0.9}{100} = \frac{0.036}{V}$$

$$= V \times 0.9 = 0.036 \times 100$$

$$V = \frac{0.036 \times 100}{0.9} = 4 \text{ ml}$$

That is 4 ml of water is added to 0.2 g of ascorbic acid to make an isotonic solution. This solution is then made up to 20 ml (final volume) with an *isotonic solution of sodium chloride, or dextrose or an isotonic buffered solution as required.*

The calculation can be given in a single step by the formula

$$V = 0.036 \times \frac{100}{0.9}$$

$$\text{i.e., } V = 0.2 \times 0.18 \times \frac{100}{0.9}$$

$$\text{or } V = 0.2 \times 0.18 \times 111.1 = 4$$

In general, the formula is $V = \boldsymbol{W} \times \boldsymbol{E} \times \mathbf{111.1}$ ... (53)

where V = volume of water required to prepare an isotonic solution with the given weight of the drug

E = sodium chloride equivalent

W = weight of the drug

10. Expression of Strengths of Intravenous Fluids

The electrolyte content of our body fluids is expressed in terms of millimoles (m.mol.) or milliequivalents (m.Eq) of ions per liter in recent times. Hence the strength of intravenous infusion solutions, prepared to correct the balance of electrolytes in body fluids are also expressed in similar terms.

The mole is now the basic international unit to specify the amount of an element, compound or an ion. One gram mole is the molecular weight of that compound or an ion expressed in grams. A millimole is one thousandth of this amount. Therefore a millimole of an ion is the sum of the atomic weights of the elements in the ion expressed as milligram.

For example,

1 mole of water	-	18
1 gram mole of water	-	18 g
1 millimole of water	-	0.018
1 gram millimole of water	-	0.018 grams (or 18 milligram)

The milliequivalent of an ion is one thousandth of 1 gram equivalent weight of the ion. Alternatively it is the ionic weight (sum of the atomic weights of the elements present) of an ion in milligrams divided by the valency of the ion. Thus, the milliequivalent is therefore the millimole divided by the valency of the ion.

Ions	Gram equivalent weight of ions (ionic weight/valency)	Weight of 1 mEq (mg)
Sodium Na^+	$\frac{23}{1}$	23
Potassium K^+	$\frac{39}{1}$	39
Calcium Ca^{2+}	$\frac{40.0}{2}$	20
Chloride Cl^-	$\frac{35.5}{1}$	35.5
Bicarbonate HCO_3^-	$\frac{61.0}{1}$	61.0
Phosphate HPO_4^{2-}	$\frac{96.0}{2}$	48.0

Suitable salts are used to provide these ions. To calculate the amount of salt required, the following formula is used

Weight in gram of salt containing one gram Eq. of an ion

$$= \frac{\text{molecular weight of salt}}{\text{valency of ion} \times \text{number of such ions in the molecule}}$$

To obtain the weight of salt in mg (milligram) containing 1 mEq of an ion, the above result is divided by 1000.

For example, the following table explains the equation given above.

Ion	Salt used	Molecular weight of salt	Valency of ion	Number of such ions in the salt	Weight of salt in mg containing 1 mEq of the ion
Na^+	NaCl	58.5	1	1	58.5
Na^+	Na_2PO_4	358.0	1	2	179.0
Ca^{2+}	$CaCl_2$	147.0	2	1	73.5
Cl^-	$CaCl_2$	147.0	1	2	73.5

The total ionic concentrations of plasma is from 300 to 320 millimoles per liter and the principal ions present are sodium (Na^+), potassium (K^+), magnesium (Mg^{++}), calcium (Ca^{++}), chloride (Cl^-), bicarbonate (HCO_3^-), and phosphate (PO_4^{3-}).

Average normal composition of blood plasma

Ions	m.Eq/litre
Cations	
Na^+	142
K^+	5
Ca^{2+}	5
Mg^{2+}	3
Total	155
Anions	
HCO_3^-	27
Cl	103
HPO_4^{2-}	2
SO_4^{2-}	1
Organic acids	6
Proteins	16
Total	155

10.1. Conversion of percentage strength to millimoles per liter

$$\text{Millimoles per liter} = \frac{10000C}{W} \quad \text{... (55)}$$

where C = percentage w/v strength of salt

W = milligrams of salt containing 1 millimole of the specified ion.

Example

Find out how many millimoles per liter of bicarbonate ions are contained in a solution of sodium bicarbonate 10% w/v?

In this C = 10% w/v

W = 84 mg

(Molecular weight of sodium bicarbonate is 84 grams and hence 1 millimole of sodium bicarbonate is 84 mg which contains 1 millimole of bicarbonate ions)

$$\therefore \text{ Millimoles per liter} = \frac{10{,}000 \times 10}{84}$$

$$= 1190.045$$

Thus 10% w/v solution of sodium bicarbonate contains 1190 millimoles of bicarbonate per liter.

10.2. Conversion of millimoles per liters to percentage strength

$$\text{Percentage strength } w/v = \frac{M \times W}{10{,}000} \quad \text{... (56)}$$

Where M = millimoles of specified ion per liter

W = milligram of salt containing 1 millimole of specified ion.

Example

Find out the percentage strength (w/v) of a solution of sodium bicarbonate containing 1190 millimoles of bicarbonate per liter.

$$\text{Percentage strength} = \frac{M \times W}{10{,}000}$$

$$= \frac{84 \times 1190}{10{,}000} = 10$$

The strength of the solution is 10% w/v of sodium bicarbonate.

10.3. Conversion of mEq/litre into weighable quantities

To convert mEq/litre to mg/litre:

$$W \times E \quad \text{... (57)}$$

To convert mEq/litre to g/litre:

$$W \times E \div 1000 \quad \text{... (58)}$$

To convert mEq/litre to % W/V:

$$W \times E \div 10{,}000 \quad \text{... (59)}$$

where W = number of milligrams of salt containing 1 mEq of the required ion.

E = number of mEq/litre.

10.4. Osmolarity and osmolality

Osmolarity is that mass of solute which when dissolved in sufficient solvent to produce a liter of solution will exert an osmotic pressure equal to that exerted by a gram molecular weight of an ideal unionised substance dissolved in a liter of solution. The unit is milliosmol (m Osm/liter). One milliosmol represent osmotic activity of one millimole of the solute or ion.

The osmolar concentration is calculated as follows.

1. For a non-electrolyte

$$\frac{\text{grams/liter}}{\text{molecular weight}} \times 1000$$

$$= \text{that many mOsm/liter}$$

2. For a strong electrolyte

$$\frac{\text{grams/liter}}{\text{molecular weight}} \times \text{number of ions}$$

$$\text{formed from a molecule} \times 1000$$

3. For individual ions if desired,

$$\frac{\text{grams of ion/liter}}{\text{ionic weight}} \times 1000 = \text{that many m.}$$

$$\text{mOsm of ions/liter}$$

The osmolar concentration of 0.9% sodium chloride is 308 m Osm/liter.

Osmolality is the mass of solute, which when dissolved in one kilogram of water, will exert an osmotic pressure equal to that exerted by a gram molecular weight of an ideal unionised substance dissolved in a kilogram of water. The Osmolality of the blood serum is 300 m mol.

Osmolarity which expresses weight/volume relationship is simpler to understand and use than osmolality which is difficult to determine. Osmolarity can be converted into osmolality and vice versa.

(Osmoticity is a general term which refers only to an osmotic state without referring to osmolality or osmolarity).

The USP requires that labels of Pharmacopoeial solutions of intravenous replenishment fluids, nutrients(s) or electrolyte(s) as well as the mannitol injections should state the osmolar concentration, in millimoles per liter except where the contents are less than 100 ml.

Example

A company supplies a lactated Ringer's 5% dextrose solution which is labelled to contain per liter

Dextrose (anhydrous)	50 g
Sodium chloride	6 g
Potassium chloride	300 mg
Calcium chloride	200 mg
Sodium lactate	3.1 g

and claims total osmolar concentration as approximately 524 m.Osm per liter. Verify the total claim.

$$\text{Dextrose} = \frac{50 \times 1000}{198.17} = 252.3 \text{ m.Osm/liter}$$

$$\text{Sodium Chloride} = \frac{6 \times 1000}{58.44}$$

$$= 205.33 \text{ m.Osm/liter}$$

i.e. 102.66 m.Osm of Na^+/liter and 102.66 m.Osm of Cl^- per liter

Potassium Chloride

$$\frac{0.3 \times 2 \times 1000}{74.55} = 8.04 \text{ m.Osm/liter}$$

(i.e. 4.02 m.Osm of K^+/liter and 4.02 m.Osm of Cl^-/liter

Calcium chloride

$$\frac{0.2 \times 3 \times 1000}{110.99} = 5.4 \text{ m.Osm/liter}$$

(that is 1.8 m.Osm of Ca^{++} and 3.6 m.Osm of Cl^- per liter)

Sodium lactate

$$\frac{3.1 \times 2 \times 1000}{112.06} = 55.32 \text{ m.Osm/liter}$$

(i.e. 27.66 m.Osm Na^+/liter and 27.66 m.Osm of lactate ion/liter)

Total osmolar concentration i.e. 252.3 + 205.33 + 33 + 8.04 + 5.4 + 55.32 m.Osmis 526.4 m.Osm/liter. It is in good agreement with the label claim. The m.Osm of potassium, calcium, and lactate are 4.02, 1.8, 27.66 m.Osm/liter respectively in this solution.

The osmolality of blood serum is approximately 300 millosmal. It is an useful factor in adjusting an injection isotonic with blood.

Example

How much sodium chloride is needed to adjust isotonicity of a solution containing 20 milliosmol of calcium per liter as calcium chloride.

Required milliosmol to get a solution isotonic with blood is 300.

The solution should contain 20 milliosmol of calcium ions per liter. For this, 60 milliosmol of calcium chloride/liter (20 + 20 + 20 for Ca^{2+}, Cl^-, Cl^- respectively) is required.

Thus already 60 m.Osm/liter is there and the milliosmol required to be adjusted is 240 (i.e. 300 – 60 = 240)

This much (240 m.Osm) of m.Osm should be provided by the addition of sodium chloride.

Then the formula for the preparation of the solution is therefore.

Calcium chloride ($CaCl_2 \cdot 2H_2O$)

$$60 \text{ milliosmols} = 20 \text{ milliosmol of } Ca^{2+}$$

$$= 20 \times 147 = 2.49 \text{ g liter}$$

Sodium chloride (NaCl)

240 milliosmols (i.e. 120 milliosmols of Na^+ and 120 milliosmols of Cl^-) of sodium chloride are to be added.

The weight of NaCl providing 120 m.Osm each of Na^+ and Cl^- ion is $120 \times 58.5 = 7.02$ gram per liter.

The final formula is

Calcium Chloride	2.94 g
Sodium chloride	7.02 g
Water for injection to make	1000 ml

Example

Calculate the quantities of salts in grams required for the preparation of 1 litre of a peritoneal dialysis solution in which the ionic concentration is as follows:

Sodium	130	m.mol.	
Acetate	35	m.mol.	
Chloride	100	m.mol.	(approx)
Calcium	1.5	m.mol.	
Magnesium	0.75	m.mol.	

Since the acetate ions will be contributed by sodium acetate, 35 m.mol. of sodium will be obtained from this source. The remainder of the sodium $(130 - 35) = 95$ m.mol. will be contributed by sodium chloride

Quantities required:

sodium chloride required for 95 m.mol of $Na^+ = \frac{95 \times 58.44}{1000} = 5.56$ g

sodium acetate of ($CH_3CO_2Na \cdot 3H_2O$) required

$$\text{for 35 m.mol. of acetate} = \frac{35 \times 136.1}{1000}$$

$$= 4.76 \text{ g}$$

calcium chloride ($CaCl_2 \cdot 2H_2O$) required

$$\text{for 1.5 m.mol. of } Ca^{2+} = \frac{1.5 \times 147}{1000}$$

$$= 0.220 \text{ g}$$

magnesium chloride ($MgCl_2 \cdot 6H_2O$) required

$$\text{for 0.75 m.mol. of } Mg^{2+} = \frac{0.75 \times 203.3}{1000}$$

$$= 0.15 \text{ g}$$

Chloride is contributed by NaCl, $CaCl_2$ and $MgCl_2$ i.e.

95 m.mol + 3 m.mol + 1.5 m.mol

= 95.5 m.mol (approx. 100 m.mol)

To this glucose is added any concentration between 1.4 percent to 7 percent depending on the requirement for dialysis (any amount from 14 g to 70 gms for 1000 ml) and the solution is made upto 1000 ml with water for injection.

10.5. Osmolality determination

Of the four colligative properties of the solutions namely osmotic pressure, elevation of boiling point, lowering of vapour pressure, and freezing point depression, the latter is easy to measure and is accurate. Semiautomatic high sensitivity osmometers that measure freezing point depressions are available.

Freezing point depression is related to osmolality. The relationship is given by the equation

$$\Delta T_f = K_f im. \quad \text{... (60)}$$

where ΔT_f = depression in freezing point of water

K_f = molal depression constant or cryoscopic constant

m = molal concentration

i = $g V$ (where g = molal osmotic coefficient and V = number of ions produced by the electrolyte

For strong electrolytes, the dissociation is complete and hence $g = 1$. The departure of g from unity (i.e. $1 - g$) is an indication of interionic attraction. This occurs in moderately concentrated solutions. For non-electrolytes $i = v = 1$ and therefore $g = i/v = 1$

Solutions for peritoneal dialysis or hemodialysis are required to contain a mixture of anions and cations in approximately physiological concentrations. The bicarbonate present in blood plasma may be replaced by lactate or acetate ions in dialysis solution to overcome some of the formulation problems.

In clinical laboratory, the term "osmolality" is generally used, but is usually reported as mosm/l.

11. Distribution Law

If two immiscible liquids are taken in a beaker, they form two separate phases. If a solute that is soluble in both the liquids is added, it will distribute or partition between the two immiscible liquids. Finally a dynamic equilibrium is set up.

The ratio in which the solute distributes itself between the two immiscible liquids is a constant at constant temperature. This is called *Nernst's distribution law* or *Nernst's partition law* or simply *distribution* or *partition law*.

When a solute 'X' is distributed between two immiscible solvents. A and B to form dilute solutions in each of the solvent and when the solute behaves ideally

$$\frac{\text{concentration of solute in } A}{\text{concentration of solute in } B} = \text{the distribution coefficient}$$

$$\text{or briefly } \frac{C_A}{C_B} = K_D \quad \text{... (61)}$$

The constant K_D or simply K is called the *distribution coefficient* or *partition coefficient* or *distribution ratio.*

If several solutes are distributed between two immiscible solvents, each solute gets distributed between the two immiscible solvents independently of the other.

The solute may exist partly or wholly associated in one of the two phases or it may exist dissociated in any one of the two phases. Thus, if a solute undergoes association or dissociation in any one of two immiscible solvents the above equation for distribution applies only to that part of the solute which is present as simple molecules in both the solvents.

Thus if the solute exists as monomers (simple molecules) in solvent A and as dimers (associated) in solvent B, the distribution coefficient is given by

$$K = \frac{C_A}{\sqrt{C_B}} \quad \text{... (62)}$$

and if 'n' molecules of the solute associate in solvent B, then the distribution coefficient is indicated by

$$K = \frac{C_A}{n \sqrt{C_B}} \quad \text{... (63)}$$

If a solute undergoes dissociation (into ions) in one of the two immiscible solvents, then the degree of dissociation should be taken into account.

Consider two immiscible solvents A and B containing a solute distributed between them. Let A be oil and B be the aqueous phase in which the solute undergoes dissociation (into ions). Then, the distribution coefficient is given by

$$K = \frac{C_A}{C_B(1-\alpha)} \text{ or } \frac{C_0}{C_W(1-\alpha)} \quad \text{... (64)}$$

where α indicates the degree of dissociation

However ionisation (dissociation) depends on the pH of the aqueous solution. Let the solute concentration (a weak acid) be represented by $[HB]$

The undissociated form of the weak acid is common to both the phases and hence the true distribution coefficient is given by

$$K = \frac{[HB]_0}{[HB]_W} = \frac{C_0}{C_W} \quad \text{... (65)}$$

The total acid concentration in aqueous phase is obtained by chemical analysis and is given by

$$C_W = [HB]_W + [B^-]_W \quad \text{... (66)}$$

where $[HB]_W$ = concentration of undissociated solute in water

$[B^-]_W$ = concentration of dissociated solute in water

The apparent or observed distribution coefficient (K') is given by

$$K' = \frac{[HB]_0}{[HB]_W + [B^-]_W} = \frac{C_0}{C_W} \quad \text{... (67)}$$

This observed distribution coefficient depends on two equilibria.

1. the distribution equilibrium with respect to undissociated solute in the two phases i.e. oil and water.
2. the dissociation equilibrium of the solute in the aqueous phase

The dissociation constant is given as

$$K_a = \frac{[H_3O^+][B^-]_W}{[HB]_W} \quad \text{... (68)}$$

The concentration of solute (C) in the aqueous phase before distribution can be given as

$$C = C_0 + C_W \quad \text{... (69)}$$

Making use of the above equations and assuming equal volumes (that is of oil and water) one can arrive at

$$\frac{K_a + [H_3O^+]}{C_W} = \frac{K_a}{C} = \frac{K+1}{C}[H_3O^+] \quad \text{... (70)}$$

This is similar to linear equation of the form $y = a + bx$. Therefore a plot of $K_a + [H_3O^+]/C_W$ versus $[H_3O^+$ yields a straight line with a slope that is equal to $(K+1)/C$ and an intercept K_a/C. The free distribution coefficient K can be obtained over the range of hydrogen ion concentration in consideration. The values required to substitute in this equation are only the hydrogen ion concentration, C_W and C and that indicates, the oil phase need not be analysed.

11.1. Applications of distribution coefficient

(a) *Extraction*

Extraction of a solute from one liquid phase into another liquid phase is used in analytical chemistry and in the extraction of solute (active principle) from extract of crude drugs. Extraction becomes more efficient if divided portions of extracting solvent are used in successive extractions than when the total amount of solvent is used in one single extraction. Consider W grams of solute are to be extracted from V_1 ml of one solvent 'A' with successive portions of V_2 ml of a second solvent 'B' that is immiscible with A. If W_1 grams of solute remain in the solvent A after first extraction with solvent B, the concentration of solute in the solvent A is W_1/V_1 and then the concentration of the solute in the solvent B is $(W - W_1/V_2)$. The distribution coefficient is

$$K = \frac{W_1/V_1}{(W - W_1)/V_2}$$

$$= \frac{\text{concentration of solute is solvent A}}{\text{concentration of solute in solvent B}} \quad \ldots (71)$$

$$\text{or, } K = \frac{W_1 V_2}{V_1(W - W_1)}$$

$$KV_1(W - W_1) = W_1 V_2$$

$$KV_1 W - KV_1 W_1 = W_1 V_2$$

$$KV_1 W = KV_1 W_1 + W_1 V_2$$

$$KV_1 W = W_1(KV_1 + V_2)$$

$$\left(\frac{KV_1}{KV_1 + V_2}\right) W = W_1$$

$$\text{or, } W_1 = W \frac{KV_1}{KV_1 + V_2}$$

After n successive extractions

$$W_n = W\left(\frac{KV_1}{KV_1 + V_2}\right)^n \quad \ldots (72)$$

This equation indicates that when n is large and V_2 is small, extraction is more efficient. Small V_2 indicates a large number of extractions with small portions of extracting liquid 'B'. W_n indicates amount left behind in the solvent A after extraction.

The distribution coefficient of isobutyric acid between water and ether is 1/3 at 25°C. What will be amount of isobutyric acid removed (or extracted) if 4 g of isobutyric acid in 100 ml of water is extracted with

(a) 100 ml of ether at 25°C

(b) two successive 50 ml portions of ether at 25°C

(c) four successive 25 ml portions of ether at 25°C.

The formula is

$$W_n = W\left[\frac{KV_1}{KV_1 + V_2}\right]^n$$

where W_n = Weight of active principle left in the original solvent (i.e. water)

W = Weight of active principle in the original solvent (i.e. water)

V_1 = Volume of liquid (i.e. solvent) containing the active principle

V_2 = Volume of extracting liquid used for extraction (i.e. ether)

n = number of extraction

(a) If 100 ml of ether is used for extraction the amount of isobutyric acid extracted would be

$$W_n = 4\left[\frac{\frac{1}{3} \times 100}{\frac{1}{3} \times 100 + 100}\right]^1 = 4\left[\frac{33.3}{33.3 + 100}\right]^1$$

$$= 4\left[\frac{33.3}{133.3}\right] = 0.1992 \text{ or nearly 1 gram}$$

Amount extracted is $4 - 1 = 3$ g

(b) If we use two successive 50 ml portions of ether, the amount of isobutyric acid extracted would be

$$4\left[\frac{\frac{1}{3} \times 100}{\left(\frac{1}{3} \times 100\right) + 50}\right]^2$$

$$= 4\left[\frac{33.33}{33.33 + 50}\right]^2 = 4\left[\frac{33.33}{83.33}\right]^2$$

$$= 4(0.399)^2$$

$$= 4 \times 0.1595$$

$$= 0.6383 \text{ gm}$$

Amount extracted is

$$4 - 0.6383 = \mathbf{3.36} \text{ gm}$$

(c) If four successive 25 ml portions of ether are used, the amount of isobutyric acid extracted would be

$$= 4\left[\frac{\frac{1}{3}\times 100}{\frac{1}{3}\times 100 + 25}\right]^4$$

$$= 4\left[\frac{33.33}{33.33 + 25}\right]^4$$

$$= 4(0.571)^4$$

$$= 4 \times 0.01062 = 0.425 \text{ g}$$

Amount extracted is $4 - 0.425$

$$= \mathbf{3.575 \text{ g}}$$

(b) Release of drugs from certain dosage forms

Suppositories and ointments contain non-aqueous vehicles. The release of drug from this involves partitioning into the aqueous body fluids or secretions. This partitioning principle is also involved in the prolonged release of drugs.

(c) *Drug absorption through living membranes*

In drug absorption, there is partitioning between the lipoidal barriers surrounding the cell and the aqueous body fluids in contact with them. Partitioning is also involved in the distribution and excretion of drugs in the body.

(d) *Preservation of Emulsions and Creams*

Deterioration is due to the enzymes (act as catalysts) produced by micro-organisms such as yeast, molds and bacteria. Hence they must be destroyed or the growth of these micro-organisms should be inhibited. For the purpose of destruction or prevention of growth, preservatives (i.e. anti-microbial agents) such as benzoic acid are added to the pharmaceutical products such as emulsions and creams which are biphasic systems containing oily and aqueous phases. One of the two phases in emulsions and creams is distributed as small globules throughout the other phase. Of these, the aqueous phase is liable to be attacked by microorganisms. Therefore, the preservative action is mostly needed in aqueous phase. This is usually accomplished by getting a proper concentration of a preservative in the aqueous phase. This is achieved by the addition of necessary amount of preservative so that enough concentration is partitioned in the aqueous phase.

It has been shown that preservative or bacteriostatic action of most preservatives is due almost entirely to the undissociated form and not to the ionic form. The total concentration needed for the preservative (*HP*) may be calculated using the formula considering the mostly used preservative benzoic acid,

$$C = qC_O + C_W = q[HB]_0 + [HB]_W + [B^-]_W \quad \text{... (73)}$$

where C = original concentration of the benzoic acid in the aqueous phase before the addition of oily phase

q = V_0/V_W, the volume ratio of the oil and the water phases

C_0 = molar concentration of benzoic acid in the oil phase existing as monomers i.e. equal to $[HB]_0$

C_W = molar concentration of benzoic acid in water $C_W = [HB]_w + [B^-]_w$

However, the distribution of benzoic acid among various phases depends on

(a) the distribution coefficient K

$$K = \frac{[HB]_0}{[HB]_w} \text{ or } [HB]_0 = K[HB]_w \quad \text{... (74)}$$

(b) the dissociation constant K_a of the acid in aqueous phase

$$K_a = \frac{[H_3^+O][B^-]_w}{[HB]_w} \quad \dots (75)$$

$$\text{or } [B^-]_w = \frac{K_a[HB]_w}{[H_3O^+]} \quad \dots (76)$$

(c) the phase volume ratio V_0/V_W

(d) pH of the aqueous phase

Substituting these values in the equation

$$C = q[HB]_O + [HB]_W + [B^-]_W \quad \dots (77)$$

We get

$$C = qK[HB]_W + [HB]_W + \frac{K_a[HB]_W}{[H_3O^+]} \quad (78)$$

$$\text{or } C = [HB]_W \left[qK + 1 + \frac{K_a}{[H_3O^+]} \right].$$

$$\text{or } [HB]_W = \frac{C}{qK + 1 + K_a/[H_3O^+]} \quad (79)$$

The above last two equations may be used to calculate the concentration of acid (benzoic acid) to be added to the biphasic system (oil and water) so as to get a final concentration $[HB]_W$ of undissociated acid in the aqueous phase which is buffered at a definite pH.

(e) *Partitioning in solubilized systems*

The principle of partition coefficient is involved in the dissolution of insoluble or sparingly soluble substances by micellar solubilization (Refer Interfacial phenomena). It may be considered that the solubilisation is a partition of the sparingly soluble substance between the interior of the micelles formed by surface active agents and the surrounding aqueous phase.

(f) *Drug action and partition coefficient*

The partitioning between the oil and water phases indicates the lipophilic or hydrophobic character of a drug molecule. The passage of a drug through lipid membranes and subsequent interaction with macromolecules at receptor sites involve partitioning of the drug. The hypothesis proposed by *Meyer and Overton* says that narcotic action of a non-specific drug is a function of the distribution coefficient of the drug between a lipoidal medium and water. Later it was found that narcosis was a function only of the concentration of the drug in the lipids of the cell. The modified rule of *Meyer* is that isonarcotic action (equal narcotic action) occurs at equal concentrations of a wide variety of drugs of different chemical types in the lipoidal phase.

(g) *Partition Chromatography*

This is a technique used for separation of components in a mixture. It depends upon the differences in the distribution coefficients of the components between two immiscible liquids. One liquid is maintained stationary by adsorption on to an inert solid support, which may be a powdered solid or a filter paper. The other liquid constitutes a mobile phase. Components of a mixture introduced into the system will move at different rates in a column or on a paper due to differences in partition coefficients of the components. This technique is used for separation, purification and identification of the components.

(h) *Equilibrium constants for complexes*

The partition coefficient technique is used to determine the equilibrium constant for a variety of complexes including drug protein complexes.

Suggestions for Practicals

1. Determination of solubility of a given solid substance (Sodium chloride)

Solubility is defined as the number of grams of solute required to produce 100 ml of saturated solution in a given solvent at a given temperature or at room temperature.

(a) *Gravimetric method*

Note down the temperature. Take approximately 100 ml of water in a clean beaker. To this add sodium chloride little by little with shaking until a portion of the salt remains undissolved. After ensuring the saturated solution has been formed, filter the solution through a filter paper over a funnel into a clean and dry vessel. Reject approximately 20 ml of the filtrate. Collect the subsequent filtrate. From this, pipette out accurately 10 ml of the solution after rinsing the pipette with the same solution into a tarred china dish. Evaporate the solution (i.e. the solvent) by heating the china dish over flame. At the final stage of evaporation, reduce the flame and continue heating until the residue is obtained. Wipe out the outer surface of the china dish to get rid of any soot formed. Cool the china dish to room temperature and weigh the china dish with the residue. Find out the weight of the residue.

Then, the solubility of sodium chloride is given as

$$\frac{\text{residue weight}}{10} \times 100$$

Report

The solubility of sodium chloride at room temperature...... g/100 ml of solution (Give the room temperature recorded)

Alternatively solubility can also be expressed as number of grams of solute required to produce a saturated solution in 100 ml of the solvent at a given temperature (or at room temperature). For this, the calculation will be as follows

Weight of 10 ml of the saturated solution of sodium chloride in water = a grams

Weight of the residue obtained after evaporation = b grams

Weight of water in 10 ml of the saturated solution = $(a - b)$ grams

The solubility of sodium chloride = $\frac{b}{a-b} \times 100$

Report

The solubility of sodium chloride is..... grams/100 ml of the solvent at room temperature (Give the room temperature recorded)

Another method of expressing the solubility is the amount of solvent required to dissolve 1 gram of solute at a given temperature. For this, the calculation is as follows.

$$\frac{a-b}{b} = \frac{\text{weight of water}}{\text{weight of residue}}$$

This gives the number of parts of water required for 1 part of solute to produce a saturated solution. Based on this Pharmacopoeias describe, the solubility of solutes as follows

Descriptive terms for solute	Parts of solvent required for 1 part of solute
Very soluble	Less than 1 part
Freely soluble	From 1 to 10 parts
Soluble	From 10 to 30 parts
Sparingly soluble	From 30 to 100 parts
Slightly soluble	From 100 to 1000 parts
Very slightly soluble	From 1000 to 10,000 parts
Insoluble/practically insoluble	More than 10,000 parts

(b) Titrimetric method

Prepare approximately 20 ml of saturated solution of oxalic acid in water by shaking at room temperature as described under sodium chloride solution preparation. (To hasten the dissolution of oxalic acid in water, use well powdered oxalic acid).

Pipette exactly one ml of the saturated solution and titrate against 0.1N sodium hydroxide solution using phenolphthalein as indicator. Find out the amount of oxalic acid present in the pipetted solution and calculate the solubility of oxalic acid in 100 ml of the solution. Each ml of $N/10$ sodium hydroxide *equiv* 0.063 g of oxalic acid.

2. *Effect of temperature on solubility of a drug in a given solvent*

Find out the solubility of potassium nitrate in water by gravimetric method at different temperatures. For example, find the solubility at 30°C, 35°C, 40°C, 45°C, 50°C, 55°C and 60°C. Everytime equilibrium at each temperature should be ensured. A thermostat is used to maintain the temperature. Draw a solubility curve taking the temperature on x axis and solubilities on 'y' axis. Observe the steep increase in solubility of potassium nitrate in water with increase in temperature.

Similarly find out the solubility of sodium chloride in water at different temperatures by gravimetric method. Draw a solubility curve for sodium chloride also. Observe the increase in solubility is very gradual with increase of temperature.

3. *Effect of solvents on solubility of a given substance*

Determine solubility of oxalic acid by titrimetric method, in water, alcohol, and glycerin at room temperature. Report the solubility of oxalic acid in different solvents.

4. *Determination of partition coefficient of oxalic acid between ether and water*

Nernst's distribution law states that if a solute 'x' distributes itself between two immiscible solvents A and B at constant temperature and 'x' is in the same molecular condition in both the solvents then, at equilibrium

Partition coefficient K_D

$$= \frac{\text{Concentration of } x \text{ in } A}{\text{Concentration of } x \text{ in } B}$$

Take 30 ml of aqueous solution of oxalic acid and transfer into a separating funnel. To this add 30 to 40 ml of ether. The system is shaken in the funnel till the oxalic acid is distributed and attains equilibrium in the two phases. Release periodically the stopper of the funnel to let out the vapour. Collect the aqueous layer and ether layer separately. Pipette out exactly 10 ml each of the aqueous portion and ether portion separately and titrate against $N/10$ sodium hydroxide solution using phenolphthalein as indicator. Find out the concentration in 10 ml. From this value find out the concentration in 100 ml of the aqueous layer and in 100 ml of ether layer. (Each ml of $N/10$ NaOH *equiv* 0.0063 g of oxalic acid)

$$= \frac{\text{Volume of NaOH} \times \text{Normality of NaOH} \times \text{Equivalent factor} \times 100}{10}$$

The partition efficient of oxalic acid

$$= \frac{\text{Concentration of oxalic acid in 100 ml of ether}}{\text{Concentration of oxalic acid in 100 ml of water}}$$

Repeat the experiment with 2% oxalic acid solution and verify whether you are getting the same values of partition coefficient or not.

5. *Determination of pK_a value of salicyclic acid*

The *Henderson-Hasselbalch* equation may be derived as follows. The dissociation of weak acid is represented as

$$HA \qquad H^+ + A^-$$

$$K_a = \frac{[H^+][A^-]}{[HA]}$$

Taking logarithms,

$$\log K_a = \log [H^+] + \log [A^-] - \log [HA]$$

Reversing the signs

$$-\log K_a = -\log [H^+] - \log [A^-] + \log [HA]$$

$$pK_a = \text{pH} + \log \frac{[HA]}{[A^-]}$$

$$= \text{pH} + \log \frac{[\text{unionised}]}{[\text{ionised}]}$$

if [unionised] = [ionised],

$$pK_a = \text{pH}$$

The pH of the solution is equal to pK_a at half neutralisation

Pipette out 10 ml of 0.6% w/v solution of salicyclic acid in methanol in a conical flask. Titrate against $N/2$ sodium hydroxide solution using methyl red as indicator till the end point of full neutralisation. Let the volume of $N/2$ sodium hydroxide be 'x' ml.

Again pipette out 10 ml of 0.6 w/v solution of salicyclic acid in methanol from the previous stock. To this add $\frac{x}{2}$ ml of $N/2$ sodium hydroxide solution used for the above titration from the stock solution. Thus, half of the salicyclic acid is neutralised (half neutralisation). Now the concentration of unionised salicyclic acid is equal to the concentration of ionised salicyclic acid. Find out the pH of the solution using a pH meter. It gives the pK_a value of salicyclic acid since $pH = pK_a$.

6. *Effect of dielectric constant on solubility of salicyclic acid*

The dielectric constant is the property of a solvent relating to the amount of energy required to separate two oppositely charged bodies in a solvent as compared with the energy required to separate the same two oppositely charged bodies in a vacuum. The dielectric constant of water at 25°C is 78.5. It means that it takes 78.5 times more energy to separate oppositely charged bodies in a vacuum than in water. This property is related to polarity of the solvent.

The dielectric constant of absolute alcohol is 30.

Prepare mixtures of alcohol and water with different dielectric constant by alligation method. For example if we want to prepare a mixture of alcohol and water with a dielectric constant of 40, we may prepare as follows taking the dielectric constant of water as 80.

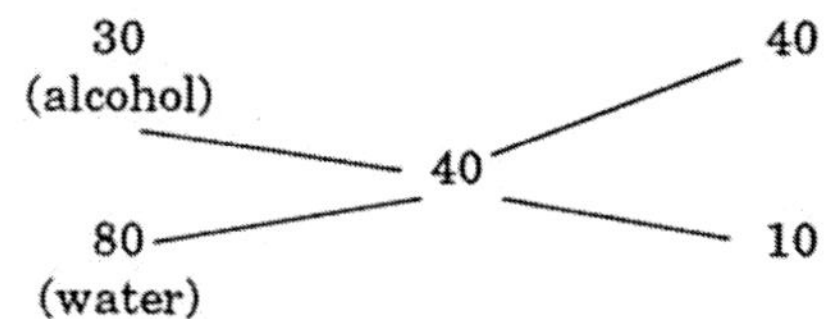

40 parts of absolute alcohol and 10 parts of water will give a mixture with dielectric constant 40.

Find out the solubility of a polar compound (say sodium chloride) in the mixture of alcohol and water with different dielectric constants and also in water and alcohol separately. Observe the solubility depends on the dielectric constants of the solvents. Similarly find out the solubility of salicyclic acid in water and in the mixture of alcohol and water with different dielectric constants and in alcohol alone. Report the result.

7. *Determination of critical solution temperature (CST) of partially miscible liquids-phenol and water*

CST (critical solution temperature) is defined as the temperature at which two conjugate solutions (or phases) merge into one another to form one layer. This is characteristic of a particular system.

Prepare 5%, 10%, 20%, 30%, 40%, 50%, 60%, 70%, 80%, and 90% w/w solutions of phenol in water. Heat the phenol-water systems on a water-bath gradually and the temperatures at which both the conjugate solutions merge into one layer are found out for each of the different concentrated mixtures using a thermometer. The percent compositions versus the temperatures are plotted. Find out the concentration which gives the maximum critical solution temperature.

Report

The upper critical solution of phenol-water system is .... °C and it occurs at a concentration of .... w/w of phenol in water.

8. *Prepare isotonic solution of cocaine hydrochloride whose amount is given for 100 ml of water. (The freezing point depression value for 1% solution of cocaine hydrochloride is* 0.11°C)

Cocaine hydrochloride	1*G*
Water	100 ml

Calculate the amount of sodium chloride needed and give the formula as shown below and the method of preparation.

Cocaine hydrochloride	1*G*
Sodium chloride	*G*
Water to	100 ml

(b) How will you prepare 500 ml of the above solution?

(Note: Always calculate for 100 ml first. After that expand the formula for the required volume).

(c) How will you prepare 90 ml of the above solution?

(Note: Always calculate for 100 ml first. After that reduce the formula for the required volume)

9. *Determination of heat of solution of a given sample*

Substances dissolve with positive heat of solution (endothermic) or with negative heat of solution (exothermic) with increase in temperature, the solubility may increase (positive heat of solution) or decrease (negative heat of solution) in accordance with *Le-chatlier's* principle.

For an ideal solution, variation of solubility of solid in a liquid (water) with temperature can be expressed as

$$-\log X_2 = \frac{\Delta H_f}{2.303R}\frac{1}{T} + C$$

$$\text{or } \log X_2 = -\frac{\Delta H_f}{2.303R}\cdot\frac{1}{T} + \text{constant}$$

where X_2 = ideal solubility of solute expressed in mole fraction

T = absolute of temperature

ΔH_f = heat of fusion. This is same as heat of solution in the case of ideal solution

R = gas constant

$= 8.314 \text{ Joules mole}^{-1}\text{ deg}^{-1}$

If log solubility ($\log X_2$) is plotted against the reciprocal of the temperature, a straight line will be obtained. ΔH_f can then be obtained from the slope which is equal to $\frac{\Delta H_f}{2.303R}$.

Take 200 ml of water in a clean conical flask. Add excess benzoic acid and heat to about 90°C. See that excess benzoic acid is present undissolved at 90°C. Withdraw 10 ml of clear saturated solution at that temperature using cotton plugged pipette. Titrate against standard sodium hydroxide using phenolphthalein as indicator. Calculate the solubility of benzoic acid.

Similarly withdraw 10 ml of benzoic acid (saturated) at 80°C, 70°C, 60°C, 40°C and 30°C separately and titrate against standard sodium hydroxide solution using phenolphthalein as indicator to determine the solubility of benzoic acid in water at different temperatures.

Obtain a plot of log solubility against $\frac{1}{T}$ and from the slope $\left(\frac{\Delta H_f}{2.303R}\right)$ of the line arrive at $°H_f$ which is the heat of solution of benzoic acid (It is assumed that benzoic acid forms an ideal solution).

Alternatively, heat of solution may also be found out by using the following equation for non-electrolytes and weak electrolytes

$$°H_b = 2.303 \log \frac{\frac{C_2}{C_1} \times R}{(T_2 - T_1)/T_1T_2}$$

(where C_1 and C_2 are mole fraction solubilities at temperatures T_1 and T_2 respectively). C_1 and C_2 can also be taken in terms of molal, molar and g/litre or percent.

Note: For electrolytes, in the above equation an extra term υ is introduced in the numerator. υ is the number of ions produced in solution.

For this, the solubility of the given substance (say benzoic acid) in water at two different temperatures are found out. Substitute the values in the above equation to find out $°H_b$ which is the heat of solution for an ideal solution.

VII. IONIC SOLUTIONS AND ELECTROLYTIC EQUILIBRIA

1. Colligative Properties

When a non-volatile solute is dissolved in a solvent such as water, a solution is formed. Such solutions acquire a number of properties which are different from that of the pure solvent. Of great importance are the colligative properties a solution possesses. The colligative properties of a solution depend solely on the number of solute particles in solution. The solute particles may be molecules or ions; large or small. The colligative properties are

1. lowering of vapour pressure,
2. elevation of boiling point,
3. depression of freezing point, and
4. osmotic pressure

Substances whose aqueous solutions do not conduct electricity are nonelectrolytes. Substances whose aqueous solutions conduct electricity are termed as electrolytes. Colligative properties of a solution of non-electrolyte are the same as that of another nonelectrolyte provided both are equimolar or equimolal (one molal solution contains one gram mole of solute in 1000 grams of solvent). For example, osmotic pressure of a one molal aqueous solution of sugar is same as that of a one molal aqueous solution of urea. However, this generalisation does not apply to electrolytes because a solution of electrolyte, in general, has greater osmotic pressure than that of a solution of nonelectrolyte of same molal concentration. This anomoly is due to the increased number of particles formed in the process of ionisation. For example, potassium chloride dissociates into two particles i.e. ions.

$$KCl \longrightarrow K^+ + Cl^-$$

Hence it might be expected that the osmotic pressure of potassium chloride would be twice that of a solution of same molal concentration of a nonelectrolyte. Similar increae in vapour pressure lowering, boiling point elevation, and freezing point depression should be expected especially in dilute solutions of electrolytes. Thus it is to be expected that an ion has the same effect as a molecule on colligative properties. Accordingly, one molal solution of potassium chloride will have double the osmotic pressure of an equimolal solution of sugar (a non electrolyte) i.e. there will be two-fold increase. In the case of calcium chloride it will be three fold increase as it dissociates into 3 ions (i.e. one Ca^{2+} and two Cl^- ions. However, two other effects are observed to be operative when the concentration of electrolyte is increased. The first effect is due to the interionic attraction between the positively charged and negatively charged ions resulting in incomplete dissociation from each other As a result the ions do not exert their full effect on the osmotic pressure or other colligative properties. This effect leads to a reduction in the 2 or 3 fold intensification of a colligative property in the case of potassium chloride and calcium chloride respectively. Therefore, it is to be understood that this deviation increases with increasing concentration of the electrolytes. The second effect is opposite to the first effect and is due to the attraction of ions for solvent molecules and is simply called as solvation or hydration if the solvent is water. This effect reduces the escaping tendency of solvent molecules. This effect also reduces interionic attraction. As a result of both the effects produced, there is an enhancement in the colligative properties.

1. Van't Hoff factor

It is the ratio of the colligative effect produced by a certain concentration of electrolyte divided by the effect produced by the same concentration of nonelectrolyte. Mathematically it may be expressed, considering osmotic presure and depression of freezing point, as

$$i = \frac{\pi}{(\pi)_0} = \frac{\Delta T_f}{(\Delta T_f)_0} \quad \text{... (1)}$$

where i = van't Hoff factor for electrolytes

π = osmotic pressure of electrolyte

ΔT_f = freezing point depression of produced by electrolyte.

$(\pi)_0$ = osmotic pressure of nonelectrolyte of same concentration

$(\Delta T_f)_0$ = freezing point depression produced by nonelectrolyte of same concentration

In the case of strong electrolyte which dissociated completely in dilute solution (i.e. 100% dissociation), the van't Hoff factor is equal to number of ions produced from the molecule. For example, for NaCl, it is 2; for Na_2SO_4, 3; and for $FeCl_3$, 4.

1.2. Applications of colligative properties

The most important pharmacetical application of colligative property is in the preparation of isotonic solution meant for intravenous and ophthalmic (eye lotions and eye drops) uses. The colligative property mostly used for this purpose is freezing point depression.

In experimental physiology, tissues are kept in isotonic salt solutions in order to prevent changes or injuries to tissues as a result of osmosis.

Colligative properties are used for the determination of molecular weight of nonelectrolytes. For example, in order to find the molecular weight of a nonelectrolyte using one of the colligative properties such as freezing point depression, one needs to determine, first, the freezing point of a dilute aqueous solution of the non electrolyte and by the method of proportion, to calculate the weight of the non-electrolyte (which is the molecular weight of the non-electrolyte) that would produce theoretically a depression of 1.855°C (sometimes 1.8 is used) when 1000 gram of water is used as the solvent. If other solvents are used, freezing point depression will be different. For example, if benzene is used, the value is 5.12°C and for carbon tetra chloride, it is 2.98°C.

In the case of electrolytes, the extent of ionisation can be determined using the colligative property. First, it is necessary to know its molecular weight (which may be determined by some other method) and then to measure one of the four colligative properties. The deviation of the results from similar values obtained for non electrolytes is found by calculation. The deviation, thus, obtained gives the extent of ionisation.

2. Strong and weak electrolytes

Electrolytes can be broadly classified into strong and weak electrolytes. Strong electrolytes dissociate completely into ions in aqueous solution of moderate concent ration and conduct electricity if the solution is connected to a battery through electrodes. *Strong electrolytes include solutions of strong acids, strong bases and most salts.*

Weak electrolytes dissociate to a lesser extent and consequently the conductivity will be less. *These include weak acids and weak bases.*

Thus an electrolyte which exists entirely or very largely as ions in aqueous solution is termed as strong electrolyte whereas a weak electrolyte in aqueous solution will have substantial proportion of molecular species (unionised form) along with ions formed as a result of dissociation of some molecules Strong and weak electrolytes can be differentiated on the basis of conductance characteristics exhibited in aqueous solutions.

2.1. Transport numbers

When an electrolyte solution taken in an electrolytic cell is connected to a battery through electrodes (anode and cathode) a direct electric current flows under the influence of a potential difference between the electrodes.

Flow of electrons through the solution occurs from right to left (Fig.94). This is accomplished by the movement of cations to cathode and anions to anode.

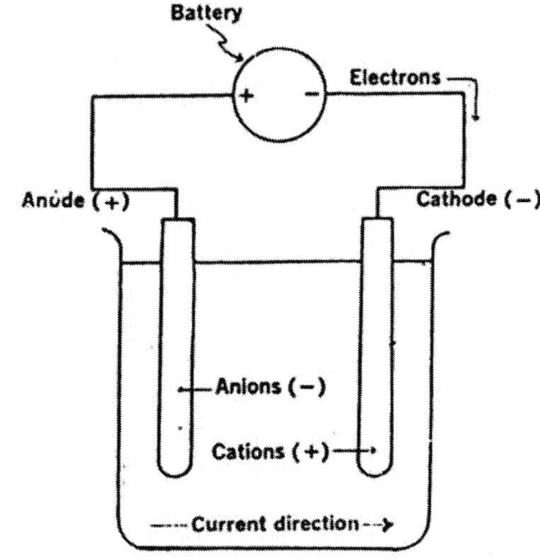

Fig. 94

The fraction of total current carried by the cations is known as the transport number of cations (t_+)

$$t_{(+)} = \frac{\text{Current carried by cations}}{\text{Current carried by cations and anions (or total current)}} \quad \text{... (2)}$$

The fraction of total current carried by the anions is known as the transport number of anions. ($t_{(-)}$).

$$t_{(-)} = \frac{\text{Current carried by anions}}{\text{Current carried by anions and cations (or total current)}} \quad \text{... (3)}$$

The transport (or transference) number is dependent on the velocity of ions. Therefore, ions that move faster carry greater fraction of current velocity of ions may be influenced by the hydration. Hydrated ions move slower.

2.2. Conductivity or conductance

The conductance of an electrolyte solution is the reciprocal of the resistance offered by the solution. While measuring conductivity, we actually measure the electrical resistance of the solution taken in a conductance cell using a Wheatstone bridge. The reciprocal of resistance gives the conductance.

The unit of conductivity is the reciprocal of ohms and is written as mhos. Since conductance varies with dimensions of the conductance cell, the conductance is calculated in terms of specific conductance. If is the conductance in a cell having electrodes of 1 sq cm cross sectional area and spaced or placed 1 cm apart. Specific conductance (κ) is computed from the formula

$$\kappa = \frac{1}{R} \cdot \frac{l}{A} \quad \text{... (4)}$$

where l/A = cell constant

l = distance between plates

A = area of electrode

It would be difficult to measure l and A. Therefore, a cell is calibrated by measuring in it the conductivity of a standard solution of known specific conductance. The cell constant is, then, calculated. This cell constant can be used to convert all measurements in that cell to specific conductance. Thus, it is simple to obtain the specific conductance just by dividing the cell constant by the resistance of the solution taken in the same ell.

2.3. Equivalent conductance

Equivalent conductance, designated as Λ, is defined as the conductance of a solution of sufficient volume to contain 1 gm equivalent of a solute when measured in a cell in which the electrodes are spaced 1 cm apart.

Equivalent conductane, Λ is obtained by multiplying the specific conductance κ by the volume (V) in *ml*, *V* of solution containing 1 gm equivalent of solute (i.e. electrolyte)

$$\Lambda_C = \kappa \times V \quad \text{... (5)}$$

$$= \kappa \,.\, \frac{1000}{C} \text{ mho cm}^2/\text{equivalent} \quad \text{... (6)}$$

Λ_C = conductance at a concentration C

2.4. Conductance of strong and weak electrolytes

When a solution of strong electrolyte is diluted, the specific conductance (κ) decreases while the equivalent conductance increases. Specific conductance decreases because of reduction in the number of ions per unit volume. Equivalent conductance increases although the quantity of electrolyte remains constant according to the definition of equivalent conductance, because there is less hindrance to the movement of ions by the neighbouring ions due to dilution.

Kohlrausch found that the equivalent conductance was a linear function of the square root of the concentration for strong electrolytes in dilute solution.

$$\Lambda_c = \Lambda_0 - b\sqrt{c} \quad \text{... (7)}$$

where Λ_c = equivalent conductance at a concentration c

Λ_0 = equivalent conductance at infinite dilution

b = a constant representing the slope of the line

When the equivalent conductance is extrapolated to infinite dilution (i.e. zero concentration), it has a special significance.

It gives the equivalent conductance of entirely dissociated ions of the electrolyte. It is inferred, at this condition, the ions are far apart and that there is no interionic interaction and the migration of ions is unhindered Kohlrausch Law states that, at infinite dilution, the equivalent conductance of an electrolyte is the sum of the equivalent conductances of the component ions and is expressed as,

$$\Lambda_0 = l_c^0 + l_a^0 \quad \text{... (8)}$$

where l_c^0 = equivalent conductance of cation

l_a^0 = equivalent conductance of anion

The significance of **Kohlrausch law** is that the conductance of any electrolyte may be obtained simply by adding the equivalent conductance of its ions.

Equivalent conductance of various ions at infinite dilution at 25°C is given below

Cation	l_c^0	Anion	l_a^0
H^+	349.8	OH^-	198.0
Li^+	38.7	Cl^-	76.3
Na^+	50.1	Br^-	78.4
K^+	73.5	I^-	76.8
NH_4^+	61.9	AC^-	40.9
$\frac{1}{2}Ca^{2+}$	59.5	$\frac{1}{2}SO_4^{2+}$	79.8
$\frac{1}{2}Mg^{2+}$	53.0		
AC^- denotes acetate ion (CH_3COO^-)			

Example: Find the equivalent conductance of acetic acid at infinite dilution if the Λ_0 for HCl = 326.1 Λ_0 for $CH_3COONa = 91$ and Λ_0 for NaCl = 126.4

$$\Lambda_0(CH_3COOH) = \Lambda_0(HCl) + \Lambda_0(CH_3COONa) - \Lambda_0(NaCl)$$

$$= 326.1 + 91 - 126.4$$

$$= 390.7$$

For strong electrolytes Λ_0 can be easily found out by extrapolation of the curve obtained by plotting $\sqrt{c}$ vs Λ_0. But for weak electrolytes such as acetic acid extrapolation is difficult because of steep rise in conductance. In such cases Kohlrausch law is very useful to find the Λ_0 for acetic acid simply by adding the l^0 of acetate ion and l^0 for sodium ion. Referring the table given, we find the equivalent conductance of acetic acid to be 390.7 which is obtained by adding l^0 for acetate ion (40.9) and l^0 for hydrogen ion (349.8).

2.5. Degree of ionisation for weak electrolytes

From conductance measurements, the degree of ionisation for weak electrolytes can be obtained by using the equation,

$$\alpha = \frac{\Lambda}{\Lambda_0} \qquad \text{... (9)}$$

where α = degree of ionisation

Λ = equivalent conductance of the electrolyte at any specific concentration of solution of the electrolyte

Λ_0 = equivalent conductance of the electrolyte at infinite dilution

The equation (9) is, however, not applicable to strong electrolytes because there is change in the mobility of ions at different concentrations.

Degree of ionisation can also be obtained from Vant Hoff factor, i, using the following equation

$$\alpha = \frac{i-1}{\upsilon - 1} \qquad \text{... (10)}$$

where i = Vanf Hoff factor for electrolyte

υ = number of ions into which the electrolyte dissociates

2.6. Theory of strong electrolytes

The ***Arrhenius theory*** is satisfactory for solutions of weak electrolytes. It does not explain the discrepancies arising when applied to strong electrolytes. In dilute and moderately concentrated solutions, strong electrolytes dissociate almost completely into ions and they fail to follow the Law of Mass action as can be applied for weak electrolytes. The degree of dissociation of strong electrolytes in aqueous solutions calculated from Vant Hoff factor differs from the value calculated from the conductivity ratio when applied to concentrations greater than 0.5 M.

These inconsistencies arise out of the influence the ions have with each other in moderately concentrated solutions of strong electrolytes through interionic attractive forces. However, this interference is negligible in dilute solutions. As the concentration is moderately increased, interference becomes operative. At high concentrations, ions associate into groups known as ion-pairs and ion triplets. eg: Na^+Cl^- and $Na^+Cl^-Na^+$. Association of higher order may also take place especially in solvents of low dielectric constant. Because of the factors mentioned above moderately concentrated solutions of electrolytes show abnormal colligative properties. Therefore, a strong electrolyte may be considered to be completely ionised, yet incompletely dissociated into free ions. It is appropriate to consider a strong electrolyte as completely ionised and to introduce a factor that accounts for the deviation of the electrolyte from 100% ionisation. To account for the deviation, *activity* and *osmotic coefficients* are used.

2.7. Activity and Activity coefficient

Due to electrostatic attraction and hydration of ions of strong electrolytes in concentrated aqueous solutions, the concentration of an ion becomes less efficient as a measure of its net effectiveness. To account for this, the term activity is introduced. It is a more efficient measure of the physical or chemical effectiveness of an ion and it may be thought of as *'effective concentration'*. This effective concentration is less than the actual or stoichiometric concentration of the electrolyte or solute.

The relationship between actual concentration and the effective concentration or activity is expressed on molal scale as,

$$a = \gamma_m m \quad \text{... (11)}$$

where m = molal concentration

a = activity

γ_m = activity coefficient on molal scale

Activity may also be expressed on molarity and mole fraction scale also

$$a = \gamma_c c, \text{ on molarity scale} \quad \text{... (12)}$$

$$a = \gamma_x x, \text{ on mole fraction scale} \quad \text{... (13)}$$

where c = molarity

x = mole fraction

γ_c = activity coefficient on molarity

γ_x = activity coefficient on mole fraction scale

At infinite dilution, the ions are widely separated and hence they do not exhibit interaction with one another. Therefore, activity equals its concentration in the solution and the equation becomes

$$a = m \text{ (on molal scale)} \quad \text{... (14)}$$

$$\text{or } \frac{a}{m} = 1 \quad \text{... (15)}$$

and the ratio is unity. When the concentration is increased the ratio is less than unity indicating the activity is less than the stoichiometric or molal concentration. Activity coefficient may be disregarded in dilute solutions (below 0.01 M) where $c \approx m$.

Activity which is a measure of an ion's effective concentration is related to its concentration at a universally accepted reference-standard state.

3. Ionic strength

Ionic strength serves as a measure of the intensity of the electrical field in a solution. It is expressed as

$$\mu = \frac{1}{2} \Sigma C_i Z_i^2 \quad \text{... (16)}$$

where μ = ionic strength

C_i = concentration of the ion (which is considered)

Z_i = valence of the ion, i

The mean ionic activity coefficient is a function of ionic strength.

The ionic strength may be found by using the equation (16) for the following solutions.

1. For 0.1 M (molar) solution of NaCl, the ionic strength is

$$\mu = \frac{1}{2}(0.1 \times 1^2 + 0.1 \times 1^2) = 0.1$$

2. For 0.1 M (molar) solution of Na_2SO_4, the ionic strength, μ is

$$= \frac{1}{2}(0.2 \times 1^2 + 0.1 \times 2^2) = 0.3$$

(With respect to Na (Na_2 in Na_2SO_4) the molar concentration is 0.2, i.e. double the quantity)

3. For 0.1 M (molar) solution of $MgSO_4$, the ionic strength is

$$= \frac{1}{2}(0.1 \times 2^2 + 0.1 \times 2^2) = 0.4$$

The ionic strength of a solution containing 0.1 M solutions of NaCl, Na_2SO_4 and $MgSO_4$ is the sum of the ionic strengths of the individual salt calculated. Thus, the total ionic strength of the solution is given as

$$\Sigma\mu = 0.1 + 0.3 + 0.4 = 0.8$$

Thus the formula may be given as below

$$\mu = \frac{1}{2}(C_1Z_1^2 + C_2Z_2^2 + C_3Z_3^3 + \text{.....} \; C_nZ_n^2) \quad (17)$$

The formula (16) is only an abbreviated form of the equation (17).

From the above discussion, the following may be inferred.

For uni-univalent electrolyte (such as NaCl), the ionic strength is equal to molarity. For uni-bivalent electrolyte (such as Na_2SO_4), and bi-univalent electrolyte (such as $MgCl_2$), the ionic strength is three times the molarity and for bi-bivalent electrolyte (such as $MgSO_4$) the ionic strength is four times the molarity.

For electrolytes which dissociate partially, the concentration of the ionised part should, first, be calculated. (Unionized part does not contribute to the ionic strength) Once the concentration of ionised part is calculated, we can find the ionic strength using the equation (16).

4. Debye-Hückel theory

This theory is applied only to very dilute solutions upto an ionic strength 0.02.

According to this theory, the activity coefficient γ_i on mole fraction scale of an ion i of valence Z_i is given by

$$\log \gamma_i = -A \, Z_i^2 \sqrt{\mu} \quad \text{... (18)}$$

The factor A depends only on the temperature and the dielectric constant of the medium. A is approximately equal to 0.51 for water.

For a binary electrolyte

$$\log \gamma_i = -A \, Z + Z - \sqrt{\mu} \quad \text{... (19)}$$

A formula that can be used upto an ionic strength of 0.1 is

$$\log \gamma_{\pm} = \frac{0.51 Z^{+} Z^{-} \sqrt{\mu}}{1 + \sqrt{\mu}} \quad \text{... (20)}$$

where $\gamma_{\pm}$ = mean ionic activity coefficient for aqueous solutions of electrolytes at 25°C on mole fraction scale

Z^{+} = valence of cation

Z^{-} = valence of anion

In the study of influence of pH on biologic action, we have to take into account, the variable salt concentration in the buffer which may obscure the results. Hence, it is necessary to adjust the buffer to a constant ionic strength in each experiment. Ionic strength may also influence solubility of drugs and rate of chemical decomposition which are discussed under the chapters Solution and Distribution Law and Kinetics respectively.

5. Osmotic coefficient

The term osmotic coefficient is introduced as a correction for the deviations of electrolytes from ideal colligative behaviour. In highly diluted solution, Vant Hoff factor '*i*' approaches v which is the number of ions into which an electrolyte dissociates. At infinite dilution $i = v$ or $\frac{i}{v} = 1$ (unity). As the concentration is increased, the value becomes less than unity.

The ratio i/v is termed as '*g*' which is *known as practical osmotic coefficient*. '*g*' indicates the degree of deviation in the case of weak electrolyte *g* has a value equal to unity for complete dissociation of strong electrolytes in a dilute solution. A value that is less than unity indicates interionic attraction and this occurs in moderately concentrated solutions of strong electrolytes.

Accounting for osmotic coefficient in a dilute solution, the cryoscopic equation may be given as

$$\Delta T_f = g\, v\, K_f\, m \quad \text{... (21)}$$

where m = molal concentration of electrolyte

ΔT_f = change in freezing point produced

K_f = molal depression constant or cryoscopic constant

g = osmotic coefficient

v = number of ions into which the electrolyte dissociates

6. Acids and Bases

Arrhenius defined an acid as a substance that yields hydrogen ions in aqueous solution and a base as a substance that yields hydroxyl ions in aqueous solution. This definition emphasizes the oppositeness of character and it does not include the behaviour of acids and bases in non-aqueous solutions. Hence, it needs a broader concept.

6.1. Proton concept - Bronsted-Lowry theory

This theory defines an acid as a substance that is capable of yielding a proton (hydrogen ion), while a base is a substance that is capable of accepting a proton.

When HCl is added to water, HCl donates the proton, H^{+} and the water which acts as a base accepts the proton donated. The protolytic reaction may be represented as

$$\underset{\text{Acid}_1}{HCl} + \underset{\text{Base}_2}{H_2O} \longrightarrow \underset{\text{Acid}_2}{H_3O^{+}} + \underset{\text{Base}_1}{Cl^{-}} \quad \text{... (22)}$$

HCl and Cl^{-} form one acid-base pair or conjugate pair and H_3O^{+} and

H_2O form another acid-base pair or conjugate pair.

The ionic species H_3O^+ is called hydronium or oxonium ion and is formed when an acid is dissolved in water. For convenience sake it is often written as H^+, though it is practically non-existent in solution.

Some other examples are:

1. $\underset{Base_1}{NH_3} + \underset{Acid_2}{H_2O} \rightleftharpoons \underset{Acid_1}{NH_4^+} + \underset{Base_2}{OH^-}$ ... (23)

2. $\underset{Base_1}{CH_3COO^-} + \underset{Acid_2}{H_2O} \rightleftharpoons$
$\underset{Acid_1}{CH_3COOH} + \underset{Base_2}{OH^-}$ ... (24)

3. $\underset{Acid_1}{NH_4^+} + \underset{Base_2}{H_2O} \rightleftharpoons \underset{Base_1}{NH_3} + \underset{Acid_2}{H_3O^+}$ ... (25)

It may be observed from the examples given above, that not only molecules but also cations and anions may function as acids or bases.

The relative strength of an acid or base depends on its tendency to give up or take up protons. HCl gives its proton H^+ readily and hence it is a strong acid whereas CH_3COOH is a weak acid as it gives up its proton H^+ only to a small extent.

Solvents in which an acid or a base is dissolved influence the strength of the acid or the base. This is due to the ability of the solvent to donate or accept the proton. For example, HCl is a weak acid in glacial acetic acid and acetic acid is a strong acid in liquid ammonia.

Solvents may be protophilic, protogenic, amphiprotic and aprotic. A protophilic solvent has the ability to accept the proton from an acid. A protogenic solvent has the ability to donate protons (e.g. formic acid, acetic acid, liquid HCl etc). Amphiprotic solvents are be proton donors and acceptors (e.g. water and alcohol). Aprotic solvents can neither accept nor donate protons (e.g. hydrocarbons)

6.2. Electron-pair concept (Lewis theory)

Proton concept of acids and bases does not indicate the basic reason for proton transfer. It is incapable of explaining how substances like boron trichloride and stannic chloride can behave like acids though they do not donate protons. To overcome these deficiencies, Lewis proposed the electron-pair concept. According to his theory, an acid is a substance that accepts a pair of electrons donated by a base to form a covalent co-ordinate bond with the base, and a base is a substance that donates a pair of unshared electrons to the acid to form a co-ordinate covalent bond.

For example, the proton H^+ accepts a pair of electrons to form a co-ordinate covalent bond with NH_3.

$$H^+ + :\overset{H}{\underset{H}{\ddot{N}}}:H \longrightarrow \left[H \leftarrow \overset{H}{\underset{H}{\ddot{N}}}:H \right]^+$$

Boron trichloride is an acid as it accepts a pair of unshared electron from NH_3.

$$Cl:\overset{Cl}{\underset{Cl}{B}} + :\overset{H}{\underset{H}{\ddot{N}}}:H \longrightarrow Cl:\overset{Cl}{\underset{Cl}{B}}:\overset{H}{\underset{H}{\ddot{N}}}:H$$

7. Ionisation of Acids and Bases

Strong acids and bases ionize extensively whereas weak acids and bases ionize only slightly in aqueous solutions. However their neutralizing power is equal. For example both 1 N solutions of HCl (a strong acid) and CH_3COOH (a weak acid) will neutralize identical quantities of alkali.

A strong acid in aqueous solution contains a greater concentration of hydrogen ion, $[H^+]$ whereas a weaker acid contains a lower concentration of hydrogen ion, $[H^+]$ in aqueous solutions. Thus, the difference between the strong and weak acid is attributed to the concentration of hydrogen ion.

7.1. Ionisation of weak acids

A reversible reaction of weak acid which ionizes incompletely in water may be given as

$$\underset{Acid_1}{HA} + \underset{Base_2}{H_2O} \rightleftharpoons \underset{Base_1}{A^-} + \underset{Acid_2}{H_3O^+} \quad \text{... (26)}$$

According to the Law of Mass action, the rate of forward reaction (R_f) is proportional to the concentration of reactants and the rate of reverse reaction (R_r) is proportional to the concentration of products

i.e. $R_f = K_1[HA][H_2O]$ ... (27)

and, $R_r = K_2[A^-][H_3O^+]$ ... (28)

At equilibrium, $R_f = R_r$

[Note: The student must understand that the concentrations of reactants and products may or may not be equal. It is the speeds of the forward and reverse reactions that are equal]

Solving for the ratio $\frac{K_1}{K_2}$, we obtain

$$K = \frac{K_1}{K_2} = \frac{[H_3O^+][A^-]}{[HA][H_2O]} \quad \text{... (29)}$$

Since $[H_2O]$ is a constant, this equation may be written

$$K[H_2O] = \frac{[H_3O^+][A^-]}{[HA]} = K_a \quad \text{... (30)}$$

where K_a = ionisation or dissociation constant of the weak acid

The equation (30) may also be written as

$$55.3K = \frac{[H_3O^+][A^-]}{[HA]} = K_a \quad \text{... (31)}$$

where 55.3 is the number of moles of 1 litre of water at 25°C. (1 litre of water weighs 997.07 g at 25°C). The number of moles for this weight is 997.07/18.02 = 55.3 moles/litre where 18.02 is the molecular weight of water. According to Brönsted-Lowry nomenclature ionisation constant is termed as ***acidity constant.***

In terms of concentration symbols, the reaction (26) may be given as

$$\underset{(c-x)}{HA} + H_2O \rightleftharpoons \underset{x}{H_3O^+} + \underset{x}{A^-}$$

where c = initial concentration of the acid HA

x = concentration of H_3O^+ or A^- since both are formed in equimolar concentration

Substituting these values in the equation (31)

$$K_a = \frac{x^2}{c-x} \quad \text{... (32)}$$

When compared to x, c is large because the dissociation is only slight Hence, the term x in the denominator may be disregarded. Then,

$$K_a \simeq \frac{x^2}{c} \quad \text{... (33)}$$

or, $x^2 = K_a c$

or, $x = [H_3O^+] = \sqrt{K_a c}$ ... (34)

[Note: The ionisation constant of a weak acid such as acetic acid is given as 1.75×10^{-5} i.e. 0.0000175 moles per liter. From this value we understand the slight extent of ionisation of the weak acid in water]

Acids which donate more than one proton are termed polyprotics. The ionisation of polyprotic acid occurs in stages. One such example may be given by the eliquibria involved in the ionisation of phosphoric acid.

$$H_3PO_4 + H_2O \rightleftharpoons H_2PO_4^- + H_3O^+$$

$$H_2PO_4^- + H_2O \rightleftharpoons HPO_4^{2-} + H_3O^+$$

$$HPO_4^- + H_2O \rightleftharpoons PO_4^{3-} + H_3O^+$$

Applying the Law of Mass action, an overall ionisation constant K_a can be obtained for the phosphoric acid by multiplying ionisation of individual reversible reaction

$$\text{i.e. } K_a = K_1K_2K_3 = \frac{[PO_4^{3-}][H_3O^+]^3}{[H_3PO_4]} \quad \text{... (35)}$$

7.2. Ionisation of weak bases

Ionisation of weak bases such as NH_3 may be considered. The reversible reaction is given as

$$NH_3 + H_2O \rightleftharpoons NH_4^+ + OH^- \quad \text{... (36)}$$

[Note: In the above reaction water acts as an acid by donating a proton to NH_3. $\ddot{N}H_3$ accepts the proton (Bronsted-Lowry definition of a base) by offering its unshared pair of electrons on the nitrogen atom (Lewis definition of a base)

Writing in a general form, the equation (36) becomes

$$B + H_2O \rightleftharpoons BH^+ + OH^- \quad \text{... (37)}$$

The ionisation constant or basicity constant may be written for the above reaction applying the Law of Mass action as for weak acid dealt above

$$K[H_2O] = \frac{[OH^-][BH^+]}{[B]} = K_b \quad \text{... (38)}$$

Using the same procedure as for weak acid, we obtain

$$[OH^-] = \sqrt{K_bc} \quad \text{... (39)}$$

7.3. Ionisation of water

Pure water ionizes slightly through a process known as autoprotolysis to yield hydrogen and hydroxyl ion. Accordingly one molecule of water acts as a weak electrolyte and it reacts with another molecule of water as solvent. The autoprolytic reaction is given as

$$H_2O + H_2O \rightleftharpoons H_3O^+ + OH^- \quad \text{... (40)}$$

$$\text{or, } 2H_2O \rightleftharpoons H_3O^+ + OH^-$$

On applying the Law of Mass action, we obtain

$$K = \frac{[H_3O^+][OH^-]}{[H_2O]^2} \quad \text{... (41)}$$

Since the concentration of molecular water exists in great excess compared to the concentration of hydronium ion or hydroxyl ion, it can be considered to be a constant.

Combining the concentration of water, $[H_2O]^2$ with K, we obtain a new constant, K_w known as ionic product of water.

$$K[H_2O]^2 = [H_3O^+][OH^-] = K_w \quad \text{... (42)}$$

The numerical value of K_w varies with temperature. At 25°C, it is approximately equal to 1×10^{-14}.

Since the concentration of H_3O^+ is equal to the concentration of OH^-.

$$[H_3O^+] = [OH^-] \doteq \sqrt{1 \times 10^{-14}} \doteq 1 \times 10^{-7} \quad \text{... (43)}$$

A solution in which $[H_3O^+]$ is equal to $[OH^-]$ is termed a neutral solution.

Consider a case where an acid is added to pure water. Because of addition of acid to water, hydronium ion concentration will be increased. This disturbs the equilibrium between $[H_3O^+]$ and $[OH^-]$ momentarily. To reestablish the equilibrium, some of the hydroxyl ions already present will combine with a part of the added hydronium ions to form nonionized water molecules until K_w has been reduced to 1×10^{-14}. However, when equilibrium is restored, $[H_3O^+]$ will not be equal to $[OH^-]$. Take for example, if the concentration of hydronium ion is 1×10^{-3} mole ion per litre of solution, the concentration of hydroxyl ion will be 1×10^{-11} mole ion per litre at reestablished equilibrium (i.e. $1 \times 10^{-3} \times 1 \times 10^{-11} = 1 \times 10^{-14}$). Since the solution contains much greater concentration of H_3O^+ than that of $[OH^-]$, the solution is said to be acid or acidic.

In a similar manner, if an alkali is added to pure water, equilibrium is disturbed momentarily. On reestablishment of the equilibrium, the concentration of OH^- will be much greater than the concentration of H_3O^+ and the solution is said to be basic or alkaline.

7.5. Relationship of K_a and K_b

A simple and interesting relationship exists between the ionisation constant of a weak acid and its conjugate base or a base and its conjugate acid.

For example, consider the ionisation constant of the base NH_3 and its conjugate acid NH_4^+ in water

The reaction of NH_3 with water is,

$$NH_3 + H_2O \rightleftharpoons NH_4^+ + OH^- \quad \text{... (44)}$$

Applying the Law of Mass action to the above equation, the ionisation constant or basicity constant is

$$K_b = \frac{[NH_4^+][OH^-]}{[NH_3]}$$

The reaction of the conjugate acid NH_4^+ with water is

$$NH_4 + H_2O \rightleftharpoons NH_3 + H_3O^+ \quad \text{... (45)}$$

Applying the Law of Mass action to the equation, the ionisation constant or acidity constant is,

$$K_a = \frac{[NH_3][H_3O^+]}{[NH_4^+]} \quad \text{... (46)}$$

Multiplying equations (45) and (46)

$$K_aK_b = \frac{[NH_3][H_3O^+][NH_4^+][OH^-]}{[NH_4^+][NH_3]} \quad \text{(47)}$$

$$K_aK_b = [H_3O^+][OH^-] = K_w \quad \text{... (48)}$$

From the above relationship, it may be deduced that

1. the strength of an base may be expressed in either of the K_a or K_b,
2. K_b of a base may be calculated if K_a of its conjugate acid is known, and
3. the stronger a base is, the weaker its conjugate acid.

The same may be deduced for an acid and its conjugate base. The equation will be same (i.e. $K_aK_b = K_w$)

Dissociation constants of some weak acids and bases in water at 25°C are given in the following table

Dissociation Constants in Water at 25°

Substance		K
Acetic		1.75×10^{-5}
Acetylsalicyclic		3.27×10^{-4}
Barbital		1.23×10^{-8}
Barbituric		1.05×10^{-4}
Benzoic		6.30×10^{-5}
Benzyl penicillin		1.74×10^{-3}
Boric	K_1	5.8×10^{-10}
Caffeine		1×10^{-14}
Carbonic	K_1	4.31×10^{-7}
	K_2	4.7×10^{-11}
Citric (1 H_2O)	K_1	7.0×10^{-4}
	K_2	1.8×10^{-5}
	K_3	4.0×10^{-7}
Dichloroacetic		5×10^{-2}
Ethyle-nediaminetetraacetic acid (EDTA)	K_1	1×10^{-2}
	K_2	2.14×10^{-3}
	K_3	6.92×10^{-7}
	K_4	5.5×10^{-11}
Formic		1.77×10^{-4}
Glycerophosphoric	K_1	3.4×10^{-2}
	K_2	6.4×10^{-7}
Glycine	K_1	4.5×10^{-3}
	K_2	1.7×10^{-10}
Lactic		1.39×10^{-4}
Mandelic		4.29×10^{-4}
Monochloroacetic		1.4×10^{-3}
Oxalic (2H_2O)	K_1	5.5×10^{-2}
	K_2	5.3×10^{-5}
Phenobarbital		3.9×10^{-8}
Phenol		1×10^{-10}
Phosphoric	K_1	7.5×10^{-3}
	K_2	6.2×10^{-8}
	K_3	2.1×10^{-13}
Picric		4.2×10^{-1}
Propionic		1.34×10^{-5}
Saccharin		2.5×10^{-2}

Substance		K
Salicyclic		1.06×10^{-3}
Succinic	K_1	6.4×10^{-5}
	K_2	2.3×10^{-6}
Sulfadiazine		3.3×10^{-7}
Sulfamerazine		8.7×10^{-8}
Sulfapyridine		3.6×10^{-9}
Sulfathiazole		7.6×10^{-8}
Tartaric	K_1	9.6×10^{-4}
	K_2	4.4×10^{-5}
Trichloroacetic		1.3×10^{-1}
Weak Bases		
Acetanilide		4.1×10^{-14}(40°)
Ammonia		1.74×10^{-5}
Apomorphine		1.0×10^{-7}
Atropine		4.5×10^{-5}
Benzocaine		6.0×10^{-12}
Caffeine		4.1×10^{-14}(40°)
Cocaine		2.6×10^{-6}
Codeine		10^{-7}
Ephedrine		2.3×10^{-5}
Morphine		7.4×10^{-7}
Papaverine		8×10^{-9}
Physostigmine	K_1	7.6×10^{-7}
	K_2	5.7×10^{-13}
Pilocarpine	K_1	7×10^{-8}
	K_2	2×10^{-13}
Procaine		7×10^{-6}
Pyridine		1.4×10^{-9}
Quinine	K_1	1.0×10^{-6}
	K_2	1.3×10^{-10}
Reserpine		4×10^{-8}
Strychnine		1×10^{-6}
	K_2	2×10^{-12}
Theobromine		4.8×10^{-14}(40°)
Thiourea		1.1×10^{-15}
Urea		1.5×10^{-14}

8. Electronegativity and dissociation constant

When acetic acid is dissolved in water, the polar molecules of the water have a greater affinity for the hydrogen of acetic acid (CH_3COOH) than the acetate ion (CH_3COO^-) has for its hydrogen. Due to this difference in affinities, the acetic acid ionises. (water is a polar molecule because of high electronegative oxygen in water and hence, it has more affinity for hydrogen ion).

Electronegativity increases the dissociation constant in the case of weak acids and it decreases the dissociation constant in the case of weak bases.

Introduction of chlorine atom into acetic acid increases the ionisation and hence the acidity. Monochloro acetic acid ($Cl-CH_2-COOH$) is more acidic than acetic acid. The reason is attributed to the highly electronegative chlorine atom which increases the dissociation constant due to *inductive* effect. As a consequence, the bond between the hydrogen and the oxygen atom in the carboxyl group ($-COOH$) is weakened. Because of this weakening, the degree of dissociation increases. Introduction of two or three chlorine atoms further weaken the bond leading to increased degree of ionisation. The ionisation constants for the acetic acid, monochloroacetic acid, dichloroacetic acid, and trichloroacetic acid are 1.75×10^{-15}, 1.40×10^{-3}, 5.0×10^{-2} and 1.3×10^{-1} respectively.

In the case of weak base, substitution of chlorine reduces the strength of the base (Increased ionisation because the affinity for hydrogen ion is reduced).

9. Ionic strength and Dissociation constant

Acidity constant or dissociation constant of a weakly acidic drug molecule is one of the most important properties as it can be related to physiologic and pharmacologic activities, solubility, rate of solution, extent of binding (i.e. protein binding) rate of absorption of the drug.

In very dilute solutions, the effect of ionic strength upon the acid-base equilibria (in the case of weak acidic or basic drugs) may be ignored. When stronger solutions are considered, the effect of ionic strength on dissociation constant must be taken note of. Most pharmaceutical solutions (elixirs and syrups) are in a concentration range where the ionic strength may influence the ionic equilibria and observed dissociation constants.

pK_a value refers to negative log of dissolution constant of the weak acid. The value may get altered by ionic strength. The altered value is called apparent $pK_a(pK_a')$.

For solutions with an ionic strength upto 0.3, the apparent $pK_a(pK_a')$ is,

$$pKa' = pK_a + \frac{0.51(2z-1)\mu}{1+\sqrt{\mu}} \quad \text{... (49)}$$

where pK_a' = tabulated thermodynamic dissociation constant

Z = charge on the acid

μ = ionic strength

9.1. Determination of Dissociation constant

The dissociation constant for a weak acid or base can be obtained by various methods such as conductivity measurements, visible or ultraviolet absorption spectrometry, potentiometry, etc. Of these methods, potentiometric pH measurement is the most widely used. The principle involved in this method is very simple. It may be understood by referring the equation (30). Rewriting the equation in the form shown

$$K_a = \frac{[H_3O^+][A^-]}{[HA]} \quad \text{... (50)}$$

When equimolar concentrations of salt $[A^-]$ and acid [HA] are present, the dissociation constant K_a numerically is equal to the hydronium ion concentration.

i.e. $K_a = [H_3O^+]$ when $[A^-] = [HA]$

What one has to do is to measure the pH of a solution containing equimolar concentrations of the acid and a strong base salt of the acid. At this concentration pH (which is the negative log of $[H_3O^+]$ is equal to pK_a. From pK_a the K_a may be calculated. (pK_a is the negative log of dissociation constant).

Though this method is simple and rapid, it is not sufficiently accurate. For a high degree of accuracy and precision, a dilute solution of the weak acid (10^{-3} to 10^{-4} M) is titrated against a strong base. After each increments of addition, the pH of the resulting solution is determined potentiometrically. The resulting data can be handled by the method proposed by Benet and Goyan. The proton balance equation (discussed latter in this chapter) for the above titration of the weak acid HA against the strong base (such as KOH) would be

$$[K^+] + [H_3O^+] = [OH^-] + [A^-] \quad \text{... (51)}$$

where $[K^+]$ represents the concentration of the base added.

Rearranging the equation and introducing Z for $[A^-]$, we obtain

$$Z = [A^-] = [K^+] + [H_3O^+] - [OH^-] \quad \text{... (52)}$$

For a monoprotic acid, the sum of concentrations of both unionised and ionised species, after equilibrium has been established, must be equal to C_a; the stoichiometric (added) concentration of the acid.

$$C_a = [HA] + [A^-] = [HA] + Z \quad \text{... (53)}$$

Substituting for HA (refer equation 50), the equation (53) can be given as

$$C_a = \frac{[H_3O^+]Z}{K_a} + Z \quad \text{... (54)}$$

Which on rearrangement yields

$$Z = C_a - \frac{Z[H_3O^+]}{K_a} \quad \text{... (55)}$$

If Z values are plotted against the values of $Z[H_3O^+]$, a straight line results with a slope. The slope is equal to $1/K_a$ and the intercept (obtained by extrapolation) gives the value of C_a. This method can be applied to a substance (weak acid or weak base) which can not be purified, or a substance which has an unknown degree of solvation.

10. pH

Hydronium ion concentration or hydroxyl ion concentration is expressed as gm.mole of ions per litre. For a normal solution of a strong acid (e.g. 1 N HCl), the hydronium ion concentration is nearly 1 while for a normal solution of a strong base (e.g. 1 N NaOH), it is approximately 1×10^{-14}. Thus, we can understand that there is a variation from 1 to 1/100,000,000,000,000. Because the calculations with these numbers are cumbersome, Sorensen (in 1909) proposed that hydronium ion concentration could be expressed in terms of negative log of hydronium ion concentration. To this value he assigned a symbol pH. Mathematically it is expressed as

$$pH = -\log [H_3O^+] \text{ or } \log \frac{1}{[H_3O^+]} \quad ... (56)$$

Autoprotolysis of pure water yields one hydronium ion for each hydroxyl ion produced. Hence, $[H_3O^+]$ must be equal to $[OH^-]$. At 25° each has a value of 1×10^{-7} moles/litre corresponding to a pH of 7. This figure is designated as the neutral point. Values below 7 represents acidity; the smaller the number, the greater the acidity. Values above 7 represent alkalinity; the larger the number, the greater the alkalinity.

The pH scale and the corresponding hydrogen and hydroxyl ion concentrations are given below

pH	$[H_3O^+]$ moles/litre	$[OH^-]$ moles/litre	
0	1	10^{-14}	↑
1	10^{-1}	10^{-13}	
2	10^{-2}	10^{-12}	
3	10^{-3}	10^{-11}	increasing
4	10^{-4}	10^{-10}	acidity
5	10^{-5}	10^{-9}	
6	10^{-6}	10^{-8}	
7	10^{-7}	10^{-7}	Neutral
8	10^{-8}	10^{-6}	
9	10^{-9}	10^{-5}	
10	10^{-10}	10^{-4}	increasing
11	10^{-11}	10^{-3}	alkelinity
12	10^{-12}	10^{-2}	
13	10^{-13}	10^{-1}	
14	10^{-14}	1	↓

Proton – Balance Equation (PBE)

In a proton balance equation, the sum of the concentration terms for species that form by proton consumption is equated to the sum of concentration terms for the species formed by the release of proton. This equation is based upon Brönsted-Lowry system in which the total number of protons released by acidic species must equal the total number of protons consumed by basic species PBE is useful in arriving at more accurate pH values by calculation.

Steps involved in obtaining PBE are:

1. Start with the species added
2. Place all species formed by the release of protons on the right side of the equation.
3. Place all the species that has taken up protons on the left side of the equation
4. Add $[H_3O^+]$ to the left side of the equation and $[OH^-]$ to the right side of the equation resulting from the interaction of two molecules of water.

10.1. pH of strong acids and bases

When HCl is added to water, the reactions that take place are

$$HCl + H_2O \rightleftharpoons H_3O^+ + Cl^-$$

$$2H_2O \rightleftharpoons H_3O^+ + OH^-$$

The PBE for this system would be

$$[H_3O^+] = [OH^-]\ [Cl^-] \quad ... (56)$$

Compared to $[Cl^-]$, the $[OH^-]$ would be negligible. In that case, the equation becomes

$$H_3O^+ = Cl^- = C_a \quad ... (57)$$

where C_a is the molar concentration of HCl in water. According to the equation (54), the hydronium ion concentration is equal to stoichiometric concentration of the acid (100% ionisation is assumed)

In a similar manner, the $[OH^-]$ for a solution of NaOH may be written as

$$[OH^-] = [Na^+] = C_b \quad \text{... (58)}$$

where C_b is the molar concentration of NaOH in water.

Eg.1: Calculate the pH of a 0.001 M solution of HCl

$$pH = -\log 0.001$$
$$= -\log (1 \times 10^{-3})$$
$$= 3$$

Eg. 2: Calculate the pH of 0.001 M solution of NaOH.

$$pOH = -\log 0.001$$
$$= -(1 \times 10^{-3})$$
$$= 3$$
$$pH = pKw - pOH$$
$$= 14 - 3 = 11$$

10.2. pH of Weak Acids

PBE for a weak acid (such as acetic acid) is given as

$$[H_3O^+] = [OH^-] + [A^-] \quad \text{... (59)}$$

Writing $[A^-]$ as a function of hydronium ion concentration and when $[H_3O^+] >> [OH^-]$ the simplified equation is given as (derivation not considered)

$$[H_3O^+]^2 + K_a [H_3O^+] - K_a C_a = 0 \quad \text{... (60)}$$

This is a quadratic equation and can be written in the following form

$$[H_3O^+] = \frac{-K_a + \sqrt{K_a^2 + 4K_aC_a}}{2} \quad \text{... (61)}$$

$[H_3O^+]$ is always positive and if it is less than 5% of C_a, the quadratic equation further simplifies to

$$[H_3O^+] = \sqrt{K_aC_a} \quad \text{... (62)}$$

If the assumption $Ca >> [H_3O^+]$ is valid the equation (59) may be used. If not, the quadratic equaiton should be used.

This, after arriving at $[H_3O^+]$ using the equation, pH can be calculated.

Salts obtained from the reaction of a strong acid with a weak base acts as acid eg. Ammonium chloride, morphine sulphate etc. If such a salt is dissolved in water, it dissociates as

$$BH^+X^- \xrightarrow[H_2O]{} BH^+ + X^- \quad \text{... (63)}$$

The protonated base BH^+ reacts like a weak acid with water to give

$$BH^+ + H_2O \rightleftharpoons B + H_3O^+ \quad \text{... (64)}$$

Equations (63) and (64) can be used to obtain $[H_3O^+]$ and the concentration of the salt in solution is equal to C_a

10.3. pH of weak bases

When a weak base (such as NH_3) is dissolved in water, it ionizes to yield the conjugate acid as

$$B + H_2O \rightleftharpoons BH^+ + OH^-$$

PBE for this system would be

$$[BH^+] + [H_3O^+] = [OH^-] \quad \text{... (65)}$$

Substituting $[BH^+]$ as a function of hydronium ion concentration and when $[OH^-] >> [H_3O^+]$, the simplified equation is given as

$$[OH^-]^2 + K_b[OH^-] - K_bC_b = 0 \quad \text{... (66)}$$

This is a quadratic equation and can be writen as

$$[OH^-] = \frac{-K_b + \sqrt{K_b^2 + 4K_bC_b}}{2} \quad \text{... (67)}$$

When $C_b >> [OH^-]$, the quadratic equation further simplifies to

$$[OH^-] = \sqrt{K_bC_b} \quad \text{... (68)}$$

Thus $[OH^-]$ is first calculated and it can be converted to pOH. The pH is then given by the equation

$$pH = pK_w - pOH \quad \text{... (69)}$$

When salts formed from strong bases and weak acids (eq. sodium sulfathiazole, sodium benzoate etc) are dissolved in water, they ionize as

$$Na^+A^- \xrightarrow[H_2O]{} Na^+ + A^- \quad \text{... (70)}$$

in which A^- being the conjugate base of the weak acid, HA reacts like a base with water to yield.

$$A^- + H_2O \rightleftharpoons HA + OH^-$$

Equations (68) or (69) can be used to obtain $[OH^-]$ and the concentration of salt in solution is ecual to C_b

10.4. Ampholytes

Ampholytes are substances which are capable of functioning both as acids and bases. eg: $NaHCO_3$ and NaH_2PO_4

When an ampholyte representing the type NaHA is dissolved in water, the following reactions may take place

$$NaHA \longrightarrow Na^+ + HA^-$$

$$HA^- + H_2O \rightleftharpoons A^{2-} + H_3O^+$$

$$HA + H_2O \rightleftharpoons H_2A + OH^-$$

$$2H_2O \rightleftharpoons H_3O^+ + OH^-$$

The PBE for the system is

$$[H_3O^+] + [H_2A] = [OH^-] + [A^{2-}]$$

On substitution for $[H_2A]$ and $[A^{2-}]$ as a function of $[H_3O^+]$ and simplification, we can arrive at the equaiton

$$[H_3O^+] = \sqrt{\frac{K_1K_2C_s}{K_r + C_s}} \quad \text{... (71)}$$

Mostly $C_s >> k_1$ and therefore the equation further simplifies to

$$[H_3O^+] = \sqrt{K_1K_2} \quad \text{... (72)}$$

The amino acid salt, glycine hydrochloride, when dissolved in water can aquire the form, $+NH_3CH_2COO^-$ and it can act both as acid and base as shown below

$$^+NH_3CH_2COO^- + H_2O \rightleftharpoons NH_2 . CH_2 . COO^- + H_3O^+$$

$$^+NH_3 . CH_2 . COO^- + H_2O \rightleftharpoons {}^+NH_3CH_2 . COOH + OH^-$$

Thus, a substance which carries both a charged acidic moiety and a charged basic moiety on the same molecule is called a zwitter ion. However the molecule acts as a neutral molecule. The zwitter ion concentration is maximum at a certain pH. The pH at which it is maximum is termed ***isoelectric point***.

Naturally, on the acid side of the isoelectric point, aminoacids and proteins are cationic (eg $^+NH_3 . CH_2 . COOH$) and hence are incompatible with anionic materials such as gum. Aminoacids and proteins which are anionic (eq: $NH_2 . CH_2 . COO^-$) on the alkaline side of isoelectric point, are incompatible with cationic materials such as benzalkonium chloride, cetrimide etc.

VIII DIFFUSION AND DISSOLUTION

1. Diffusion

Diffusion is a process of migration of solute molecules from a region of high concentration to a region of low concentration and is brought about by random molecular motion. This process is due to concentration gradient of solute across a solution or a partitioning membrane. The migration of solute molecules is a measure of escaping tendency of the solute in the environment to attain equilibrium.

The process of diffusion can be observed visually by placing a crystal of potassium permangnate in a beaker of water. A concentrated zone forms around the crystal and then the colour gradually diffuses until there is uniform concentration throughout. An identical situation arises when two solutions of different concentrations are separated by a semipermeable membrane.

The passage of solute molecules through a barrier may occur by

1. *simple molecular diffusion* (or permeation) or

2. *by movement through pores and channels.*

Simple molecular diffusion involves dissolution of the solute in the bulk membrane (eg. diffusion of theophylline through a polymeric membrane). The passage through pores and channels involves the movement of solute molecules through solvent filled pores of a membrane.

A barrier may be considered to be composed of fine individual membranes or component films

1.1 Fick's First Law of Diffusion

Fick's first law states that the quantity of solute dq diffusing through a unit cross section 'S' of a barrier in time dt (unit time) is termed flux, J and is represented as

$$J = \frac{dq}{S \cdot dt} \qquad \text{... (1)}$$

Flux is the rate of transfer of solute (molecules) per unit area of surface. The flux in turn is proportional to the concentration gradient $\frac{dc}{dx}$ in the plane of the area (barrier area)

$$J = -D \frac{dc}{dx} \qquad \text{... (2)}$$

where c = concentration

x = distance of movement perpendicular to the surface of the barrier and

D = diffusion coefficient.

Combining the above two equations (1) and (2)

$$dq = J \cdot S \cdot dt \qquad \text{... (3)}$$

$$dq = -D \frac{dc}{dx} \cdot S \cdot dt$$

$$\text{or } dq = -D \cdot S \cdot \frac{dc}{dx} \cdot dt. \qquad \text{... (4)}$$

The D is diffusion coefficient of the solute (or diffusant). The negative sign (–) denotes that diffusion takes place in the direction of decreasing concentration. D is also affected by temperature, pressure, solvent properties and the chemical nature of the diffusing solute.

1.2. Fick's Second Law

The second law is derived from the first law by disregarding the dependent variable dq and it emphasizes the rate of change of concentration at a definite location. Assuming unidirectional diffusion, the law is given as

$$\frac{dc}{dt} = D \cdot \frac{d^2c}{dx^2} \qquad \text{... (5)}$$

Fick's second law states that the change in concentration with time at a particular region is proportional to the change in the concentration gradient at that location in the system.

Thus, the first law gives the *amount of mass transported* across unit area of barrier in unit time whereas the second law emphasizes *the rate of change of concentration* (i.e. change in concentration with time) at a definite location. However the concentration changes only as a result of net flow of diffusion molecules to the other side. A difference in concentration results from a difference in input and output.

1.3. Steady State Diffusion

First law refers to a steady state of flow. That is, it gives the rate of diffusion across unit cross section in the steady state of flow. Second Law gives the change in concentration with time at any distance x and hence it is referred to as a non-steady state of flow. However, a *quasi-stationary state* may be described and this introduces little error when steady state under these conditions is assumed.

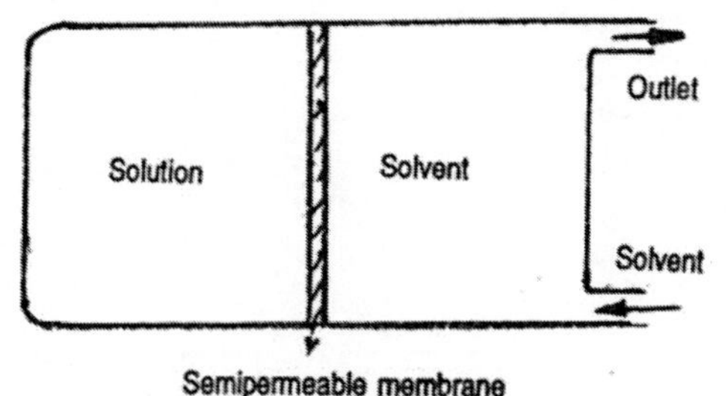

Fig. 95

Consider two compartments separated by a barrier Fig. 95. Let the left compartment contain the solution and the right compartment only the solvent. The left compartment, then, acts as the donor compartment and the right compartment as the receptor compartment.

During diffusion, the solute molecules diffuse through the barrier to reach the receptor compartment which is kept under sink conditions i.e. the solution is replaced with fresh solvent to keep the concentration at a low level. When the system has been left as such for a sufficient time, the concentrations in the solutions at the left and right of the barrier are constant with respect to time i.e. in the solutions at the surfaces of the barrier on either side. This denotes that there is no change in dc/dx and it can be said that the concentration gradient across the membrane is constant. It signifies a liner relationship between the concentration c and distance x. Such a condition is shown in the figure. Though the concentration is not rigidly constant, the condition may be referred to as a "*quasi-stationary state*".

1.4. Simple Diffusion

Consider a barrier with cross sectional area 'S' that separates two compartments (a donor and a receptor compartment). Let the thickness of the barrier be 'h', the concentration in the left compartment (donor compartment)

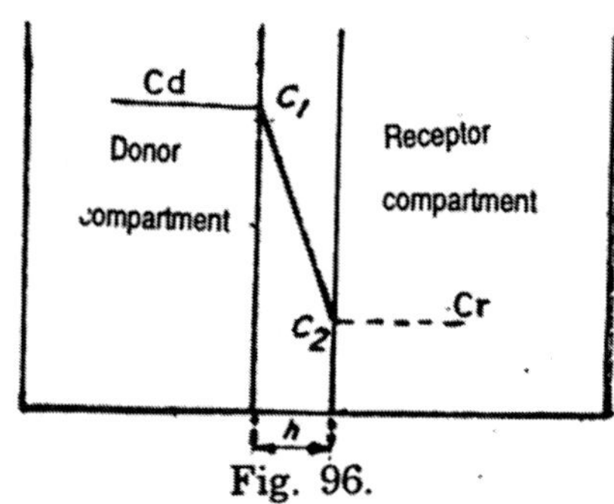

Fig. 96.

be C_1 and in the right compartment (receptor compartment) be C_2. Fig. 96

Applying Fick's first law

$$J = \frac{dq}{S \cdot dt} \text{ or } \frac{dq}{dt} = S \cdot J \qquad \ldots (6)$$

$$\frac{dq}{dt} = S.D \frac{(C_1 - C_2)}{h} \qquad \ldots (7)$$

$$\left(\text{where } J = D \cdot \frac{dc}{dx} \text{ and } \frac{dc}{dx} = \frac{C_1 - C_2}{h} \right)$$

The concentration within the barrier is assumed to be constant for a quasi-stationary state. C_1 and C_2 may be replaced by the partition coefficient K and is given by

$$K = \frac{C_1}{C_d} = \frac{C_2}{C_r}$$

or $KC_d = C_1$ and $KC_r = C_2$

Substituting in the above equation

$$\frac{dq}{dt} = D.S\, KC_d - KC_r$$

$$= D.S\, K(C_d - C_r) \qquad \ldots (8)$$

If sink conditions are provided for the receptor compartment, $C_r = 0$

$$\text{Then, } \frac{dq}{dt} = \frac{DSKC_d}{h} \qquad \ldots (9)$$

$$\text{or } \frac{dq}{dt} = PSC_d \qquad \ldots (10)$$

where $\frac{DK}{h} = P$ (permeability coefficient).

Since it is not possible to determine D, K and h independently, it is usual to combine these membrane factors into a single constant P, permeability coefficient.

Rearranging,

$$dq = PSC_d\, dt \qquad \ldots (11)$$

For a finite diffusion

$$q = PSC_d t \qquad \ldots (12)$$

It is relatively simple to obtain surface area 'S', donor concentration C_d and the amount of permeant q in the receptor sink. P can be obtained from the slope of linear plot of q versus t.

The release rate from a delivery dosage from follows zero-order release provided the dosage form delivers the drug through a saturated solution in the presence of excess solid drug. When the excess solid drug has been exhausted or if the excess solid drug is not present in the delivery form, the release rate falls exponentially and then the process is referred to as first order release.

1.5. Time lag

This is the time required for a diffusant (that which diffuses) to establish a uniform concentration gradient within the membrane that separates the donor

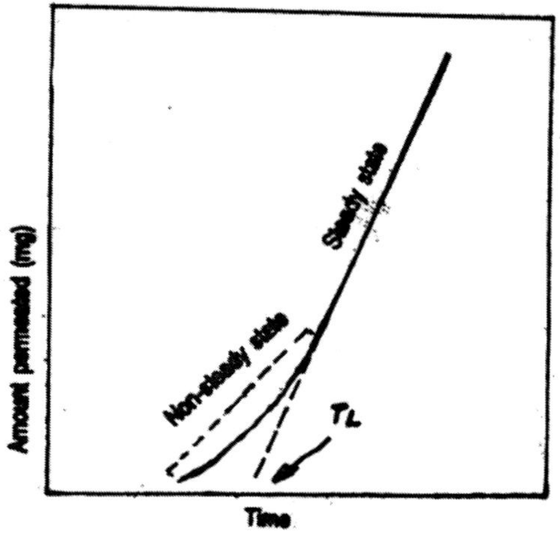

Fig. 97

and receptor compartments. This may be represented by t_l.

A steady state process is not observed for a constant activity dosage form in the initial stage of release. The initial stage is the non-steady state condition. At later stages, the concentration gradient within the membrane through which the drug diffuses becomes constant. Consequently the rate of diffusion is constant and the system is at a steady state. Thus the time required to attain the steady state is termed the lag time. This may be obtained by extrapolating the steady state portion of the line to the time axis as shown in the Fig. 97.

$$\text{The lag time } t_l = \frac{h^2}{6D} \quad \text{... (13)}$$

1.6. Electrochemical diffusion

Drug transport properties are modified if the drug is ionized. The permeation, then, depends on the concentration and potential difference across the membrane. The drug diffuses along its electrochemical gradient. The electro chemical gradient is the sum of the influences of electrical field and the concentration difference across the membrane.

1.7. Diffusion Study

Aquair and Weiner have reported cells of simple construction for diffusion work as shown in the figure.

The apparatus (Fig.98) consists of two cells A and B separated by a barrier through which diffusion can occur. It is provided with an automatic sample collection device. The drug solution is taken in the upper cell and the solvent in the lower cell. The whole set-up is thermostated.

The sample solutions are collected periodically and analysed spectrophotometrically or any other suitable method may be used.

Sorption of gas or vapour by polymers can be studied with a microbalance enclosed in a temperature controlled and evacuated chamber. The gas or vapour is introduced at controlled pressures into the chamber containing the polmer or biologic film suspended on one arm of the balance. The mass of gas or vapour sorbed at various pressures is recorded directly. From the rate of approach to equilibrium, the diffusion coefficient for the gas or vapour through the polymer or biologic film may be calculated.

The kinetics and equilibria of liquid and solute sorbed into plastics, skin, or other biologic materials can be determined by a simple method. It involves putting the sample sections of plastic or skin film in a constant temperature bath of the pure solvent or a solution having known quantity of the solute. The sections are withdrawn at various intervals of time, excess liquid is removed with absorbent tissue, and the sections are accurately weighed in

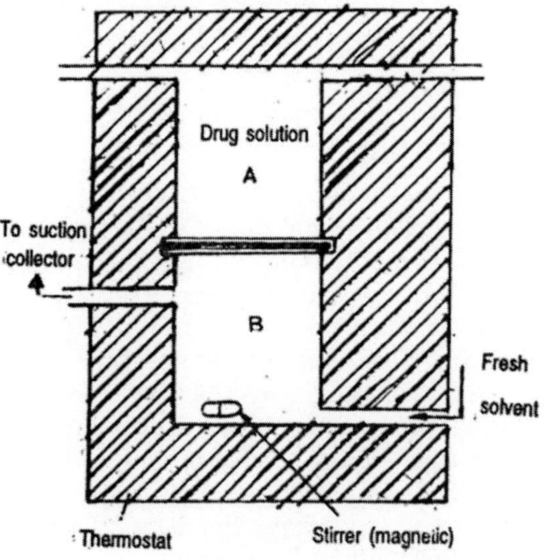

Fig. 98. Simple Diffusion Cell

tarred weighing bottles. The amount of solute (or drug) in the remaining solution is also determined by a suitable method (radio-active technique). Then, by difference, the amount of solute sorbed into the sample films is determined.

Other requirements such as partition coefficient and drug solubility may be obtained using suitable methods.

1.8. Percutaneous absorption study

For this study, animal or human skin is obtained by autopsy. This skin may be supported on a perforated plate. The skin with the perforated plate is introduced between two pyrex glass champers of which one is the donor compatment and the other, the receptor and the set up may be shown in Fig. 99 developed by Wurster et al.

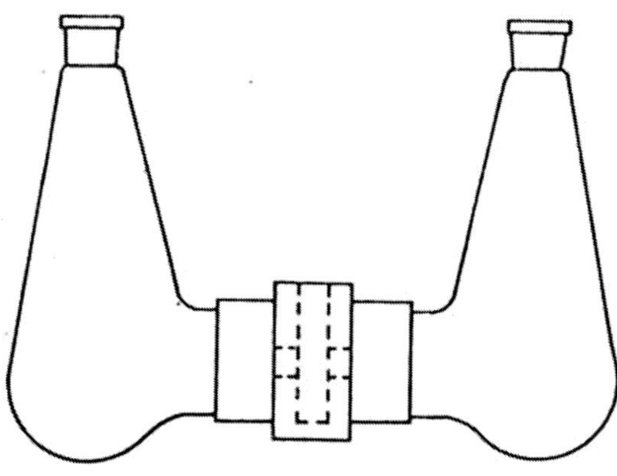

Fig. 99

The sample solution of the drug is taken in the donor compatment and the solvent in the receptor. The whole set up is placed in a constant temperature bath. The liquid in the receptor compatment is stirred by the use of a Teflon-coated bar magnet to obtain uniformity in the liquid. Samples are withdrawn periodically and assayed by a suitable method and from the results obtained, diffusion may be known.

Franz Diffusion Cell

It is a modified and improved version of the diffusion cell described earlier for in vitro studies.

Excised human skin or epidermis (which acts as semipermeable 'membrane') is inserted in between the two compartments shown in Fig.99-A.

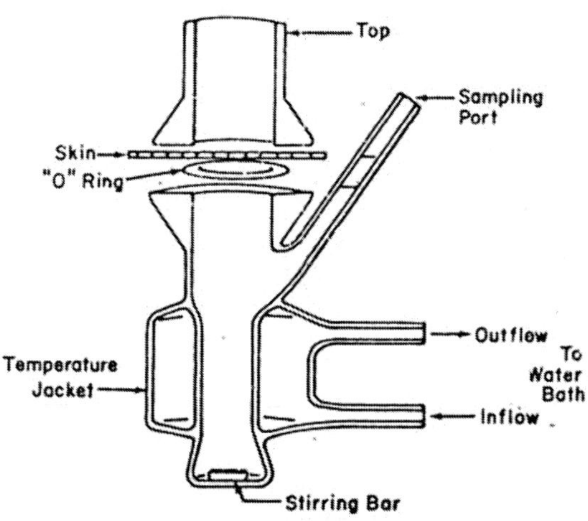

Fig. 99A

The stratum corneum side of the 'membrane' should be towards the top compartment. The top compartment, the 'membrane' and the lower compartment are arranged as shown in Fig. 98-A. Drug in solution is filled in the top compartment (solution is on the stratum corneum side of the 'membrane') Water is filled in the lower compartment till it makes contact with the opposite side of the 'membrane' completely. Body temperature 37°C ± 1°C is maintained in the lower compartment by circulating warm water through the water jacket of the lower compartment. The top compartment is kept open to ambient laboratory environment. Through the sample port in the lower compartment, samples are withdrawn periodically and analysed for the drug content by a suitable technique. The transport (or diffusion) rate of the drug through the membrane' is, then evaluated

2. Theory of dissolution

Dissolution is a process of separation of solute molecules from the solid solute and the dispersion of the separated molecules into the solvent to which the solute has been added. It is the transfer of mass from solid phase to a liquid phase. Dissolution rate refers to the rate at which a solid dissolves in a solvent.

In 1897, Noyes and Whitney developed an equation based on Fick's second law to describe dissolution process of drugs.

$$\frac{dc}{dt} = K(c_s - c_t) \quad (14)$$

where $\frac{dc}{dt}$ = dissolution rate of drug

k = proportonality constant

c_s = saturation concentration of drug

c_t = concentration of drug at time t

$c_s - c_t$ = concentration gradient

Noyes and Whitney maintained a constant surface area for their study on dissolution. But such a condition is not always possible. Hence Bruuner and Tolloczko modified the equaiton (14) by introducing the surface area, S which is variable

$$\frac{dc}{dt} = k_1 S(c_s - c_t)$$

(a) Diffusion Layer Model Theory

In 1904, Nernst proposed film theory (i.e. *diffusion-layer model theory)* According to this theory, dissolution of solid immersed in a liquid is con-

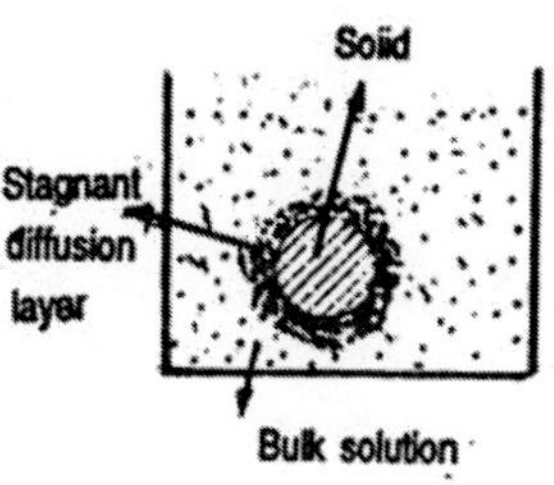

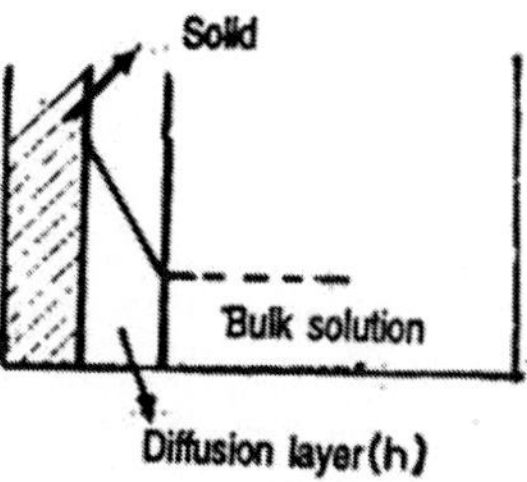

Fig. 100

sidered to be composed of two steps. (Fig.100)

1. Liberation and solution of solute molecules from the solid surface forming a thin stagnant layer or film 'h' around the solid particle.

2. Transport or diffusion of the molecules from the stagnant layer at the boundary to the bulk of the liquid under the influence of concentration gradient.

The overall rate of mass transfer is dependent on the step which is slower. In film theory the first step is faster and the second step diffusion is much slower. Therefore, diffusion is the rate-limiting step.

Brunner in the same year expanded the equation based on the above facts and included the diffusion coefficient D, the thickness of the stagnant layer 'h' and the volume of the dissolution medium, v producing.

$$\frac{dc}{dt} = k_2 \frac{DS}{vh}(c_s - c_t) \quad ... (16)$$

where k_2 = intrinsic dissolution rate constant which is dependent on the nature of the drug.

Sink condition

Gastro intestinal tract is supplied with blood vessels through which absorbed drugs are carried from the site of absorption to various tissues of the body due to movement of blood within the blood vessels Moreover, the drug concentration on either side of the epithelial layer of intestinal wall approaches equilibrium in a short time and thus the gastrointestinal wall acts as a 'natural sink'. That means the drug is transported into the blood stream instantaneously once it gets into or dissolves in the gastrointestinal tract. Therefore under *in vivo* conditions, there is no concentration buildup and hence concentration gradient has no retarding effect on dissolution rate.

In order to simulate the '*in vivo*' sink conditions, *in vitro* testing is conducted using large volume of dissolution medium or else the dissolution medium is replinished constantly with fresh solvent (i.e. it is to be assumed that the concentration of the solute in the disolution medium never reaches more than 10 to 15%)

Assuming that $\overline{c_s >> c_t}$ the equation (16) becomes

$$\frac{dc}{dt} = k_2 \frac{DS}{vh} \cdot c_s \quad \text{... (17)}$$

For a given chemical substance c_s and D are constant. The equation becomes

$$\frac{dc}{dt} = k_2 \frac{S}{vh} \quad \text{... (18)}$$

If the volume of the dissolution medium and the surface area are **kept** constant during dissolution testing.

$$\frac{dc}{dt} = K \text{ where } K = k_2 \frac{S}{vh} \quad \text{... (19)}$$

The equation predicts a constant dissolution rate under sink condition and it represents a zero-order kinetic process. This is possible by using a non-dissintegrating disc containing the chemical substance. (i.e. the drug)

But for a dissolving crystal or a regular solid dosage form like tablets and capsules, surface area changes gradually. In such cases, dissolution is expressed by Hixson and Crowell Cubic Root Law. It is given as

$$w_0^{1/3} - w^{1/3} = Kt \quad \text{... (20)}$$

where w_0 = original mass of the drug

w = mass of the drug remaining to dissolve at time t

K = dissolution rate constant.

(b) Penetration or Surface Renewal Theory (Danckwert's model)

This theory disapproves the existence of stagnant layer and approves turbulance in the dissolution medium and so on solid-liquid interface. Eddies or packets of agitated fluid (macroscopic mass) reach solid-liquid interface at random due to eddy current. They absorb solute by diffusion and carry it to the bulk of the solution. The eddies or pack-

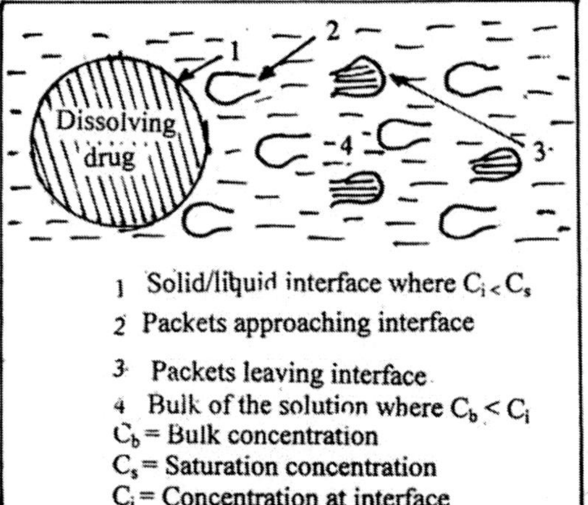

Fig. 101 Surface renewal theory

ets are replaced by fresh eddies. Because of this, drug concentration at the solid/liquid interface never reaches C_s (maximum solubility) and has lower limiting value of c_i. It is mathematically expressed as

$$\frac{dq}{dt} = A\,(C_s - C_i)\,\sqrt{\gamma D} \quad \ldots (21)$$

where r = rate of surface renewal or interfacial tension and C_i = concentiation at the interface

The model is depicted in Fig.101

(c) Double Barrier or Unlimited Solution Theory (Interfacial barrier model)

As per this model, an intermediate concentration can exist at the interface as a result of solvation mechanism rather than diffusion. Taking crystals as examples, each crystal will have a different interfacial barrier. It is given by an equation,

$$G = K_i\,(C_s - C_i) \quad \ldots (22)$$

G = dissolution rate per unit area

K_i = effective interfacial transport constant.

2.1. Factors affecting dissolution rate

(a) *Surface area*

The improved *Noyes-Whitney* equation shows that the rate of dissolution is increased by an increase in the surface area of the solids. The reduction in particle size of a given mass of powder particles leads to an increase in surface area of the powder and this is given by an equation

$$S = \frac{6m}{d\rho} \quad \ldots (23)$$

where S = surface area

m = mass of powder particles

d = diameter of particles

ρ = density of powder particles

The surface area increase of powders may be achieved by particle size reduction and solid dispersion techniques. The increased surface area offers more contact with solvents and as a result, the powders go into solution very fast. This concept is used widely for achieving faster rate of dissolution in the preparation of liquid dosage forms. It is also used in the preparation of *aromatic waters* such as *Camphor water*. Drug is dispersed as very fine powders in water soluble inert carriers by solid dispersion techniques to get more surface area and more solubility. Urea, PVP, PEG are examples of carrier substances.

Two types of surface area of interest

(a) Absolute surtace area: It is the surface area of solid surface of any particle

(b) Effective surface area: It is the area of solid surface exposed to the dissolution medium.

The dissolution rate is directly proportional to effective surface area only. Micronization of poorly aqueous soluble drugs like griseofulvin, chloramphenicol and salts of tetracycline resulted in superior dissolution than simple milled forms due to increase in surface area. This may lead to reduction in dose. Micronized griseofulvin dose is twice less than milled form because of increased absorption efficiency.

(b) *Porosity*

Increased surface area may be achieved by producing porous materials (i.e. with more porosity). Through the pores, the solvent enters and brings about easy dissolution of porous materials. The effect of porosity ceases to be of importance when the pores are of molecular dimensions because the entry of solvent molecules becomes difficult.

Lyophilisation (freeze drying) is a process by which porous and friable mass of drug powder is obtained and this brings about faster dissolution.

(c) *Temperature*

For most of the solids which dissolve with positive heat of solution, the solubility is increased with increase in temperature. The dissolution rate of such a solid can be increased at a higher temperature and brought down to original temperature (or room temperature) provided solubility of the solid at the room temperature is not exceeded.

This principle is utilized to extract most of the heat stable drugs from crude drugs by using warm or hot solvents. When complete dissolution has been achieved, the solution is cooled to room temperature.

The rate of dissolution of solids with negative heat of solution is increased with a decrease of temperature (For example, paraldehyde dissolution rate is increased with lowering of temperature)

(d) *Agitation*

The dissolution of a solid in a solvent is a mass transfer phenomenon from the solid to the bulk of the liquid through the stagnant boundary layer. Any attempt to quicken the process of mass transfer from the solid to the boundary layer or from the boundary layer to the bulk of the liquid will increase the rate of dissolution. Also that any attempt which reduces the thickness of the boundary layer brings more and more solvent in contact with the solid surface. This will increase the rate of dissolution. All the above could be achieved by agitating or stirring the system provided that the mass transfer from the solid solute is not the slower process. That is, it is not the rate determining step.

In large scale manufacture, variety of agitators are used to quicken the process of dissolution in liquid formulations.

(e) *Positioning of the solute*

Since the solution is more denser than the solvent, keeping the solid solute at the top portion of the solvent in a container, the rate of dissolution can be increased. In this method, the denser solution formed near the solute will sink and as a result fresh solvent comes in contact with the solute. This process is used in extraction of soluble materials from crude drugs. A combination of positioning and agitation provides added effect that causes still greater rate of dissolution.

(f) *Polymorphism*

Different polymorphic forms of a substance show different dissolution rates. For example predisolone shows three polymorphic forms with different dissolution rates and aspirin shows two polymorphic forms with different dissolution rates.

Of the various polymorphic forms of a substance, one of the forms is more stable with less energy (i.e. high melting point, least aqueous solubility). The other forms are metastable with more energy (i.e. low melting point, more aqueous solubility) Meta stable forms have a tendency to convert to stable form. Metastable form show more bioavailability because of greater aqueous solubility Eg. chloramphenicol palmitate shows three polymorphic forms A, B, C of which B form shows the best bioavailability and A form is virtually inactive biologically.

Polymorphs differ from each other in their solubility, density, and melting point also.

(g) *Hydrates / solvates (pseudo polymorphism)*

Dissolution is directly related to solubility of drugs. The dissolution rate can be predicted from the solubility of a drug as

$$\frac{dq}{dt} = 2.24\, c_s \qquad \text{... (24)}$$

A crystalline form of a drug can either be a plymorph or a molecule adduct or both. In an adduct, solvent molecules are incorporated in the crystal lattice of the solid and are called as solvates. The entrapped solvent is called solvent of crystallisation The solvates can exist in different crystalline forms called pseudo polymorphs.

The anhydrous form of a drug has greater aqueous solubility than the hydrates. For example, anhydrous forms of theophylline and ampicilline have higher water solubilities, dissolve at a faster rate and show better bioavailability than their monohydrate and trihydrate forms respectively.

(h) *Salt form of the drug*

Most drugs are either weak acids or weak bases. Easiest approach to enhance their dissolution rate and solubility is to convert them into their salt forms. Eg. Barbiturates and sulphonamides are converted into their sodium/potassium salt and alkaloids are converted into their salt form by reaction with hydrochloric acid or sulphuric acid.

(i) *Viscosity*

An increase in the viscosity of a solvent interferes with the dissolution rate of solutes. This interference slows down the diffusion of drug molecules from the boundary layer to the bulk of the liquid. Therefore, an increase in viscosity of the solvent decreases the dissolution rate of solids.

(j) *Surface active agents*

They increase the dissolution rate by increasing the wettability of solutes by solvent, by increasing the penetration of solvent into solutes and by facilitating greater etching of crystal surfaces by solvent. Eg. Tween 80 is used as wetting agent

2.2. Dissolution study

Many methods have been described for the *in vitro* dissolution study of granules, tablets and capsules. The dissolution study is insisted in Pharmacopoeias for tablet and capsule dosage forms to know the dissolution pattern of a drug which will ensure subsequent bioabsorption and bio availability of the drug. Bioabsroption refers to the drug absorption through biological membranes i.e. through gastro intestinal tact membrane whereas bioavailability refers to the rate and ex-

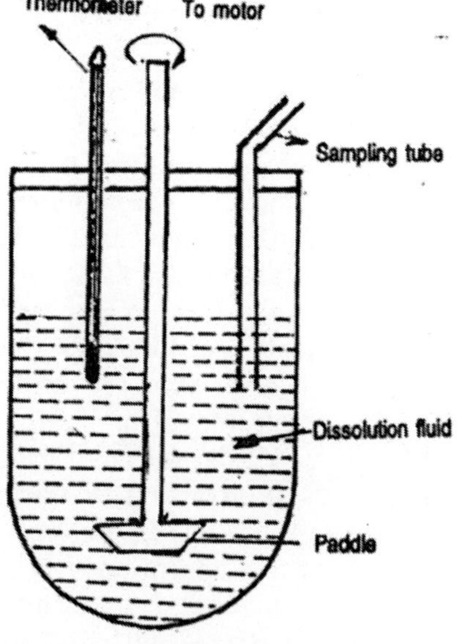

Fig.102. Dissolution Apparatus (Schematic)

tent of drug absorption into the systemic circulation.

The mostly used apparatus for the study of dissolution rates of active drugs from solid dosage forms such as tablets and capsules is the **basket** or paddle type dissolution apparatus.

The USP basket type apparatus (*Apparatus I*) (Fig.102) consists of a 40 mesh stainless steel basket attached to the end of a stirring shaft which in turn is attached to a variable speed motor. A tablet or a capsule is placed within the basket and immersed in the dissolution fluid and rotated at a speed specified or desired. The dissolution fluid may be water, buffer solution or dilute hydrochloric acid solution simulating the gastric pH. The dissolution fluid is maintained at a temperature of 37°C. During the run, samples are withdrawn at different times for analysis. The volume of the dissolution fluid is maintained constant by replacing the amount of sample removed with fresh dissolution fluid. The analysis of the sample withdrawn at different specified times is undertaken to obtain the dissolution rate.

The USP paddle type apparatus (*Apparatus-2)* consists of a round bottomed 1000 ml container to hold the dissolution fluid. This container is placed in a constant temperature bath to maintain the temperature at 37°C. (body temperature). The cover for this container has three openings for the stirring shaft, thermometer and the third one for the removal of samples and replacement of dissolution fluid. The stirring shaft is attached to variable speed motor and the other end to a paddle. During the operation, a tablet is dropped into the dissolution fluid and the fluid is stirred with the paddle positioned vertically near the bottom of the container at the specified speed (50 or 100 rpm). Samples are withdrawn at various intervals of time, replacing at the same time with the fresh dissolution fluid equal to the amount of sample withdrawn. Samples are analysed to obtain the dissolution rates of the drug from the dosage form (capsule or tablet).

In near future dissolution study may be insisted for suspensions, ointment, suppositories etc.

3. Drug Release

The release of a drug from a dosage form involves both dissolution and diffusion. Fig. 103. In recent times, sustained action tablets and capsules are made in which drugs are dispersed in a polymeric matrix. Hence drug release from polymeric matrices may be considered.

3.1. Drug release from homogeneous polymer matrices

The drug release from a homogeneous polymer matrix tablet dosage from (Fig. 103) that gradually erodes and releases the drug in the bathing medium is given by *Higuchi.*

$$Q = \left[D\,(2A - C_s)C_s t \right]^{1/2} \quad \text{... (25)}$$

$$\frac{Q}{t^{1/2}} = \left[D\,(2A - C_s)C_s \right]^{1/2} \quad \text{... (26)}$$

where Q = quantity of drug released or depleted at time t

D = diffusion coefficient

C_s = the solubility or saturation concentration of drug in the matrix

A = total concentration of drug (dissolved and undissolved) in unit volume of the matrix.

If $A > C_s$, the equation reduces to

$$\frac{Q}{t^{1/2}} = \left[2(ADC_s \right]^{1/2} \quad \text{... (27)}$$

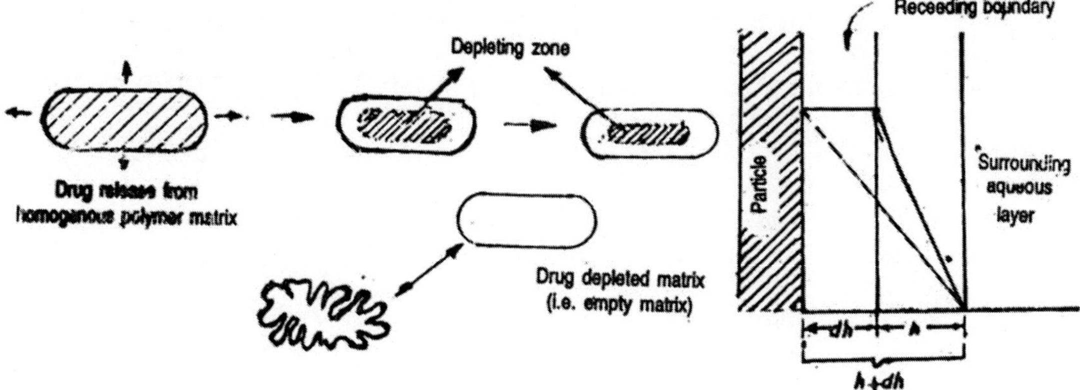

Fig.103

Drug release is assumed to involve dissolution of the drug in the polymer matrix of an erodable tablet and diffusion out from the surface of the tablet. As the drug is getting released diffusion distance is also getting increased and the depletion zone moves to the center of the tablet.

The equation indicates that the quantity of drug released is proportional to the square roots of A, D, C_s and t The rate of release can be altered by in creasing or decreasing C_s in the polymer. The release rate is also affected by A.

3.2. Drug release from granular matrix

Drug release from granular matrix is based upon the mechanism in which the surrounding liquid enters into the granular matrix, dissolves the drug and the dissolved drug is leached out leaving a sheet of polymer and empty pores. Hence the volume and length of the openings (pores or channels) are accounted for in the second from of *Higuchi* equation

$$Q = \left[\frac{D\varepsilon}{\tau} (2A - \varepsilon C_s) C_s t \right]^{1/2} \quad \text{... (28)}$$

$$\frac{Q}{t^{1/2}} = \left[\frac{D\varepsilon}{\tau} (2A - \varepsilon C_s) C_s \right]^{1/2} \quad \text{... (29)}$$

where e = total porosity of the matrix after the drug has been released

τ = tortuosity – length of the opening with branching and bending. The length is increased due to branching and bending as compared to the shortest straight through pores. A straight pore has a tortuosity of unity.

This equation has been adapted to describe the kinetics of lypophilisation (freeze-drying)

Equations (25) and (28) can be conveniently reduced to

$$Q = Kt^{1/2}$$

where K is a constant. Once the data have been collected from the diffusion study, the amount of drug released (Q) versus square root of time ($t^{1/2}$ i.e. $\sqrt{t}$) is plotted. The plot will be linear if the drug release from the matrix is diffusion controlled.

For the preparation of matrix devices, three major type of materials are used They are:

(i) insoluble plastics (eg. Methyl accylate - methyl methacrylate, polyvinyl chloride and polyethylene.

(ii) hydrophilic polymers (eg. Methyl cellulose, sodium carboxyl methyl cellulose, and hydroxy propyl methyl cellulose and

(iii) Fatty compounds (eg. carnauba wax and glyceryl tristearate)

The most common method is to prepare matrix material and then compress the mixture into tablets. Matrix embedding technique is used for making sustained release formulation.

3.3. Multilayer diffusion

Multilayer diffusion is involved in diffusion across biologic barriers and in the diffusion of gas molecules or liquid molecules across the walls of containers and plastic packaging material.

In the case of multilayer diffusion, the resistance R to diffusion in each layer is equal to the reciprocal of the permeability coefficient P of that particular layer

$$\text{i.e. } R = \frac{1}{P} \qquad \text{... (30)}$$

The total resistance is the sum of resistances offered by individual layers

$$R = R_1 + R_2 + \ldots + R_n$$

$$\text{or } R = \frac{1}{P_1} + \frac{1}{P_2} + \ldots + \frac{1}{P_n}$$

$$\text{or } R = \frac{h_1}{D_1K_1} + \frac{h_2}{D_2K_2} + \ldots + \frac{h_n}{D_nK_n}$$

$$\left(\text{hence } P = \frac{DK}{h}\right)$$

where h = thickness of the layer, D = diffusion coefficient, K = distribution coefficient

The total resistance for a multilayer (two-ply) barrier is given by

$$R = \frac{1}{P} = \frac{h_1}{D_1K_1} + \frac{h_2}{D_2K_2}$$

$$= \frac{h_1D_2K_2 + h_2D_1K_1}{D_1K_1D_2K_2}$$

$$\text{or } P = \frac{D_1K_1D_2K_2}{h_1D_2K_2 + h_2D_1K_1} \qquad \text{... (31)}$$

In multilayer diffusion, lag time is additive for a series of layers and is not discussed.

In multilayer diffusion, the rate of diffusion is controlled by the layer which offers the greatest resistance. Considering a membrane separating the donor and receptor sides containing the aqueous phases, the membrane with the two stagnant liquid layers one on either side constitute a multilayer (three-ply) barrier. This may be represented as shown in Fig.104

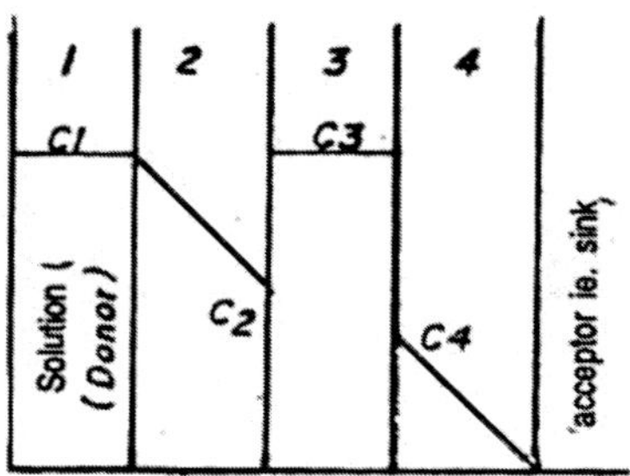

2 and 4 static diffusion layers

3 membrane layer

Fig. 104. Multilayer diffusion (in three-ply layer)

The permeability of this multilayer comprising one membrane and two static diffusion layers one on either side is

$$P = \frac{1}{R} = \frac{D_mKD_2}{h_mD_a + 2h_a D_mK} \qquad \text{... (32)}$$

where $K = \frac{C_3}{C_4} = \frac{C_3}{C_2}$

and hence, only one coefficient K appears in the denominator in the equation.

The flux through the membrane and the two aqueous diffusion layers (a three-ply barrier) is given as

$$J = P(C_1 - C_5) \quad \text{... (33)}$$

When receptor serves as sink $C_5 = 0$, and C_1 being donor compartment concentration, it may be represented as C_d.

$$\text{then, } J = PC_d \quad \text{... (34)}$$

$$J = \frac{D_m D_a K C_d}{h_m D_a + 2h_a D_m K} \quad \text{... (35)}$$

where D_m = diffusion coefficient across the membrane

D_a = diffusion coefficient across aqueous layers

K = partition coefficient

h_m = membrane thickness

h_a = aqueous diffusion layer thickness

C_d = donor concentration

The overall diffusion through this multilayer barrier is controlled by slower of the two (i.e. either the membrane layer or the two aqueous diffusion layres). That is diffusion may be under membrane control or under aqueous diffusion layers.

When the membrane offers more resistance than that is offered by the resistances of the aqueous diffusion layers i.e. $P_m << P_a$. Then the diffusion across the membrane is the rate determining step.

i.e. when $h_m D_a >> 2h_a D_m K$

the equation

$$J = \frac{D_m K D_a C_d}{h_m D_a + 2h_a D_m K} \quad \text{... (36)}$$

reduces to

$$J = \frac{D_m K D_a C_d}{h_m D_a}$$

$$\text{or } J = \left(\frac{D_m K}{h_m}\right) C_d \quad \text{... (37)}$$

This means that the concentration gradient that controls the flux resides in the membrane.

When the aqueous diffusion layers offer more resistance than that offered by the membrane layer i.e. $P_a << P_m$, then the diffusion across the aqueous diffusion layers is the rate determining step. In otherwords diffusion is controlled by diffusion across aqueous diffusion layers.

i.e. when $2h_a D_m K >> h_a D_a$

$$\text{the equation, } J = \frac{D_m K D_a C_d}{h_m D_a + 2h_a D_m K} \quad \text{... (38)}$$

reduces to

$$J = \frac{D_m K D_a C_d}{2h_a D_m K}$$

$$= \left(\frac{D_a}{2h_a}\right) C_d \quad \text{... (39)}$$

This means that the concentration gradient that controls the flux now resides in the aqueous diffusion layers.

3.4. Release of drugs soluble in topical vehicles and matrices

When the drug is soluble significantly in the ointment base, *Higuchi* equation does not provide satisfactory results with the experimental data. Then a quadratic expression introduced by *Bottari et al* is used.

$$Q^2 + 2DRA^*Q - 2DA^*C_s t = 0 \quad \text{... (40)}$$

in which $A^* = A - \frac{1}{2}(C_s + C_v)$

where Q = amount of drug released per unit area of the dosage form

D = effective diffusivity of the drug in the vehicle

A = total concentration of the drug

C_s = solubility of the drug in the vehicle.

C_v = concentration of the drug at the vehicle barrier interface

R = resistance afforded to diffusion by the barrier

The equation proposed by *Botteri et al* is useful to determine diffusion of drugs in ointment vehicles or homogeneous polymer matrices when C_s becomes significant when compared to A.

4. Diffusion principles in Biologic systems

Drug molecules pass through living membranes mainly by passive transport and active transport. In passive transport, diffusion occurs through gastrointestinal membrane from a region of high concentration in the gastrointestinal tract to a region of low concentration on the side of systemic circulation i.e. from mucosal side to serosal side. In active transport, drug molecules are carried across the membrane by an enzyme or biological carrier. It can occur against concentration gradient.

The rate of drug transport is influenced by the physiochemical properties of the drug, the nature of the membrane and the concentraion gradient of drug across the membrane. The net movement of drug is towards

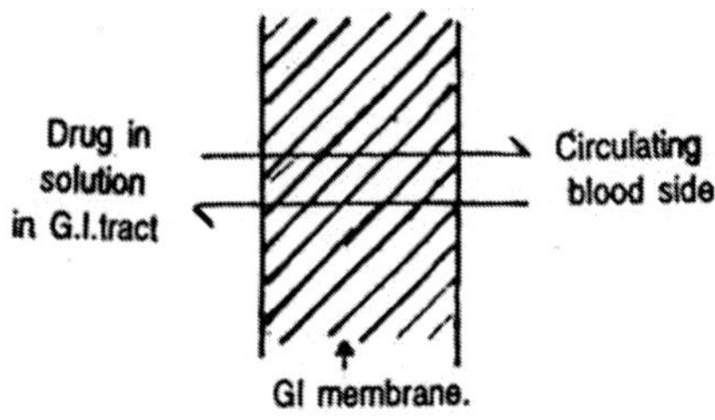

Fig. 105

blood (Fig.105) because of sink condition provided on the serosal side.

Many drugs are weakly acidic or basic. They exist in aqueous solutions as ionized and unionized species. The fraction of drug that exists as ionized or unionized is determined by the dissociation constant of the drug. (K_a value) and the pH of its aqueous environment in accordance with ***Henderson-Hasselbalch*** equation for weak acids and bases.

For weak acid $pH = pK_a + \log \frac{[A^-]}{[HA]}$

For weak base $pH = pK_a + \log \frac{[B]}{[HB^+]}$

where [HA] = is the concentration of the non-ionized weak acid

$[A^-]$ = is the concentration of the conjugate base and pK_a = dissociation exponent for the weak acid

[B] = is the concentration of the base and

$[BH^-]$ = is the concentration of its conjugate acid.

For the weak base,

$$pK_a = pK_w - pK_b \qquad \text{... (41)}$$

The proportion of ionisation **for a** weak acid is given by

$$= \frac{1}{1 + \text{antilog}\,(pK_a - pH)} \quad \ldots (42)$$

and for a weak base

$$= \frac{1}{1 + \text{antilog}\,(pH - pK_a)} \quad \ldots (43)$$

Equal amounts of ionized and unionized forms of a drug will be present when $pH = pK_a$

4.1 pH Partition Principle

Gastrointestinal membrane being predominantly lipophilic, it is permeable to unionized species of a drug in preference to ionized species of the drug. Therefore the rate of passive transport of a weak acid or base is related to the fraction of the drug that exists in the unionized form in the gastrointestinal fluids at the site of absorption. Consequently, according to pH *partition hypothesis,* the absorption of weakly acidic or weakly basic drugs will be determined chiefly by the concentration of unionzed drug form at the site of absorption.

The degree of ionization of a drug in a solution can be calculated using *Henderson-Hasselbalch* equations for weak acids and bases if pK_a of the drug and pH of the solution are known

However this principle has been found to be only partly applicable in biologic systems as evidenced from *in vivo* and *in vitro* studies. That is, both the ionized and unionized forms are significantly transported in contradiction with this simple pH *partition hypothesis.*

4.2. Modification of pH partition principle

According to Ho and *Hugachi,* the pH partition principle for the absorption of drugs is only approximate. They proposed that absorption of relatively small ionic and nonionic species through the *aqueous spores* within the membrane and aqueous diffusion layer in front of the membrane should also be considered. Other physiological factors must also be accounted for in the process of absorption.

Absorption is also influenced by the bulk flow rate (it indicates the rate of movement through intestinal tract) and the lipophilicity of the drug. Effect of flow rate on transit time influences differences in absorption. The transit time refers to the time of displacement of a volume of solution within the intestinal segment and is given by the volume divided by the flow rate. As the small intestine present a large surface area for the absorption process, this region serves as the major site of absorption for weak electrolyte drugs though the drugs are ionized.

4.3. Percutaneous absorption of tropically applied drugs

Percutaneous absorption involves three steps –

1. dissolution of drug in the vehicle

2. diffusion of the dissolved drug to the surface of the skin form the vehicle and

3. penetration of drug molecules through the skin layers.

Of the above three steps, the slowest one determines the rate of absorption of the drug through percutaneous route. Usually the rate limiting step is the passage of drug molecules through skin layers principally the *stratum corneum* (i.e. third step). Therefore this step controls the permeation of drugs into the systemic circulation.

In general the factors which affect permeation (or penetration) of drug molecules are governed by

1. concentration of the dissolved drug

2. partition coefficient between the skin and the vehicle and

3. diffusion coefficients in the vehicle and the skin barriers.

Diffusion of drug molecules through skin layers can be influenced by the components of the dosage form (mainly solvents and surfactant) hence proper choice of vehicle plays an important role in ensuring bioavailability of topically applied drugs.

4.4. Buccal absorption

Buccal absorption occurs in accordance with pH partition principle. The drug absorption is related to pK_a of the drug compound and its lipid-water partition coefficient. Buccal absorption is considered to be a first order process due to non-accumulation of drug on the blood side.

IX. COLLOIDS

Colloidal dispersions consist of two distinct phases – a dispersed phase and a dispersion phase or medium. The dispersed phase is also called as internal or discontinuous phase and the dispersion medium, as external or continuous phase

Colloidality is due to a state of subdivision of the dispersed phase. Thus, it is the particle size that distinguishes colloidal dispersions from solutions and coarse dispersions. Dispersed phase in the colloidal state may have the dimensions in the range of 0.001 μ to 0.5 μ.

Solids may be dispersed in colloidal state into solid (zinc oxide paste zinc oxide and starch in petrolatum; Tooth paste containing dicalcium phosphate or calcium carbonate with sodium carboxy methyl cellulose binder) or liquid (bentonite magma) or gas (smoke, dust etc.). Liquids may also be dispersed into solid (absorption bases), in aqueous medium (Hydrophilic Petrolatum USP) or in liquid (mineral oil emulsion) or in gas (mist, fog etc.) Gases form colloidal dispersion with solids (solid foam) and with liquids (carbonated beverages).

Molecular dispersion, colloidal dispersin and coarse dispersion from one another may be distinguished as follows:

	Molecular/ dispersions (true solution)	**Colloidal dispersions**	**Coarse dispersions**
Size	0.001 micron	> 0.001 micron to 0.5 micron	> 0.5 micron
Visibility	Invisible even in electron microscope	Detected in an ultramicroscope and visible in an electron microscope	Visible to naked eye and in light microscope
Retension	Pass through ultra filter and ordinary filter paper	Pass through ordinary filter paper but are retained by dialysis or ultrafiltration membrane	Do not pass even through ordinary filter
Diffusion	Undergo rapid diffusion	Diffuse very slowly	Do not diffuse

Note: 1 micron or micrometer
(1μ) = 10^{-6} meter = 10^{-3} mm

The size of colloidal particles contributes to optical and kinetic properties and the charges present on the particles account for their electrical properties. They usually carry a charge either positive or negative on their surface.

1. Types of colloids

Colloidal dispersions can be broadly classified into two types – lyophilic and lyophobic. A third type is the association colloid with both the tendencies (i.e. lyophilic and lyophobic). This classification is based on the affinity or interaction between the dispere phase and dispersion medium. (*lyo* means solvent, *philic* means loving, and *phobic* means hating)

1.1. Lyophilic colloids

When there is considerable interaction (or affinity) between the disperse phase and the dispersion medium, a lyophilic colloid is formed. In this dispersion, the colloidal particles are solvated and they are mostly solids in liquids. Lyophilic colloid may be hydrophilic or lipophilic. If water is the dispersion medium, it is hydrophilic. With lipophilic colloids, non-aqueous vehicle forms the dispersion medium.

Hydrophilic colloids may be further subdivided as follows:

(a) Some true solutions, for example: Water-soluble polymers such as acacia and povidone (polyvinyl pyrrolidone) form molecular dispersion in water. The molecules are of colloidal dimensions and hence are classified under colloids. b) Gelled solutions are solutions of polymers at high concentrations, They are also formed at temperatures at which their solubility in water is low. Solutions of gelatin and starch set to gels on cooling whereas solution of methyl cellulose sets to a gel on heating. If water is the dispersion meidum, they are called hydrogels. c) Particulate dispersion do not form molecular dispersions but they are present as minute particles of colloidal dimensions. Bentonite forms hydrosol with water.

Lipophilic colloids exhibt affinity for oils and hence are called olephilic. Oils are non polar and some examples are mineral oil, vegetale oils such as cotton seed oil and essential oils such as lemon oil.

Thus, lipophilic colloids may be true solutions, gelled solutions or particulate dispersions.

Polystyrene and gum rubber form colloidal solutions with benzene. Aluminium sterate dissolves or disperese in cotton seed oil. Activated charcoal forms particulate dispersion or sol in all oils.

Lyophilic colloidal dispersions are thermodynamically stable. Lyophilic substances form colloidal dispersions spontaneously with the dispersion medium. They are also reversible i.e. they can be formed after the dispersion medium has been removed. ((ie.) the residue obtained after the removal of dispersion medium forms again a colloidal dispersion on adding to the dispersion medium.

1.2. Lyophobic colloids

Lyophobic means solvent-hating. In lyophobic dispersions, the colloidal particles exhibit little interaction or affinity with the dispersion medium. Hence in lyophobic collidal dispersions, the particles are not solvated.

Lyophobic colloids may be hydrophobic and lipophobic. Hydrophobic dispersion have water as dispersion medium and the particles are not hydrated. Hydrophobic colloids may have lipophilic substances as disperse phase in water. For example, polystyrene (or gum rubber), steroids, magnesium stearate form hydrophobic colloidal dispersions with water. Hydrophobic colloids are formed with substances like gold, silver and sulphur which are not lipophilic. Lipophobic dispersions are water-in-oil emulsions.

1.3. Association colloids

Association colloids result from the formation of 'micelles' (a micelle is formed by a group of surfactant molecules) when a surfactant in sufficient amount is added to the dispersion medium (water). As a surfactant has two distinct portions of opposing solution affinities (polar and non polar) within its molecule, the molecules tend to associate to form groups called micelles within the medium. The micelles are of colloidal dimensions. Such micelles are formed at and above a concentration called *critical micellar concentration* of the surfactant. Some 50 or more molecules aggregate together to form micelles which are of the order of 50Å (0.005 μ) in diameter. They are thermodynamically stable and also reversible.

Various colloids are differentiated as follows:

	Lyophilic colloid	**Association colloid**	**Lyophobic colloid**
Disperse phase	Consists of large organic molecules of colloidal dimensions or particulate substances.	Consists of aggregate (micelles) of small organic molecules or ions of subcolloidal sizes. eg: surfactants form associated colloids (micelles) in water.	Consists of inorganic particles (i.e. aggregate of atoms; eg. gold colloid.)
Solvation	Disperse phase particles are solvated with dispersion medium	Hydrophilic portions of the molecule is solvated i.e. hydrated	No solvation (i.e. little interaction between disperse particles and the dispersion medium)
Spontaneity	Spontaneously formed once the disperse phase comes in contact with dispersion medium. They are thermo-dynamically stable and are also reversible.	Spontaneoulsy formed at and above the critial micellar concentration (CMC). They are thermo-dynamically stable and are reversible.	Does not form spontaneously but it needs special methods for the formation. Hence they are thermodynamically unstable and are irreversible.
Viscosity due to disperse phase	Viscosity of the dispersion medium is increased. At sufficiently high concentrations they may become a gel. Viscosity is related to the solvation effects and gel formation to the shape of the disperse phase molecules.	Viscosity increases as micelles increase in number and become asymmetric.	Viscosity is not increased.

	Lyophilic colloid	Association colloid	Lyophobic colloid
Effect of electrolytes	Dispersions are stable generally in the presence of low concentrations of electrolytes. But at high concentrations, the disperse phase may be salted out (coagulation)	Electrolytes reduce CMC and at higher concentrations salting out of the disperse phase occurs.	Sensitive even to low conentrations of electrolytes. This is due to neutralisation of the charge on the colloidal particles. Lyophilic colloids exert a protective effect on lyophobic colloids.

2. Properties of Colloids

Properties of colloids may be classified into optical properties, kinetic properties and electric properties.

2.1. Optical properties

The optical properties may be discussed under Faraday Tyndall effect, electron microscope and light scattering.

(a) The Faraday Tyndall effect

When a narrow strong beam of light is passed throught a colloidal dispersion, the path of the light can be observed at right angles under an ultramicrocope. This colloidal particles appear as bright spots against a dark background due to the scattering of light by the colloidal particles on the path of the beam. This optical property is actually due to discrete variations in the refractive index caused by the presence of particles (or by a small scale density fluctuations.)

(b) Electron Microscope

The ordinary light microscope cannot reveal the structural details of particles which are separated by smaller distanes since the resolving power is

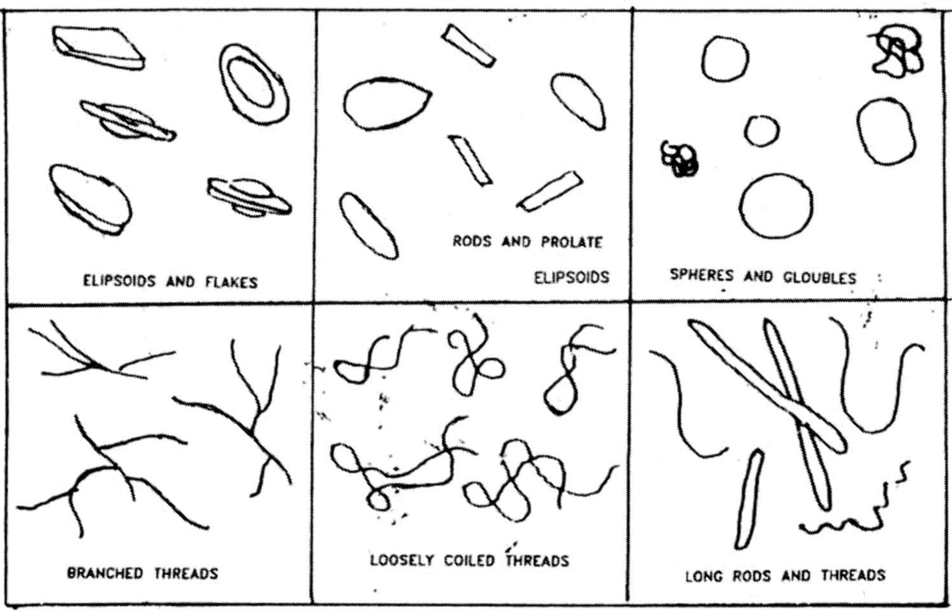

Fig. 106. Different Shapes of colloidal particles

about 2000 Å (0.2 μ). The electron microscope has a higher resolving power of about 5 Å as it employs electron beam with wavelength of about 0.1 Å. The resolving power is directly related to the wavelength of the radiation. The shorter the wavelength, the more efficient is the resolving power.

The electron microscope is used to get pictures of actual particles. It is used to study the size, shape and structure of colloidal particles.

c) Light Scattering

The scattering of light and the intensity of the scattered light depend upon the following factors.

1. wavelength of the incident beam
2. intensity of incident beam
3. difference in the refractive inded between the particles and he medium
3. difference in the refractive index between the particles and the medium

The intensity of light scattered may vary at different angles and can be used to obtain some indication as to the shape of the macromolecules (collidal particles). It may be used to obtain the molecular weight and the equation giving the relationship is given as

$$\frac{Hc}{\tau} = \frac{1}{M} + 2Bc \qquad \text{... (1)}$$

where τ = turbidity measured at 90° to the incident beam.

c = concentration of the solute in grams/litre

M = molecular weight.

B = interaction constant related to the degree of nonideality of the solution.

H = a constant for a particular system and is given by

$$H = \frac{32\pi^3 n^2 \left(\frac{dn}{dc}\right)^2}{3\lambda^4 N} \qquad \text{... (2)}$$

where n = refractive index

$\frac{dn}{dc}$ = change in refractive index with concentration

N = Avogadro's number

λ = wavelength

A plot of $\frac{Hc}{\tau}$ versus c yields a straight line at low concentration with a slope of 2B. The intercept on the $\frac{Hc}{\tau}$ axis will give the value of 1/M and hence the molecular weight.

Light scattering, apart from the molecular weight determination is used for the study of proteins, synthetic polymers, association colloids and lyophobic sols. Light scattering may be used to study the pattern of self association and thus, it showed that bile salts associate to form dimers, trimers and tetermers. Colloids may exhibit colour due to the wavelength of the scattered light. For example a colloidal dispersion of gold chloride is deep red in colour and that of silver iodide is yellow.

2.2 Kinetic properties

Kinetic properties may be classified as follows:

	Thermally induced	Gravitationally induced	Externally induced
(a)	Brownian movement	Sedimentaion	Viscosity
(b)	Diffusion		
(c)	Osmosis		

(a) Brownian motion (or movement)

The macromolecules or the colloidal particles are engaged continuously and randomly in motion within the medium. These molecules or particles are buffeted by the molecules of the dispersion medium. This random movement and bombardment with the molecules of the dispersion medium are unceasing and erratic and such a movement of colloidal particles (zig-zag movement) within the medium is termed *Brownian motion.* Brownian motion is decreased by an increase in viscosity of the medium and the motion may also be stopped by increasing this viscosity to a certain level.

(b) Diffusion

Diffusion is a process where the solute molecules move from a region of higher concentration to one of lower concentration until the concentration of the system attains equilibrium and it is due to Brownian motion.

Diffusion is given by Fick's law

$$dq = -DS\frac{dc}{dx} \cdot dt \qquad \ldots (3)$$

D = diffusion coefficient and is defined as the amount of material diffusing (dq) per unit time acros 'nit area 'S' when concentration grdient $\frac{dc}{dx}$ is unity. Diffusion coefficient is a measure of mobility of the dissolved molecules of colloidal dispersion in a liquid medium.

It is possible to compute the molecular weight of approximately spherical particles from the diffusion coefficient by substituting the data obtained from diffusion experiments in Fick's law. The expression to calculate the molecular weight is given as

$$D = \frac{RT}{6\pi r\eta N}\sqrt[3]{\frac{4\pi N}{3M\bar{v}}} \qquad \ldots (4)$$

where M = molecular weight

$\bar{v}$ = partial specific volume (volume in cm^3 of 1 g of solute)

η = viscosity of the solvent

R = molar gas constant

T = absolute temperature

r = radius of spherical particle

N = Avogadro's number

Using this method, the molecular weight of egg albumin and haemoglobin have been obtained.

(c) Osmotic pressure

Using osmotic pressure, it is possible to estimate the molecular weight and this is based on *Vant Hoff's* equation (The osmotic pressure of colloidal solutions is usually very small, since it is one of the colligative properties).

$$\pi = cRT \qquad \ldots (5)$$

Replacing the c (concentration) with $\frac{c_g}{M}$ the equation is

$$\pi = \frac{c_g}{M} \cdot RT \qquad \ldots (6)$$

where c_g = gram of solute per liter of solution

M = molecular weight

This equation is valid for very dilute solutions in which the interaction between the solute and the solvent molecules is little and the partcles are spherical.

When the solute molecules become solvated (i.e. there is interaction between solute and solvetn molecules) there is deviation and the plot of $\frac{\pi}{c_g}$ versus c_g will not be linear and it is necessary to extrapolate the curve to infinite dilution to obtain $\frac{RT}{M}$. The equation is then written as given below when there is interaction between the solvent and the solute molecules.

$$\frac{\pi}{c_g} = \frac{1}{M}RT + Bc_g \quad \text{... (7)}$$

where B = a constant and is the slope for any particular system and it gives the degree of interaction between the solvent and the solute molecules.

Using this method, the molecular weight of polymers have been obtained.

(d) Sedimentation

Brownian motion keeps the dissolved molecules of colloidal dimensions (macromolecules) or colloidal particles in continuous random motion. Hence it offsets sedimentaion due togravity. Therefore, stronger force must be employed to bring about sedimentation of colloidal particles. Even the usual laboratory centrifuges cannot cause sedimentation. This can be undertaken by the use of *ultracentrifuge.* This producessedimentation at a reasonable rate.

In this method, the colloidal dispersion is placed in a glass cell in the ultracentrifuge rotor and arranged in such a way that light passing through the cell may be photographed. The centrifuge is rotated at 50,000 rev/min and higher. The rate of sedimentation is derived from the change in the light absorption or a change in refractive index during centrifugation. The change in refractive index is translated into peaks on a photographic plate. The peaks obtained are termed as *Schlieren patterns* and the peak gives the position of boundary at each time. The boundary (x) refers to the boundary between the solvent and the high molecular weight component (dispersed in the medium) in the centrifuge cell. The boundary and hence the sedimentation is located by a change in refractive index.

Svedberg sedimentation coefficient as it is called is given by

$$S = \frac{\ln\left(\frac{x_2}{x_1}\right)}{\omega^2 (t_2 - t_1)} \quad \text{... (8)}$$

where x_1 and x_2 are measured on the *Schlieren photographs* obtained at times t_1 and t_2. ω is equal to 2π times the speed of the rotor in revolutions per second.

The molecular weight of a polymer is obtained by using the expression.

$$M = \frac{RTS}{D(1 - \bar{v}\rho_o)} \quad \text{... (9)}$$

where R = gas constant

T = absolute temperature

$\bar{v}$ = partial specific volume of the polymer

ρ_o = density of the solvent

S = *Svedberg sedimentaion coefficient* determined at 20°C.

D = diffusion coefficient obtained by calculation from diffusion data collected at 20°C.

With ultracentrifugation (sedimentaion rate method) it is possible not only to determine the molecular weight but also to determine the relative homogeneity of a polymer with respect to molecular wight. If a sample consists of a component of definite molecular weight, the *Schlieren pattern* yields a single sharp peak at any moment during the run. If several peaks appear on the *Schliern pattern,* it indicates components with different molecular weights. Thus, insulin is found to be a monodisperese (homogeneous) sysem with a molecular weight of about 6000 and gelatin, a polydispere system with fractions of molecular weight from 10,000 to 1,00,000.

(e) Viscosity

Viscosity studies provide not only the molecular weight of polymers but also information regarding the shape of the particles in a colloidal dispersion.

Einstein equation provides a quantitative expression for the flow of disperse systems consisting of spherical particles.

$$\eta = \eta_o(1 + 2.5\ \varphi) \quad \text{... (10)}$$

where η = viscosity of thedispersion

n_o = viscosity of the dispersion medium

φ = volume fraction ofthe disperse phase (It is the volume of disperse phase divided by the total volume of the system)

The following viscosity coefficients as applied to colloidal dispersions may be defined with respect to Einstein equaiton.

Relative viscosity η_{rel}) is defined as:

$$\eta_{rel} = \frac{\eta}{\eta_o} = 1 + 2.5\varphi \quad \text{... (11)}$$

Specific viscosity (viscosity ratio incremnet) may be defined as the relative increase in viscosity produced by the presence of dispersed phase.

$$\eta_{sp} = \frac{\eta - \eta_0}{\eta_0} = \frac{\eta}{\eta_0} - 1 \quad \text{... (12)}$$

hence $\eta_{sp} = 2.5\ \phi$

In addition, since the volume fraction is directly related to the concentration of the disperse phase, the above equation may be given in the form.

$$\eta_{sp} = Kc \quad \text{... (13)}$$

where K = constant

c = concentration (weight of disperse phase in 100 cm^3 of total dispersion)

The above equation applies to dilute systems only. The equation is usually written as a power series for more concentrated dispersions.

$$\eta_{sp} = \alpha c + \beta c^2 + \ldots$$

Reduced viscosity is obtained by dividing the above equation through 'c' and the ratio of specific viscosity to concentration is

$$\frac{n_{sp}}{c} = \alpha + \beta c + \ldots \quad \text{... (14)}$$

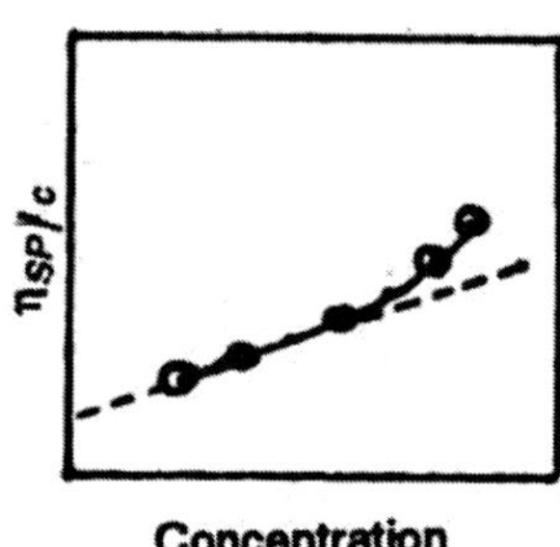

Fig. 107

Intrinsic viscosity [η] is the intercept on 'y' axis obtained by extrapolating the line obtained by plotting $\frac{n_{sp}}{c}$ versus 'c' to definite dilution. (Fig. 107)

The intrinsic viscosity is used to calculate the approximate molecular weight of a polymer and the equation relating this [η] is given

$$[\eta] = KM^a \quad \text{... (15)}$$

where K and a are constant for a given polymer solvent system and are obtained from other experiments at fixed temperatures.

This method is used to determine the average molecular weights of starch, dextran and gelatin preparations which are used as plasma extenders. The determination of intrinsic viscosity is used as a test in the BP (British Pharmacopoeia) for the standardisation of Dextran injection, a plasma substitute.

The shape of the colloidal particles (disperse phase) influences the viscosity of the dispersion. Spherocolloids produce dispersions of relatively low viscosity where linear particles produce dispersions of relatively high viscosity. Viscosity increase is due to salvation effect. When the degree of solvation is more, the dispersion becomes more viscous. Thus if a linear colloid is placed in a solvent for which it has a low affinity, the linear particles tend to aasume a spherical shape and as a result, the viscosity falls. Therefore, the viscosity studies provide a means of detecting changes in the shape of flexible colloidal particles and macromolecules.

2.3. Electric properties of colloids

The colloidal particles are either negatively charged or positively charged. The particles are negatively charged in kaolin, sulphur, and arsenious sulphide colloidal dispersion while in ferric hydroxide and other metal hydroxide colloidal dispersions, the particles are positively charged. In some other colloidal dispersions such as proteins, the charge of the particles may be positive, negative or neutral depending upon the pH of the medium.

The particles in a colloidal dispersion acquire charges from several sources mainly by ionisation or by adsorption

Ionisation

A fatty acid soap (sodium stearate), which forms micelles of colloidal size in aqueous solution, ionises to Na^+ and $C_{17}H_{35}COO^-$ so that the micelle particle carries a negative charge.

Proteins contain both basic and acidic groups in the molecule ($NH_2 - R - COOH$). In alkaline solution, the acidic group – COOH ionises to $-COO^-$ carrying a negative charge. In acid solution the basic group $-NH_2$ ionises to $-NH_3^+$ so that the particle now carries a positive charge. At an intermediate pH known as isoelectric point, the protein molecule exists as zwitter ion when the net charge is zero provided no other ions are adsorbed. It can be depicted as

$R\begin{smallmatrix} NH_2 \\ COO^- \end{smallmatrix}$	$R\begin{smallmatrix} NH_3^+ \\ COO^- \end{smallmatrix}$	$R\begin{smallmatrix} NH_3^+ \\ COOH \end{smallmatrix}$
negative ion	zwittter ion	positive ion

(A protein is least soluble at its isoelectric point and can be readily precipitated.)

Adsorption

A non-ionising colloidal particle may preferentially adsorb ions and thus the particle may acquire a positive or negative charge depending upon which ion (that is anion (–) or cation (+)) is adsorbed. This adsorption of ions through which particles acquire electric charges usualy occur in hydrophobic colloids.

(a) Electric double layer (refer under suspensions also)

The presence of electric charges on the dispersed particles influences the distribution of positive and negative ions in the vicinity of the solution that surround each particle. (Fig. 108) Thermal motion also has some influence over the distribution of charges. The resultant effect is that each particle is surrounded by an electric double layer.

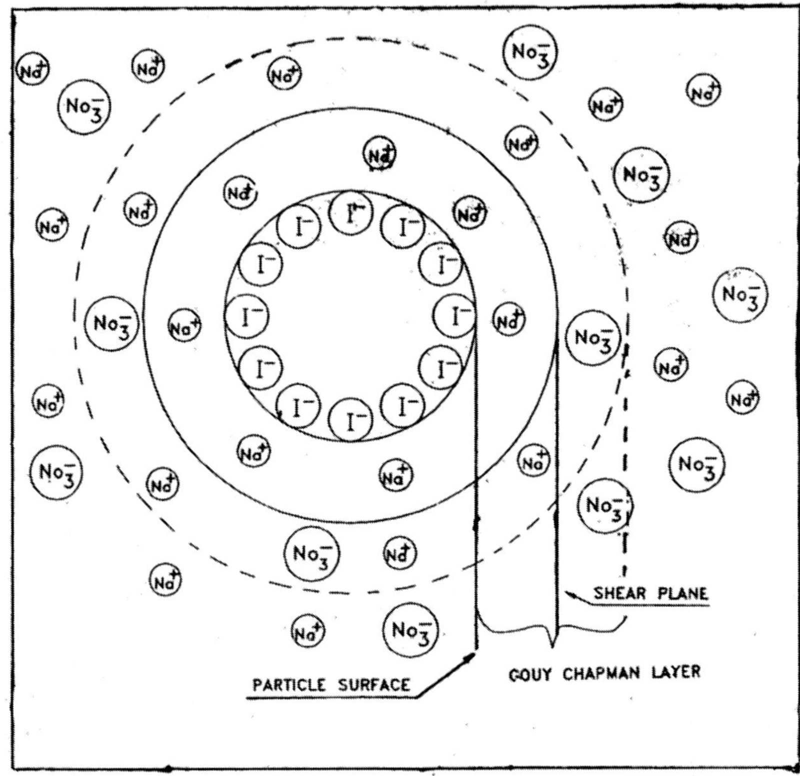

Fig. 108

Consider the colloidal dispersion of silver iodide prepared by chemical reaction.

$$AgNO_3 + NaI \longrightarrow AgI + NaNO_3$$

The colloidal dispersion in water as such will contain Ag^+, I^-, Na^+, NO_3^- and traces of H^+ and OH^- ions.

If the reaction is conducted with an excess of sodium iodide, the surface layer of silver iodide contains more I^- ions than Ag^+ ions and the aqueous solution contains relatively high cocentration of Na^+ and NO_3^-, a lower concentration of I^- and traces of H^+, OH^- and Ag^+ ions.

As the silver iodide particles contain more of I^- ions on their surface, each of the silver iodide particles is negatively cahrged and it attracts positive ions from the solution and repels **negative ions. As a result, the aqueous** solution in the vicinity of the surface (of the AgI particle) contains a much higher concentration of Na^+ ions (called *counter ions* or *gegenions*) and much lower concentration of NO_3^- ions than in the bulk of the solution. The counter ions Na^+ are pulled closer to its surface and these counter ions tend to stick to the surface as closely as possible as the hydration sphere (the solvated layer on the particle) permits. At the same time, thermal motion (of water molecules) tends to disperse the Na^+ ions throughout the solution. As a consequence, the layer of counter ions surrounding the particle is spread out and however the Na^+ concentration is highest in the immediate vicinity of the negative surface forming a compact layer called. Stern layer and the concentration of Na^+ ions decreases with distance from the surfae throughout a diffuse layer called *Gouy-Chapman* layer. Thus the negatively charged surface layer is surrounded by a cloud of Na^+ ions (counter ions) required for electroneutrality. The combination of the two layers of oppositely charged ions constitutes an electric double layer. The thickness of the double layers usually ranges from 10 to 100 Å (0.001 to 0.1 μ)

The presence of electrical double layer around each particle in a colloidal dispersion gives rise to electrokinetic effect. They are electrophoresis, electro-osmosis, sedimentation potential, and streaming potential.

(b) Electrophoresis

When an electric field is applied to a colloidal dispersion, the particles carying the charge (+ or –) move towards the electrode of opposite charge. When the particles move, the counter ions within the hydration shell (i.e. solvation layer) are dragged along with (the surface of the hydration shell is the plane of shear) and the counterions in the free or mobile solvent (i.e. medium) move towards the other electrode. This phenomenon is termed *elecrophoresis.*

Electrophoretic mobility may be observed using electrophoresis cell. The cell is fitted with two electrodes. After taking a colloidal dispersion in the cell, an electric potential is applied across the electrodes. Under the influence of electric field, the colloidal particles move towards the oppositely charged electrode. The velocity of the particles can be measured by timing their movement. This maybe undertaken by observing through an ultramicroscope (and hence called microelectrophoresis) which is fitted along with.

The rate of movement of individual colloidal particle is a function charges on the particle and is directly related to the *zeta potential.* The equation relating zeta potential to the mobility of ion is

$$\zeta = \frac{v}{E} \cdot \frac{4\pi\eta}{\varepsilon} \times (9 \times 10^4) \quad \text{... (16)}$$

where ζ = zeta potential in volts

v = velocity of movement of colloidal particles in cm/sec. in an electrphoresis cell of definite length in cm.

η = viscosity of the medium in poises

ε = dielectric constant of the medium

E = externally applied potential gradient in volts/cm.

$\frac{v}{E}$ = mobility

(9×10^{14}) converts electrostatic units into volts.

When the dispersion medium is water and all the measurement are carried out at 20°C, the equation reduces to approximately

$$\zeta = 150\frac{v}{E} \quad \text{... (17)}$$

The electrophoretic mobility of colloidal particles can be obtained from the rate of movement of the boundary of a sol using a simple 'U' tube apparatus. This method is calleld *moving boundary electrophoresis* and is used when the particles cannot be observed individually with an ultramicroscope. In moving boundary electrophoresis a sharp bounary is formed between the sol and the pure dispersion medium and its movement in an electric field is obseved visually if the disperse phase is coloured. If the disperse phase is colourless, the boundary is observed by a change in refractive index along the column using special optical equipment (*Schlieren method*).

This method permits the dentification of different colloidal components in a mixture, to study the electrophoretic mobility of the components in the mixture (eg. proteins) and to estimate the relative amounts present.

(c) Electro-Osmosis

If the charged colloidal particles are rendered immobile, the counterions in the free water (dispersion medium) move towards the electrode of opposite charge dragging the water along with. This flow of liquid meidum under the influcence of electric field is called *electro-osmosis* and is considered to be opposite in principle to that of electrophoresis. The pressure produced by the process of electro-osmosis is called *electro-osmotic pressure*.

The atmosphere of counterions around the particles (apart from the counterions present within the hydration shell of the charged colloidal particles) confers a charge on the dispersion medium. This causes the liquid medium to move towards the opposite electrode under the influence of electric field. This phenomenon can be observed if the tube containing the colloidal dispersion is plugged in the middle with a porous material and across which a potential is applied. This method also provide for obtaining zeta potential.

(d) Streaming potential

It is the converse of electro-osmosis. In this a potential difference is created, if the liquid is forced to flow past a plug or bed of cahrged particles by applying hydrostatic pressure. The potential differene is created because of the displacement of counterions in the free water. This method too can be used to determine the zeta potential.

(e) Sedimentation potential

This is the reverse of electrophoresis. When the colloidal particles are caused to undergo sedimentation, a potential difference is created.

(f) Donnan Membrane Effect

The presence of charged macromolecules (colloid) on one side of a semipermeable membrane (impermeable to macromolecules) will affect the diffusion of smallions (may be drug ions) through the semipermeable membrane. This effect is due to the electrical gradient across the membrane and as a consequence, the charged drug ions of the same charge as the macromolecules are driven to the opposite side of the membrane altering the concentration of the drug ions. This is termed *Donnan membrane equilibrium* or simply *Donnan effect* and may be demonstrated as follows.

Suppose a colloidal solution, the colloidal particles of which carrying negative charges, together with its counterions say R^-Na^+ contained in a semipermeable membrane sac is placed in a solution of a drug (such as sodium salicylate) which has ionised into positive and negative ions say Na^+D^-. Considering the volumes of solutions on the two sides of the membrane (i.e. inside and outside) are equal, the system at quilibrium is represented as follows

Outside (o)	Inside (i)	
Na^+	R^-	$\begin{bmatrix} Na^+ \\ D^- \end{bmatrix}$ Permeable ions
D^-	Na^+ D^-	R^--Non Permeable ion

In acccordance with the principle of escaping tendencies (refer chemical potential under *Thermodynamics*), the conentration of the drug (Na^+D^-) must balance on both sides of the membrane.

i.e. $[Na^+]_o [D^-]_o = [Na^+]_i[D^-]_i$ ... (18)

where o and i indicate outside and inside respectively.

Applying electroneutrality on both sides,the concentration of positively charged ions must balance the concentration of negatively charged ions

i.e. outside: $[Na^+]_o = [D^-]_o$

and inside: $[Na^+]_i = [R^-]_i + [D^-]_i$

Substituting these in the equaiton (18) we obtain

$$[D^-]_o [D^-]_o = \left([R^-]_i + [D^-]_i \right)[D^-]_i$$

$$[D^-]_o^2 = [R^-]_i [D^-]_i + [D^-]_i [D^-]_i$$

$$[D^-]_o^2 = [D^-]_i^2 + [R^-]_i [D^-]_i$$

$$= [D^-]_i^2 \left(1 + \frac{[R^-]_i}{[D^-]_i} \right)$$

$$\frac{[D^-]_o^2}{[D^-]_i^2} = 1 + \frac{[R^-]_i}{[D^-]_i}$$

$$\text{or } \frac{[D^-]_o}{[D^-]_i} = \sqrt{1 + \frac{[R^-]_i}{[D^-]_i}} \quad ... (19)$$

From the above equation which represents the ratio of concentrations of diffusiable drug anion outside and inside the membrane at equilibrium, it may be understood that a charged polyelectrolyte (i.e. macromolecules of colloidal dimensions) inside a semipermeable membrane sac would affect the equilibrium concentration ratio of a diffusible anion. That is it tends to drive the ion (drug ion) of like charge on its side to the opposite side through the semipermeable membrane. It is simple mathematics that when $[R^-]_i/[D^-]_i$ is equal to 15, the ratio of $[D^-]_o/[D^-]_i$ is equal to 4 and when $[R^-]_i/[D^-]_i$ is equal to 120, the ratio $[D^-]_o/[D^-]_i$ will be equal to 11. Thus the addition of an anionic polyelectrolyte such as sodium carboxy methyl cellulose to a diffusible drug anion such as potasium benzyl penicillin and sodium salicylate enhances the difusion of drug and thereby increases the absorption. The presence of charged electrolyte not only influences the distribution of drug ion acording to *Donnan equilibrium* but will bring about an increse in the rate of transfer of the drug across the membrane.

It was also found that ion exchange resins, sulphate and phosphate ions which do not diffuse through intestinal wall, will drive anionic drug from the intestinal tract into the blood stream.

[Note: Charges on the membrane also influence the permeability of anions and cations. For example, a collodion membrane which posseses fixed anions and mobile cations will be selectively permeable to cations and the anions being repelled by negatively charged membrane. Conversely, a membrane with fixed cations and mobile anions will be selectively permeable to anions).

3. Preparation of Colloids

3.1. Lyophilic colloids

Owing to the affinity of lyophilic colloids for the dispersion medium, these colloidal sols are formed with relative ease.As there is considerale interaction between the disperse phase and the liquid dispersion medium, (i.e. there is extensive solvation) lyophilic dispersions are formed spontaneoulsy when the material is placed in contact with the liquid. They are thermodynamically stable and reversible.

Acacia and povidone will readily disperse if added to water forming a colloidal solution. Gelatin and starch form colloidal sols spontaneously (especially in hot water) with water.

3.2 Lyophobic collids

Most of the lyophobic dispersions are hydrophobic dispersions. They include aqueous dispersions of insoluble organic and inorganic compounds which have a low degree of hydration (i.e. less interaction).

Because, hydrophobic dispersions are intrinsically unstable and there is little interaction between the disperse phase and the dispersion medium (water), preparation of hydrophobic colloids need special methods. They can be prepared by dispersion or condensation. Dispersion methods involve breaking up of disperse phase to small particles of colloidal dimensions through comminution (particle size reduction) or peptisation. Condensation methods involve the aggregation of small molecules or ions to produce particles of colloidal dimensions.

(a) Dispersion methods

Colloid mills, ball mills and micronizers can be used to reduce the size of particles to colloidal range. In a colloid mill, the coarse material is sheared in a narrow gap between a static cone and a rapidly rotating cone.

In electrical dispersion method (*Bredig's arc method*) the dispersions of metals are prepared by producing an electric arc by keeping close together two electrodes made of the metal immersed in water containing traces of KOH as stabiliser in a container cooled by ice externally. The intense heat vaporises some of the metal and the vapor condenses into colloidal particles in water. Eg. silver, gold, platinum hydrosols.

Colloidal dispersions of many materials such as sulpur and graphite can be obtained by means of ultrasonic waves. Emulsification by ultrasound waves is the method of choice for the preparation of soyabean oil in water emulsions for intravenous injection.

Peptization is a process of dispersion of a precipated material (flocculated or aggreagated) into smaller aggregates of colloidal dimension.

It can be effected by the addition of deflocculationg or peptizing agents. Peptizing agents may be surfactants, water soluble polymers, or ions which are adsorbed at the particle surface and they do not allow aggregation and keep the particles in the colloidal dimensions. Peptization can also be brought about by the removal of flocculating agents (electrolytes) and their removal results in the disintegration of floccules into small particles of colloidal dimensions. Even washing the gelatinous precipitate of aluminium hydroxide with water bring about peptization. Ferric hydroxide yields a sol when ferric chloride (Fe^{3+} being common ion) is added to it.

(b) Condensation methods

A change in solvent may bring about the formation of colloidal particles by condensation. If an alcoholic solution of resin is poured slowly into water, a colloidal dispersion of resin in water is obtained. In the same manner, when an alcoholic solution of sulphur is mixed with water a bluish white colloidal dispersion of sulphur is produced. This is usually undertaken in the presence of a stabilising agent to prevent precipitation.

Colloidal dispersion may be obtained by chemical reaction also. Colloidal sulphur may be obtained by bubbling hydrogen sulphide gas into an aqueous sulphur dioxide solution

$$2H_2S + SO_2 \longrightarrow 3S + 2H_2O$$

Colloidal dispersions of aluminium hydroxide may be prepared by hydrolysing aluminium chloride

$$AlCl_3 + 3H_2O \longrightarrow Al(OH)_3 + 3HCl$$

By double decomposition of sodium chloride with silver nitrate, a colloidal dispersion of silver chloride may be obtained.

$$NaCl + AgNO_3 \longrightarrow AgCl + NaNO_3$$

A colloidal dispersion of ice in ether or chloroform can be obtained by freezing saturated solution of organic solvent in water.

4. Purification of colloidal dispersion

Most of the hydrosols contain low molecular weight water soluble impurities. Presence of electrolytes as impurities in hydrophobic dispersion has to be avoided as it may coagulate such dispersions. These dissolved impurities are removed by dialysis, electrodialysis and ultrafiltration. However traces of electrolytes are needed to stabilise the collidal system.

(a) Dialysis

It is a process based on unequal rates of passage of solutes and solvent through microprous membrane.

Dialysis can be simply carried out by placing the colloidal sol in a *cellophane sac* and immersing this sac into a large vessel of water. Low molecular weight solute molecules diffuse out into water while the colloidal particles remain inside the sac entrapped. Dialysis rate may be increased by increasing the area through which diffusion occurs, by stirring, and by maintaining a high concentration gradient across the membrane. To maintain a high concentration gradient, the water is replaced continuously or changed repeatedly. Diffusion is continued until the colloidal sol is substantially free form the low molecular weight solute molecules.

Ordinary dialysis is relatively slow and if electrolytes of low molecular weight are the impurities to be removed, the process of dialysis can be speeded up by applying an electric potential. This technique is called *electrodialysis*.

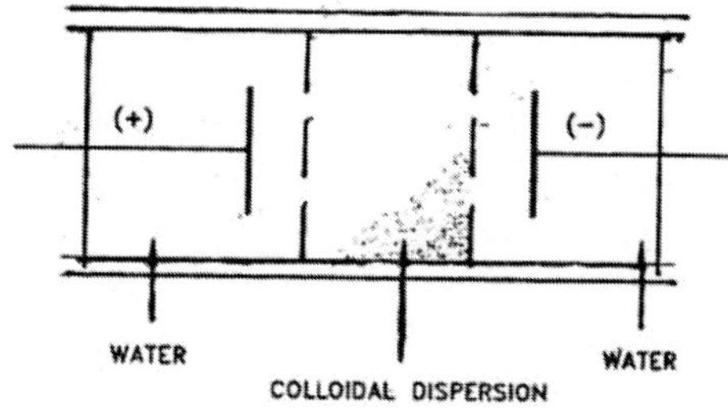

Fig.109 Electro-dialysis cell

An electrodialysis cell consists of three compartments two outer and one center compartment. (Fig. 109) The center compartment is separated from the two other compartments on either side by two dialysis membranes supported by screens. The two outer copartments contain water and also the electrodes and the center compartment the colloidal sol. When an electric potential is aplied, the anions move from the sol into the anode compartment while the cations move from the sol into the cathode compartment. The collidal particles in the center compartment move towards one of the membranes according to the charge they carry. Non electrolyte solute molecules (impurities) diffuse into both the outer compartments. As the density increases due to the accumulation of colloidal particles, they settle to the bottom of the center compartment as shown in Fig.109. The supernatant liquid can be changed be decantation and thus the purified colloidal sol is prepared by electrodialysis and decantation. This process is called *electrodencantaiton.*

(b) Ultrafiltration

Keeping the colloidal sol in a compartment that is closed by a dialysis membrane pore size 0.003 μ and applying pressure, the liquid and the low molecular weight solute molecules are forced through the membrane. The colloidal particles are retained within the compartment. This separation process is called *ultrafiltration.* Ultrafiltration differs from dialysis only in that the passage of the small molecules of low molecular weight through the membrane is enhanced by applying usually high positive pressures. As the process uses high pressure, the membrane is usually supported by a fine wire screen.

In order to avoid the increase in the concentration of colloidal particles and to remove the dissolved impurities completely the water is replaced continuously or repeatedly by equal amounts of deionised water. To maintain uniform concentration throughout the colloidal sol, the sol is stirred.

Ultrafiltration has been used to separate and purify colloidal sols. An ultrafilter may be an ordinary filter paper impregnated with collodion (Cellelose tetranitrate dissolved in a mixture of ether and alcohol in the ratio of 3:1) or cellophane (a regenerated cellulose in swollen gel sheet) or cellulose acetate.

5. Stability of Colloids

The stability of a colloidal dispersion depends on two factors

1. presence of charge (+ or –) on the dispersed colloidal particles

2. Solvent sheath surrounding each dispersed particle

When the colloidal particles collide as a result of *Brownian movement*, the above two factors will prevent mutual adherence. It may be said that the stability of lyophobic colloid is largely due to the electric charges on the surface of the dispersed particles and for lyophilic sols it is the solvent sheath that is significant in stabilising the system.

In a lyophobic sol as already mentioned, the particles are stabilised by the presence of electric charges on their surfaces. The like charges present on their surfaces prevent the coagulation of the particles. Coagulation is a process where the colloidal particles aggregate together resulting in the precipitation of the dispersed particles and ultimately the colloid dispersion breaks up i.e. becomes unstable. Coagulation may be brought about by the addition of electrolytes which reduce the zeta potential (the sign and magnitude of charge on the particle). The coagulating power of electrolytes depends on the valency of the active ion (ion causing coagulation). The higher the valency of the ion, the greater is the precipitating power. This is known as the *Schulze-Hardy* rule.

The stability of lyophobic colloids is described by DLVO theory *(Derjaguin, Landau, Verwey and Overbeek)*. The forces operating on colloidal particles in a dispersion are the repulsive and attractive forces. The repulsive forces are due to overlapping of electrical double layer and the attractive forces are due to London type *van der Waals* forces. The potential energy of repulsion (V_r) is shown in Fig. 110 and also the potential energy of attraction V_a. V_0 indicates the composite potential energy, (i.e. interaction curve).

As two particles approach each other in the medium a weak attractive

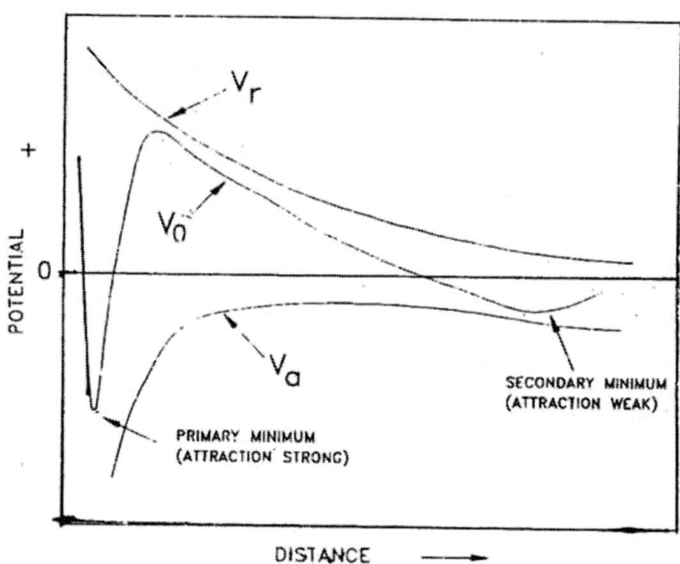

Fig. 110

force exists beyond the range of electrical double layer repulsive forces. This attractive region is called the *secondary minimum*. It is responsible for flocculation. This is significant in the controlled flocculation of suspended particles in a coarse dispersion (a suspension). If the thermal energy is equal or greater than the repulsive barrier (V_r) the particles come closer and encounter strong attraction in the *primary minimum* shown in the figure. When the particles get into the primary minimum, they coagulate.

At low electrolyte concentration, the repulsive forces predominate so that the particles experience only a repulsive force upon approach. The particles remain individually and the system is called dispersed or peptized. At a high concentration of electrolyte, the electrical double layer forces are greatly diminished. As a result, *van der Waals* forces of attraction predominate and the particles encounter net attractive forces ending in coagulation.

Lyophilic and association colloids are thermodynamically stable and they exist in true solution. Hence, they do not coagulate on the addition of moderate amounts of electrolytes. However they coagulate if sufficient amount of electrolyte is added. This is termed 'salting out'. The coagulating power in lyophilic colloids amy be given by *Hofmeister or lyotropic series*. Anions of Hofmeister series in decreasing order of precipitating power are citrate, tartrate, sulfate, acetate, chloride, nitrate, bromide and iodide. The precipitating power is due to their ability to dislodge solvent sheath from the colloidsl particles.

Even the addition of solvents such as alcohol and acetone which are having greater affinity to water causes coagulation of colloidal particles. Addition of such solvents lowers the dielectric constant of the medium which is unfavourable for the colloidal particles.

When oppositely charged hydrophilic colloids are mixed, the particles may separate from the dispersion medium to produce a layer rich in the colloidal aggregates. This colloidal rich layer is known as *coacervate* and the phenomenon is termed *coacervation*. Such a coacervation is enountered when solution of gelatin carrying positively charged gelatin particles below its isoelectric point is mixed with a negatively charged acacia particles (pH-3) in solution in a certain proportion (Coacervation of gelatin may also be brought about by the addition of alcohol, sodium sulfate or starch solution). The mutual coagulation of two sols of oposite charge is due to mutual attraction, adsorption and precipitation.

If the coacervate is formed in a stirred suspension of insoluble drug particles, the coacervate will surround the drug particles. The particles thus coated can be separated and dried. This technique forms the basic of one method of microencapsulation.

6. Sensitisation and Protection

When a small amount of hyrophilic or hydrophobic colloid is added to a hydrophobic colloid of opposite charge, the hydrophobic colloid becomes sensitive.

Sensitisation is attributed to a reduction in zeta potential below the critical value (the value below which coagulation occurs). It is also reasoned that it is due to a reduction in the thickness of the ionic layer surrounding the colloidal particles.

However, addition of large amounts of hydrophilic colloid tends to stabilise the system because of adsorption of hydrophilic colloid particles forming a protective cover on the hydrophobic collid particles. This phenomenon is called *protection*. The hydrophilic sol used for the purpose of protecting the hydrophobic colloid is known as protective colloid. This protective power of hydrophilic colloid may be given in terms of "*gold number*".

The *gold number* is the weight in milligrams of the protective colloid (on dry basis) needed to prevent a colour change from red to violet in 10 ml of gold sol on the addition of 1 ml of 10% solution of sodium chloride. Gold numbers of some protective colloids are given below.

Protective colloid	Gold number (mg)
Gelatin	0.006 – 0.01
Albumin	0.1
Acacia	0.1 – 0.2
Tragacanth	2

7. Micellar solubilisation

Surfactants are amphiphiles i.e. they have both polar and non-polar groups. This dual nature confers a surfactant with a property to get adsorbed at the interface (air-water, oil-water, or solid-water interfaces) in which the hydrophilic group (polar group) is oriented towards the aqueous phase and the hydrocarbon group (non-polar group) is oriented towards air or oil in contact with the aqueous phase.

Consider a beaker in which water is taken. If a surfactant in increasing amount is dissolved, its concentration in the solutions increases. The molecules of the surfactant form adsorbed monolayers at air-water and glass water inter-surfaces. the monolayers at the interfaces, as more surfactant is dissolved, become more and more crowded until they are so tightly packed that further accommodation needs excessive compression of the surfactant molecules. At this stage beyond this concentration in the bulk of the solution what occurs is the formation of micelles. This process starts at a certain concentration called *critical micellar concentration* (CMC)

The shape of micelles formed in dilute solutions of surfactants is approximately spherical and the micelles are of colloidal dimension. The polar groups of the surfactant molecules are arranged in the outer sphere in an aqueous solution and non-polar groups are oriented towards the center forming the spherical core of the micelle. The micelles are spherical. When the concentration of the surfactant is increased,the micelles may regroup into cylindrical or rod-shaped structures whose diameter may be slightly less than twice the fully extended length of the monomers (single molecules).

A solution of surfactant forming micelle at critical micellar concentration has a different dielectric constant from the interior of the micelle. Such solutions of surfactants have the ability to dissolve substances that are normally insoluble or only slightly soluble in the solvent alone (i.e. dispersion medium). This is known as *micellar solubilisation.* The solubilized substance is called *solubilizate.*

The location where the solubilizates get solubilized depends on the balance between polar and non-polar properties of the molecule (Fig. 111). Saturated hydrocarbons are dissolved in the non-polar part of the micelle (i.e. micelle interior) in aqueous solutions. If the solubilizate itself is amphiphilic (eg. n-alcohols), it forms mixed micelles i.e. the molecules are incorporated into the palisade layer of the micelle. weakly polar groups of substances are drawn deeper into the palisade layer. Water soluble polar substances are considered to be adsorbed on the surface of the micelle. It is believed that in the micelles formed from non-ionic surfactants, hydrogen bonding substances such as phenol and *p*-hydroxybenzoic acid are taken up between the polyoxyethylene groups. It is considered that they undergo inclusion within the polyoxyethylene exterior.

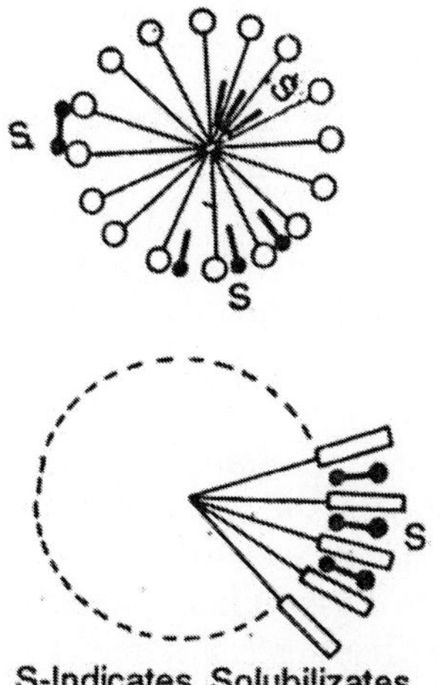

Fig.111. A Micelle with Solubilizates

The micellar solubilisation has been used to bring into solution a wide range of poorly soluble materials. They may be volatile oils, coal tar, phenobarbital, sulphonamides, vitamins, hormones, and dyes. Solubilization may bring changes in absorption and biologic availability. The stability of drugs which undergo oxidation and hydrolysis may be altered by solubilisation.

8. Kraft and Cloud points

Micelle forming surfactants exhibit a temperature related *Kraft point* (K_t) and *Cloud point* (C_t).

At low temperatures, the solubility of surfactants show a small increase with rising temperature. Beyond a particular temperature, called Kraft point, there is a rapid increase in solubility. The increase in solubility indicates that there is micelle formation at Kraft temperature (K_t).

Above a definite temperature (Kraft Point) there is rapid increase in the concentration of the micelle forming surfactants. It is the temperature at which the solubility and critical micellar concentration are equal. (This is something like upper critical temperature found for phenol water systems). An increase in the concentration of surfactant below K_t results in the precipitation of the surfactant. On the otherhand if the temperature is increased above K_t, the solubility of the surfactant increases. At K_t the surfactant (crystal) melts and associates into micelles and hence the solubility is rapidly increased on increasing the temperature above the K_t.

A temperature analogous to lower critical temperature is also observed for many non-ionic polyoxyethylated surfactants in solution. In this case above a definite temperature, the solubility decreases and cloudiness appears and then on further increase in temperature, the surfactant separates as a precipitate. If the concentration is high, it forms a gel. Thus, the temperature above which cloudiness suddenly appears is known as *cloud point* (C_t).

9. Pharmaceutical applications of colloids

Colloidal state of medicinal drugs seems to have an increased therapeutic properties with reduced side effects. Thus, the colloidal silver, silver iodide and silver protein (used in the eye infection) are effective germicides and they do not cause irritation as ionic silver salts. Colloidal copper has been used in cancer and colloidal mercury in syphilis.

The adsorption of toxins from the gastrointestinal tract by kaolin and the rate of neutralisation of excess acidity in the stomach by aluminium hydroxide may be increased by using these compounds in colloidal state.

Proteins are important natural colloids and are found in the body as components of muscle, bone and skin, Hydroxyethyl starch which is a colloid is used as a plasma substitute. Synthetic polymers which form colloidal solutions are used as coating material for solid dosage forms to protect against atmospheric moisture or from acid in the stomach (*enteric coating*).

Hydrophilic colloids are used as suspending agents and as protective colloid for hydrophobic colloids.

Association colloids are used to increase the solubility, stability, absorption of drugs, and to improve the taste of certain compounds in pharmaceutical preparations.

Radioactive colloids are used as diagnostic aids. Colloidal gold is used as diagnostic and therapeutic aids.

Artificial Kidney: Blood is a colloidal dispersion. It is purified from unwanted electrolytes and small molecules by dialysis through membranes in the kidney. In the case of kidney failure, the blood can be purified externally by dialysing through semipermeable membrane in a device which is called artificial kidney. This process is called haemodialysis.

Many foods are colloidal in nature. Milk is an emulsion of butter fat in water stabilised by a protein, caesin. Gelatin deserts, fruit jellies and whipped creams are also colloids.

GELS

Dispersions of lipophilic colloids form semisolid masses at certain concentration and are called gels. Any system to be called as a gel should satisfy the following criteria.

(a) They are coherent colloidal system having at least two components namely gelling agent and a fluid component.

(b) Each component is continuous throughout the other

(c) They exhibit mechanical properties characteristic of a solid state.

The gelling agent may be small inorganic particles or large organic molecules. The fluid component may be water (hydrogel) or organic liquids (organogel).

The various forms of gels are

(a) Two phase system gel

(b) One phase system gel

Two-phase system gel

Aluminium hydroxide gel is a two-phase system. In this the gel consists of a net work of small discrete particles of aluminium hydroxide in water as shown in Fig. 112.

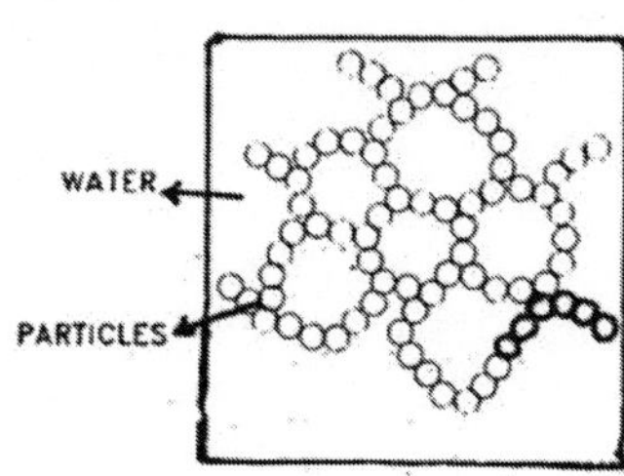

Fig. 112.

If the gelling component is inorganic and the particle size of the insoluble component is relatively large and the fluid component is water, the gel is referred to as Milk or magmas. They are thick and viscous and there is no need to add suspending agent. Bentonite magmas and Milk of Magnesia are examples.

The gels and magmas are thixotropic forming semisolids on standing and becoming liquid on agitation. They should be shaken before use and to be labelled accordingly.

One phase gel

They contain organic macro molecule uniformly distributed in a liquid in such a manner that no apparent boundaries between dispersed molecules and the liquid occur.

A single or one phase gel is made by dispersing synthetic macro molecules carbomer or natural gums (tragacanth) in water. The gels prepared with gums are called mucilages. Apart from water, alcohol and oils may also be used as a fluid component. For example mineral oil can be combined with polyethylene resins to get oleaginous ointment base.

If the gel contains a higher proportion of fluid component, usually water, the gel is referred to as a jelly. The consistency of jellies is less compared to gels. The jellies are used as lubricants for surgical gloves, catheters and rectal thermometers. Lidocaine hydro-chloride jelly is used as topical anaesthetic. Vaginal jellies with medicaments are available as contraceptives. They may contain some surfactants to increase the spermicidal action of the drug. A typical base contains sodium alginate, glycerin, calcium gluconate and water. The calcium ions cause cross linking with sodium alginate to give a jelly. This base may be used to prepare medicated jelly. Jellies are prone to microbial attack and therefore contains preservatives like methyl paraben or ethyl paraben. Tragacanth gum is used in the preparation of Ephedrine sulphate Jelly. Other compounds like acacia, chondrous, gelatin and carboxymethyl cellulose may be used to get jellies with water.

Method of preparation of gels

a) By reducing the solubility of a colloidal material by change of temperature, gelation may be induced. For example, solutions of gelatin or agar sets as a gel on cooling. In contrast to this, cellulose ethers which are soluble in water due to hydrogen bonding sets to a gel in water on raising the temperature. This is because of reduction in solubility resulting from the disruption of hydrogen bonding.

b) By flocculation of hydrophilic colloids with electrolytes or precipitating liquids, gelation can be brought about. In this, gelatin is induced by adding just sufficient precipitant to produce a gel but insufficient precipitant to bring about complete precipitation. For example, a solution of ethyl cellulose in benzene is gelled by adding petroleum ethers.

c) Evaporation of certain colloidal solution leads to gelation. For example, collodion (solution of tetra nitro cellulose in alcohol and ether) forms a gel when the solvents are evaporated.

d) Chemical reaction that leads to change in the shape of lyophilic molecules causes gelation. (denaturation). For example, denaturation of albumin on heating leads to gelling, silica gel is produced by the interaction of sodium silicate and acid in aqueous solution and Milk of magnesia is produced by chemical reaction.

e) Hydration and swelling of dry colloid in contact with a liquid produce a gel. Examples are xerogels. Such as gelatin sheet, acacia tears, tragacanth strips, starch grains, etc. Xerogels result from shrinkage when the fluid component is removed by evaporation or freeze drying and swell and reform into gel on contact with the fluid component.

Structure of gels

The nature of the gelling agent and the type of force that is responsible for the linkages of the gelling agent determine the structure, rigidity and other properties of the gel.

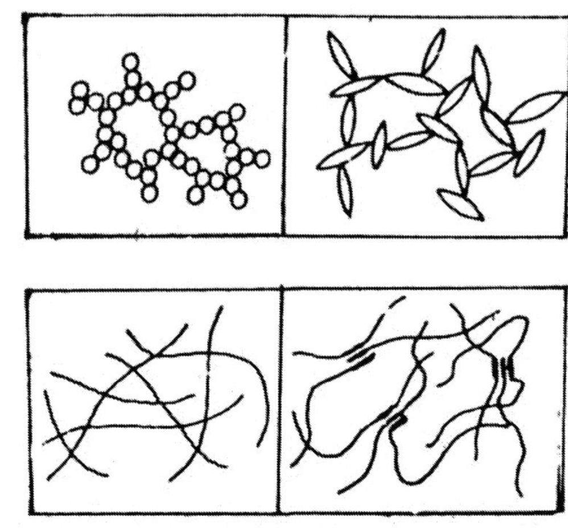

Fig. 113. Representation of gel structure

The gel may contain spherical or anisomeric aggregates of small molecules, linear macromolecule entangled into network with lesser points of contact or several molecules aligned in a crystalline order as shown in Fig. 113.

The force of attraction responsible for the linkages may be 1. a weaker attraction such as *van der Waals* force or weaker hydrogen bonds and dipole interaction as in agar, pection, and gelatin. Such a gel has elastic property and are called elastic gels. or 2. stronger primary valency as in silica gel which consists of three dimensional network of – Si – O – Si – O – bonds having pores scarcely larger than a few molecules diameters in width. Because of the resultant large surface area, the gel is useful adsorbent for water vapour and hence used as desiccant.

Either temperature or agitation is just sufficient to overcome the weaker forces. For example, agar or gelatin gel on heating liquefy and are called thermogels. Bentonite and aluminium hydroxide gels will reduce their viscosities on agitation and converted back to gel on removal of the stress. This isothermal transition of gel to sol and sol to gel is called thixotropy and the gel is called thixotropic gel.

Measurement of elasticity of gels

An assessment on the stability of gels is important to control the quality of gelling agent such as gelatin, agar and pectin.

a) British Gelometer

It is used for the determination of jelly strength of gelatin. The strength is expressed as a Bloom number which is equivalent to the weight in grams necessary to produce a 4 mm depression in a jelly of 6.66%. w/w matured at 0°C by means of a plunger 12.7 mm in diameter. The bloom number is dependent on the average molecular weight of gelatin. For gelation, the BP prescribes a jelly strength of not less than 150. The solubility of gelatin glycerin (glyco gelatin) supository and its solution time depends upon the bloom number.

b) The rigidity of modulus gelatin gels Saunders and Ward

A cylinder of gelatin set in a glass tube is subjected to shearing stresses by applying a known pressure at one end of the tube. The rigidity of the gel is calculated from the volume displacement which is measured by causing mercury to move along a calibrated capillary tube. This method was used for measuring rigidities of gelatin gels over the range 5×10^3 to 5×10^5 dyne/cm^2 and was suitable for gelatin concentrations upto 10%. It was also found that presence of glycerin upto 40% increased the modulus of rigidity of gelatin gels.

Properties of gels.

1. Swelling

If a xerogal is placed in contact with a liquid, the gel solvates and the volume of the xerogel increases. It is referred to as swelling and the pressure that develops if a xerogel is confined is known as swelling pressure. If a gel takes water without increase in volume, it is called "imbibition". Swelling of protein gel is influenzed by pH and electrolytes.

2. Syneresis

Gels will often contract spontaneously and exude some of the fluid medium with consequent squezing out effect and it is called syneresis. eg. clotting of blood. The degree of syneresis decreases usually as the concentration of gelling agent increases. The syneresis indicates that the system is thermodynamically unstable. The syneresis may also occur slowly during storage period. In deficient gel ointment base, water is 'bleeding' out without syneresis.

3. Aging

Colloidal system usually exhibits slow aggregation called aging. The aging results in the gradual formation of denser network of gelling agent.

4. Adsorption of vapors by xerogels

Xerogels provide larger surface area because of its porous nature. The porosity provides for uptake of vapour by capillary condensation. Xerogels specially silica gel are therefore used as drying agents.

5. Rheological properties

Gels show the following mechanical properties similar to solids namely rigidity, tensile strength and elasticity. In thixotropic gels, these properties are observed below yield value.

6. Chemical reaction in gels

Chemical reaction may be carried out within the gel structure avoiding disturbances caused by mechanical influences or convection current. For example precipitation of silver chromate in a rhythmic pattern occurs throughout the gel.

7. Diffusion in gels

The net work of gels contains continuous pores filled with a liquid. Any component that is soluble in the liquid component can diffuse through the gel. The diffusion is effected by such factors that normally affect simple diffusion and in addition the factor due to the presence of gel net work.

The rate of diffusion of a solute in a simple solution is given by

$$\frac{dm}{dt} = -DA\frac{dc}{dx} \quad \ldots (5)$$

where dm is the amount of solute diffusing in time dt across an area A under the influence of concentration gradient $\frac{dc}{dx}$ (refer under diffusion). If the size of diffusing particles becomes comparable with the pore diameter of the gel, the diffusion is retarded considerably and ceases when the particles are larger than the widest pores in the gel. It is called "sieve effect" of the gel. An electrical double layer will exist at the liquid interface. When electrolyte diffuses through the gel, the following effect is noticeable. The electrolyte ions that possess a similar charge to the mobile gegenions of the gel are able to enter the pores easily and the mobile gegenions are displaced along the pores. However, the charged framework of the gel will tend to prevent the entry of other electrolyte ions since both carry same charges. This effect gives rise to a selective permeability of the gel either to positive or negative ions. For example, gelatin gel that carries negative charge in alkaline medium is selectively permeable to cation (positure charges) Conversely, the same gelatin gel caries a positive charge in acid medium and hence selectively permeable to anion (negative changes)

8. Adsorption of a solute on gels

The diffusing solute may get adsorbed on the walls of the gel. The solutes may have different adsorption affinities on the walls. This will retard the movement of the various solutes at different level in a column of a gel when a mixture of solutes are poured on the top of the gel in a column. The adsorbed solutes may be eluted with different solvents. This is the principle in adsorption chromatography.

Application of Gels

a) **Dosage Forms:** Gelatin gels are used in the preparation of hard or soft gelatin capsules and glycogelatin suppositories

Mineral oils gelled by warming with insoluble soap, aluminium monostearate are used to suspend drug substances in oily injections. Liquid paraffin gelled with polythene forms a proprietary ointment base. Organic solvents gelled with aluminium stearate is used in the preparation of slow release dosage forms. This may be undertaken as follows: A suspension of drug particles in a volatile organic solvent (vehicle) is prepared. To this aluminium monostearate is added and warmed. This produces a gel, the matrix of which enmeshes the drug particles. dry gel is then obtained by evaporating the solvent. The dried gel is broken up into granules and used for tablet making.

b) **Microbiological Media** Agar and gelatin gels are used in the preparation of culture media for micro organisms and also in microbiological assay of antibiotics, antiseptics etc.

c) **Gel filtration** It is a technique of separation of solutes of different molecular sizes. Sephadex resin is a cross linked polysaccharide material when it is dispersed in water in a column a gel is formed. If a solution containing mixed solutes (solutes with different molecular weight and sizes) are passed through the gel, the largest solute molecules will come out first followed by decreasing sizes of solute molecules. Hence the process is called molecular sieving.

d) **Dialysing Membrane** It is made up of cellulose acetate or cellulose nitrate. It is one of the xerogels The membrane is microporous network of macromolecule. The molecules are usually aggregated into bundles or micelles by secondary forces like hydrogen bonding. The gel is prepared in such a way that it allows only diffusion of ions or small molecules but prevents escape of colloidal particles. The permeability coefficient of the membrane is

$$\frac{Q}{t} = \frac{TA \Delta C}{d} \quad \text{... (6)}$$

where Q is the amount of material passing through a membrane of area A and thickness d under the influence of concentration gradient ΔC in time t. Factors affecting permeation are (a) pore size (b) charges in the membrane (c) Donnan membrane effect. (refer under colloids).

The membrane is usually prepared as follows: Ether or acetone solution of the polymer is prepared. The solution is cast on flat surface or on a rotating mould. Several layers are applied and each layer is allowed to evaporate under controlled conditions of humidity and temperature. The membrane is finally rigidised by dipping in a liquid like petroleum ether in which it is insoluble.

AEROSOL

An Aerosol is defined as colloidal dispersion of liquids or solids in gases. Particle size is usually within colloidal range. If the particle size exceeds 1 μm the physical stability is affected.

Aerosols may be prepared by either dispersion or condensation methods. The dispersion method is usually used in the preparation of pharmaceutical products. In this, a solution or suspension of one or more medicaments is dispersed in the liquid propellant or in a mixture of liquid propellants. This is then contained in a pressurized container. When the valve in the container (i.e. Pressurized pack) is opened, the vapour pressure of the propellant forces the mixture out of the container. The expansion of the propellant at room temperature and at atmospheric pressure produces a dispersion of the medicament in air. In addition to liquid propellants (i.e. Fluorinated hydrocarbons), the pressure packs often use Nitrogen, Nitrous oxide and Carbon dioxide to expel the contents from their containers.

Suggestions for Practicals

Preparation and study of some properties of colloids

I. Preparation of Ferric hydroxide colloid:

Boil 250 ml of pure water in a beaker. Add 5 ml of 30% ferric chloride solution to this with constant stirring. A dark reddish brown colloidal dispersion is produced. It is an example of positive colloid. The particles carry positive charges because of preferential adsorption of ferric ions onto colloidal particles.

II. Preparation of Arsenious sulphide colloid:

Pass hydrogen sulphide gas into 100 ml of 0.01 M arsenious oxide solution in water to produce arsenious sulphide colloid. It is an example of negative colloid.

By using paper chromatographic technique, whether the colloidal particles in a colloid are positively charged or negatively charged can be known.

Perform the following:

(a) **Effect of ageing:** Observe the colloidal preparations for one week. Report any color change and/or precipitation during this period.

(b) **Effect of centrifugation:** Centrifuge the colloids and observe the effect of centrifugation on the stability of the colloids.

Mutual Coagulation

(c) Mix two oppositively charged colloids and observe the effect due to the mutual neutralisaiton of the charges on the colloidal particles.

(d) **Effect of electrolytes on the stability of colloids:** Prepare 100 ml of 0.1 N NaH_2PO_4, Na_2HPO_4 and Na_3PO_4 solutions in water. Titrate 10 ml of ferric hydroxide colloid with each of the electrolyte solution separately. Find out the volume of electrolyte solution required to induce precipitation. From the value obtained calculate the number of millimoles of the electrolyte required to induce precipitation per 100 ml of the colloid. Report the effect of electrolytes to induce coagulation in the decreasing order.

X. SUSPENSIONS AND EMULSIONS

Coarse dispersions include suspensions and emulsions.

1. SUSPENSIONS

A suspension is a heterogeneous (biphasic) system consisting of a solid phase in a liquid phase. The solid phase is subdivided into small particles and dispersed in the liquid medium in which the solid is insoluble or sparingly (or slightly) soluble. Suspensions being coarse dispersions, the size of the greater number of particles may exceed 0.1μ.

A pharmaceutical suspension may be defined as a coarse dispersion of finely subdivided insoluble solid drug suspended in a suitable liquid (usually aqueous) medium. A suspension may be for internal, external or parenteral use.

Suspensions for oral administration is a better means of administration than of solid dosage forms such as tablets and capsules especially when swallowing is difficult. Thus, they prove more useful for administering for infants and old patients. As suspensions contain subdivided solid particles, surface area is large and this is taken advantage of for drugs which are adsorptives or antacids. Examples may be kaolin, magnesium trisilicate etc. Often drugs which are bitter in soluble form are administered in their insoluble form as a suspension to mask the taste. For example insoluble chloramphenicol palmitate is used in the form of suspension to reduce the bitter taste of the chloramphenicol base.

Suspensions for external use are mainly lotions. This facilitates the drug application in the form of liquid which provides a fine coating of the drug to promote the action of the drug on the affected part of the skin. It is not messy to use in the form of suspensions as in the case of ointments. Calamine lotion is a good example.

Parenteral suspensions are of particular importance in the field of *depot* therapy. This is based on the slow release of the drug for extended action. This is made possible due to the size of the particle whose solubility is low and the particles take more time to dissolve providing for sustained action. *Insulin zinc suspension* is an example.

1.1. Desirable properties of suspensions

A suspension is required to satisfy certain desirable properties so that it is acceptable. The desirable qualities are:

1. There should not be rapid settling of suspended particles
2. If the particles do settle, they must not form a hard cake at the bottom of the container and

should be easily redispersible into uniform mixture when shaken.

3. The suspension should be easily pourable.
4. In the case of parenteral preparations, it should flow through the syringe needle
5. In the case of external preparation, it should spread easily on the surface of the skin and it must not be too fluid to run off the skin surface
6. The colour and odour should be acceptable and pleasing for oral and external uses.

We are mainly concerned with the physical stability. The physical stability may be defined as the condition in which the particles do not aggregate and should remain uniformly distributed throughout the dispersion medium. Even if the particles settle, redistribution must be easy with moderate amount of agitation.

1.2. Interfacial properties

When the interfacial properties between the solid phase and the liquid are considered, two factors must be taken into account. They are the *surface free energy* increase resulting from increase in surface area of suspended particles due to reduction in size of particles and the *presence of electrical charges* on the surface of the dispersed solid particles in a liquid medium.

Surface free energy

The increase in surface free energy due to a reduction in size of the particles is given by the relation

$$\Delta G = \gamma \Delta A \qquad \text{... (1)}$$

where ΔG = increase in surface free energy in ergs.

ΔA = increase in surface area in cm^2

γ = interfacial tension in dynes/cm.

With excess free energy (i.e. when $\Delta G > 0$) due to increase in surface area, the system tends to approach a stable state by reducing the surface free energy spontaneously. When $\Delta G = 0$ the system is thermodynamically stable. It may be said that smaller the ΔG, the more thermodynamically stable is the suspension. A reduction in γ can be brought about by adding a wetting agent (surfactant). The molecules of the wetting agent get adsorbed between the particle and the medium and cause a reduction in interfacial tension. This produces a reduction in ΔG making the suspension stable. However, the interfacial tension cannot be made equal to zero and therefore the suspended particles in contact with liquid medium possess a finite positive interfacial tension and as a result the particles tend to flocculate or aggregate. This may be desirable or undesirable in a pharmaceutical suspension. In the event of particles remaining deflocculated, they settle relatively slowly. The settled particles tend to form eventually a hard cake at the bottom of the container. When such a sediment (a hard cake like) is formed, it becomes extremely difficult to redisperse uniformly the particles throughout the medium.

Be it a solid or liquid, when reduced greatly in size, there is a tendency for the particles or the globules to agglomerate or stick together. This agglomeration can occur either in air or in a liquid medium. This tendency for the agglomeration is due to excess free energy resulting out of size reduction (or comminution). When there is excess free energy, the system is thermodynamically unstable. Then, regrouping of particles to form agglomerates occurs in an attempt to reach a thermodynamically stable state. Hence, the process of agglomeration is spontaneous. In an agglomerate, the particles are held together by weak *vander Waals* forces of attraction. In a liquid medium they settle and ultimately form a hard sedimented cake.

Electrical Properties at the surface of the dispersed particles

Both attraction and repulsion forces exist between particles dispersed in a liquid medium.

The particle-particle interaction (due to attraction and repulsion) may be given as follows.

1. *The various electrostatic contributions:* They may be ion-ion, ion-dipole, dipole-dipole and dipole-induced dipole. They have both attractive (between dissimilar charges) and repulsive forces (between similar charges)
2. The *London dispersion forces* (between atoms of one particle with those of the other. It is induced dipole-induced dipole interaction (attraction)
3. The covalent bonds (attractive)
4. *Born repulsion forces* (repulsive). It is due to overlapping of electron clouds of the atoms present in a molecule or ion.

The attractive forces due to covalent bonds and *Born repulsion forces* have an effect only when the particles are actually in touch with each other.

The London dispersion forces and hydrogen bonding forces are generally more important in describing interparticulate behaviour of non-ionic compounds in suspensions. The surface properties of the particles depend on the balance achieved between these attractive and repulsive forces.

In general, the particles in a suspension have forces of attraction which are of the London *vander Waals* type and the forces of repulsion due to the interaction of the electric double layer surrounding each particle (See under Interfacial phenomena).

The region in which the influence of the surface charge (i.e. potential) of the particle is appreciable is termed the electric double layer region. The electric double layer is considered to comprise.

1. **The Stern layer consisting of counterions:** The thickness is of the ionic dimension. The potential drop across the stern layer from the surface of the particle is sharp.
2. **The diffuse double layer:** The potential drop across this layer is somewhat gradual and it drops to zero at the end of its surface where it meets electro-neutral region.

The charged particles suspended in a liquid medium migrate towards the oppositely charged electrode under the influence of electric field. When a particle moves the counterions in the Stern layer and the solvent molecules in the solvated layer (solvent-sheath or layer called solvated layer) also move intact with the particle. That is, the plane of shear occurs at the surface of the solvated layer. This solvated layer is slightly thicker than the Stern layer.

The potential energy of the two particles (as they approach each other) may be plotted as a function of the distance of separation (Fig. 114). The energy of attraction (due to *London dispersion forces*) and the energy of repulsion (due to overlapping of electrical double layer) are represented in the graph as V_A and V_R respectively. The net energy (due to interaction between attractive and repulsive forces) is represented as V_n which is also the energy barrier

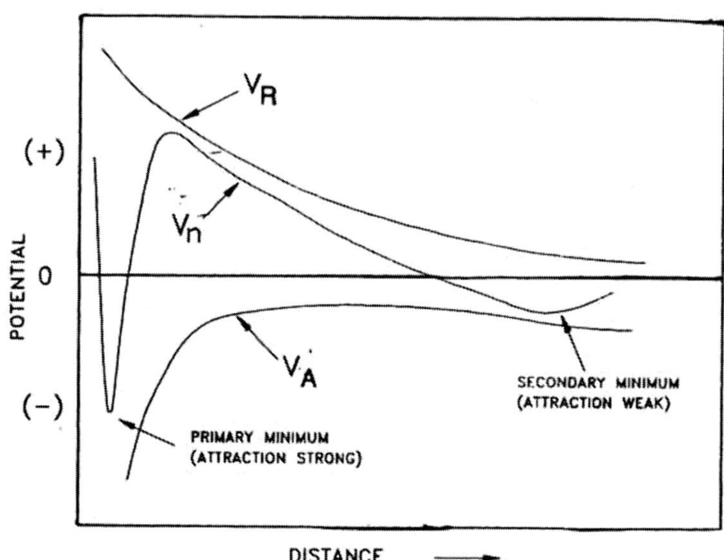

Fig. 114

curve. This curve has two minima and a peak. The minimum occuring at longer distance is called secondary minimum and that occuring at negligible distance is called primary minimum.

In the presence of high repulsive energy, the potential barrier energy is also high and it prevents the collision of the approaching particles and hence, they remain deflocculated. When the sedimentation of such deflocculated particles is complete, they tend to be closely packed and the particles at the bottom gets compressed by the weight of the particles in the upper layer as well as by the dispersion medium. At this stage, the energy barrier is overcome and the particles come closer and closer and they enter into primary minimum. As a result, they experience attractive forces and ultimately form a hard cake like sediment. To regain the original energy barrier, or to get the particles dispersed a high energy is required. Hence even on vigorous agitation, the redispersion of the particles is not achieved and the particles remain as a cake.

When the particles flocculate in the secondary minimum where the attractive forces reach over the range of repulsive forces, the particles remain flocculated but are separated by a distance approximately from 1000 to 2000Å. In the secondary minimum the particles are loosely held in floccules and are not able to enter into primary minimum since the energy barrier is too large to be surmounted.

It may be said that flocculated particles are weakly bonded and settle rapidly. The flocculated particles on sedimentation do not form a cake and are easily redispersed on shaking the container.

1.3. Flocculation and Deflocculation in suspensions

The overall (or resultant) charge existing on the suspended particle is called as *zeta potential* and it is a measurable indication of the charge. Therefore, flocculation and deflocculation may be considered in terms of zeta potential. When the zeta potential is high, the particles remain dispersed and

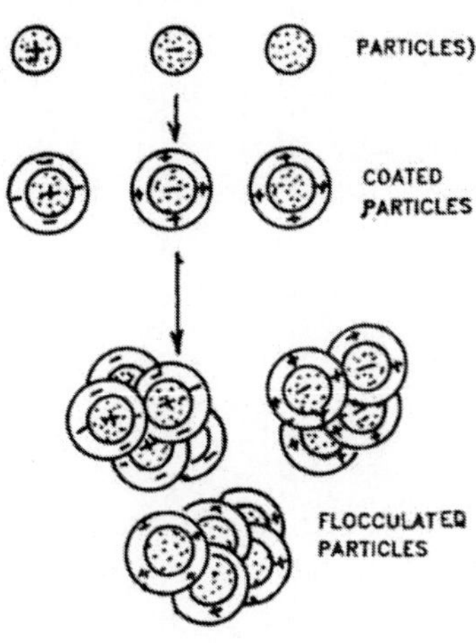

Fig. 115

The zeta potential can be progressively lowered by the addition of an electrolyte (whose ion which is oppositely charged to that of the suspended particles is preferentially adsorbed). At some concentration of the electrolyte, the forces of attraction dominate over the electrical forces of repulsion slightly. Under these conditions (i.e. when the zeta potential is sufficiently lowered), the particles when they approach each other, form loose aggregates commonly called *flocs*. (Fig.115) Then such a suspension is said to be *flocculated*.*

*Flocculation is a term used by some workers as aggregation in the secondary minimum and the coagulation as aggregation in the primary minimum.

are said to be *deflocculated*. These particles resist collision due to the high zeta potential even if the particles are brought close by way of random motion or agitation.

The difference between *deflocculated* and *flocculated* suspensions may be given as follows (Fig. 116).

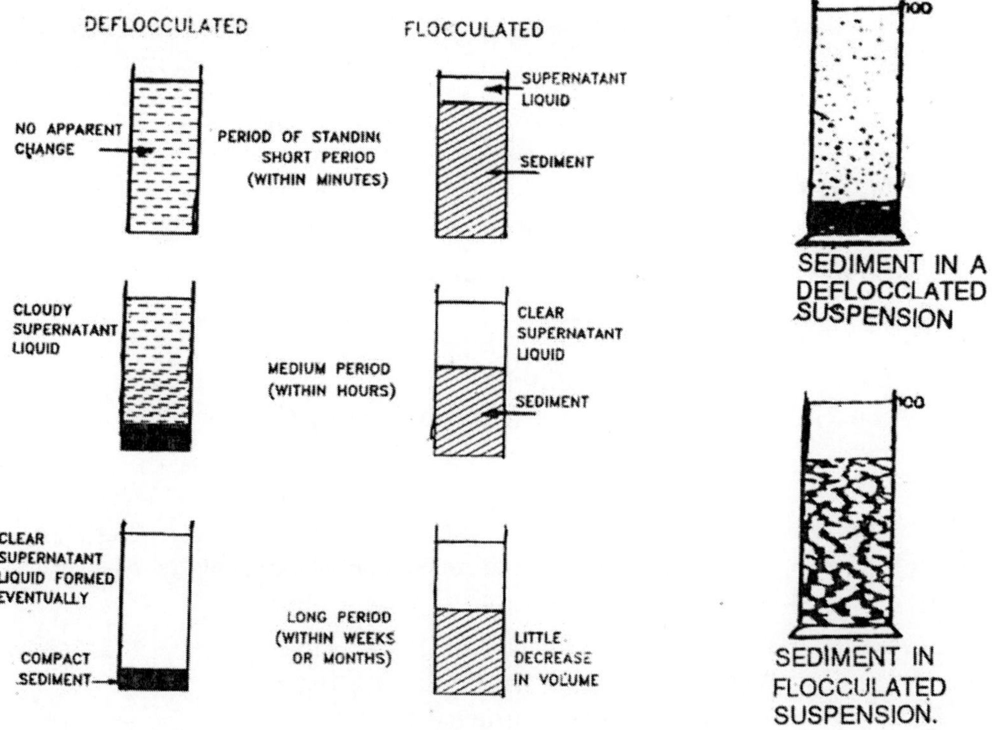

Fig. 116

	Deflocculated Suspension	Flocculated Suspension
1.	The particles in the suspension remain individually.	Particles form light fluffy conglomerates called flocs.
2.	Since the particles are small and remain separately, the rate of sedimentation is slow	Since the flocs are groups of particles, rate of sedimentation is fast.
3.	Formation of sediment at the bottom of the container takes a long time	Formation of sediment is quick.
4.	The sediment formed becomes eventually a hard cake	The sediment is loosely packed and presents a scaffold like structure with entrapped liquid. The sediment does not form a dense hard cake.
5.	Sediment volume is *small*	Sediment volume is *large*
6.	The supernatent liquid remains cloudy for a longer time as very small particles (approaching colloidal dimensions) take very long time to settle.	The supernatent liquid becomes clear at a shorter time since small particles are entrapped within the flocs and settle along with flocs rapidly.
7.	Redistribution of the sedimented particles by shaking the container is difficult.	Redistribution of the sedimented particles by shaking the container is easy.
8.	The suspension has a pleasing appearance	The suspension is somewhat unsightly unless the sediment volume and the volume of the original suspension are equal.

Settling and its control

The sedimentation velocity of particles in a suspension is related to

1. size of the particles
2. density of the particles
3. viscosity of the dispersion medium.

The effect of these factors can be given by *Stoke's law*

$$v = \frac{d^2(\rho_s - \rho_l)g}{18\eta_l} \quad \ldots (2)$$

where v = average velocity of sedimentation of particles (cm/sec)

d = diameter of the particle in cm.

ρ_s and ρ_l = densities of the dispersed phase (solid) and the dispersion medium (liquid) respectively

g = acceleration due to gravity

η_l = viscosity of the dispersion medium.

Stoke's law is applicable to dilute suspensions containing spherical particles and the settling of particles should be slow with less turbulence i.e. the settling should be streamline. Pharmaceutical suspensions being concentrated, there is disturbance for the settling of particles and hence *Stoke's law* cannot be effectively applied. However, these factors may be expected to influence the rate of settling.

According to *Stoke's law*, settling rate for the particles may be reduced by decreasing the particle size provided the particles are deflocculated.

The rate of sedimentation may be delayed by increasing the viscosity of the medium (by adding suitable suspending agents) as it is inversely related to the viscosity of the dispersion medium. This approach to reduce the rate of sedimentation is frequently used. However there is an optimum level for this approach as too much increase in viscosity may hinder the flow of the suspension out of the container. That is, pourability is affected and the viscosity increase may also make the redistribution of the particles uniformly throughout the dispersion medium difficult.

The other approach that may be applied is to narrow down the density difference between the dispersed particles and the dispersion medium. This is seldom possible as the density of solid particles is always greater than the liquid.

Brownian movement

When the size of the dispersed particles approach that of colloidal dimensions, *Brownian motion* sets in. Such a *Brownian motion* may be observed if the size of the particle is reduced approximately to 2μ. However the Brownian movement depends on the density of the particles and the density and viscosity of the dispersion medium. Considering the size of the particles normally found in most of the pharmaceutical suspensions it is unlikely that the particles will undergo *Brownian movement.*

Effect of flocculation on sedimentation rate

In a deflocculated suspension, the larger particles settle relatively at a faster rate than the smaller particles. As a result, a clear boundary is not easily decernable and the supernatent liquid remains cloudy for a considerable period of time. In the case of flocculated suspension, groups of particles are aggregated into flocs and the flocs tend to fall together while settling and there is a clear boundary formed between the sediment and the supernatent liquid. Settling in a flocculated suspension depends on size and porosity of the flocs. However, the rate of settling in a flocculated suspension is faster.

1.4. Sedimentation volume and degree of sedimentation

In order to assess a formulation of suspension in terms of amount of flocculation, two parameters namely *sedimentation volume* and *degree of sedimentation* are useful.

Sedimentation volume

The sedimentation volume is the ratio of ultimate volume of the sediment to the total volume of the suspension.

$$F = V_u / V_0 \qquad \ldots (3)$$

where F = sedimentation volume

V_u = ultimate volume of the sediment

V_0 = total volume of the suspension

The sedimentation volume (F) normally ranges from less than 1 to 1 and it may exceed 1. For example, if the sedimentation volume is 0.85, it means that 85% of the total volume of the suspension is occupied by the sediment (usually flocculated suspension will occupy that much of volume). When $F = 1$, the sediment volume and the total volume are equal and such a suspension is pharmaceutically acceptable. It is possible for the sedimentation volume to exceed the total volume of the suspension i.e. $F > 1$. It indicates that the network of flocs formed in the suspension is loose and fluffy that it encompasses a volume greater than the original volume of the suspension.

Degree of flocculation

Degree of flocculation is a better parameter to compare different formulations in terms of flocculation. It is the ratio of the sedimentation volume of the flocculated suspension (F) to the sedimentation volume of the suspension when deflocculated (F_α).

$$\beta = \frac{F}{F_\alpha} \qquad \text{... (4)}$$

The degree of flocculation refers to the increased sediment volume because of flocculation. For example, if $\beta = 4$, the sediment volume in the flocculated suspension is increased by four times the volume of sediment in the deflocculated state. A suspension with a higher degree of flocculation is to be preferred.

1.5. Formulation of suspensions

The formulation of suspension is aimed at producing a suspension with optimal physical stability. A physically stable suspension may be produced either by

(a) the use of structured vehicle to keep the deflocculated particles in suspension, or

(b) the use of the principles of flocculation in order to assure an easy uniform redispersion of particles with minimum of agitation.

In the first approach using structured vehicles, the deflocculated particles are entrapped. This reduces the settling time and as the structured vehicle (non-Newtonian type) has shear-thinning property, redispersion is somewhat easier by shaking the container. However, when the particles ultimately settle, they form a cake at the bottom of the container making it difficult to redisperse the settled particles.

The second approach is the preparation of flocculated suspension. In this, the particles settle rapidly and the redispersion is easy. Within the time gap between the shaking of the container and the consumption the drug particles may settle rapidly allowing only a dose that is subtherapeutic. As a consequence, in the formulation of suspensions, optimum physical stability may be obtained by producing suspensions with controlled flocculation in a structured vehicle

Dispersion of particles

The first step in the formulation of suspension is the dispersion of the (drug) powder in a liquid medium. Before dispersion can be effected, the particles should be properly wetted. Wetting is a problem with hydrophobic particles. This can be brought about by the use of wetting agents. They act by lowering the contact angle between the surface of the particle and the wetting liquid (the dispersion medium). Wetting agents are surfactants whose *HLB* values lie within the range of 7 to 9. The powder may be prepared as a slurry in a solution of wetting agent and then the required amount of vehicle may be added to disperse the powder. Alcohol and glycerin may also be used to disperse the powder. Glycerin and similar hydrophilic substances flow into void space between the particles, coat the particles, and separate the particles bringing about dispersion. Wetting agents in smaller amounts promote wetting and deflocculation.

Controlled flocculation

The next step is to produce controlled flocculation in the suspension. Flocculation in a suspension prevents formation of a hard cake, when the particles settle down. Flocculation in a suspension may be brought about by adding

(a) electrolytes

(b) surfactants

(c) polymers

The most widely used flocculating agents are the electrolytes. When added in sufficient quantity to a well wetted and dispersed particles suspension, they (electrolytes) cause a reduction in electrical forces of repulsion bringing about flocculation in the suspension. Electrolytes reduce the electric barrier and thereby produce a reduction in zeta potential on the dispersed particles. The addition of electrolyte must be judicious so that zeta potential is reduced to a level which brings about flocculation resulting in maximum sedimentation volume.

Consider a suspension in which the particles are dispersed in an aqueous medium and the particles carry positive charges with high zeta potential (Fig. 117). The particles in the suspension remain deflocculated due to high zeta potential. If monobasic potassium phosphate is added to the suspension, the negatively charged phosphate ions get adsorbed on the particles bringing down the potential. This effect causes the particles to flocculate and the sediment volume is increased. On the addition of increased amounts of the electrolyte (i.e. monobasic potassium phosphate), the zeta potential gradually falls to zero and then the charge on the particle becomes negative (i.e. overall charge gets reversed). Until now, the suspension remains flocculated. But on increasing the negative charge with further addition of the electrolyte, the particles again get deflocculated since the zeta potential is increased on the negative side. The results of these effect

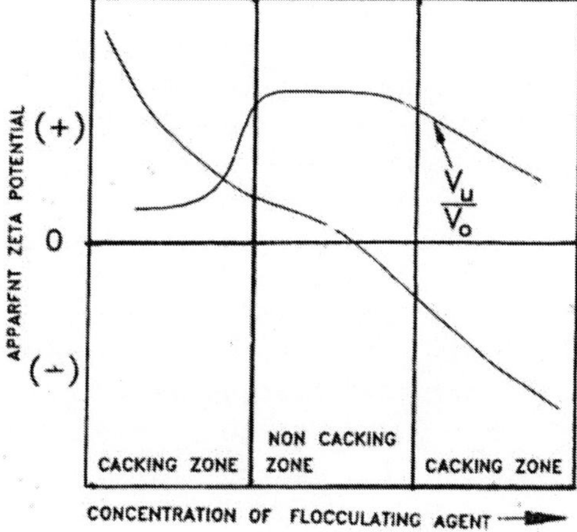

Fig. 117

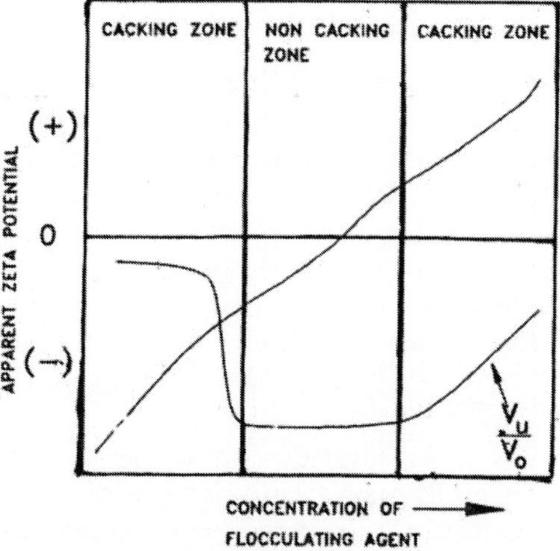

Fig. 118

mentioned above may be presented in Fig. 117 and 118.

Similarly if the particles in a suspension are negatively charged initially, the addition of aluminium chloride brings about the effect shown (Fig. 118). That is the negative charge is progressively reduced by the addition of aluminium chloride as the aluminium ions (positively charged) get adsorbed on the particles. On sufficient addition of aluminium chloride, the zeta potential reaches zero and then increases in the positive direction.

In both the cases when zeta potential is high, the particles remain deflocculated and the sediment volume is less. This sediment eventually forms a hard cake making redistribution of the suspension difficult on shaking the container. On reduction in zeta potential by the addition of the electrolyte, the particles form flocs. It may be observed that the onset of flocculation is coincident with the maximum sedimentation volume. This volume virtually remains constant until the zeta potential becomes sufficiently high on the opposite side. At this stage the sedimentation volume starts to fall indicating deflocculation and the sediment eventually forms a cake.

These effects have been demonstrated with bismuth subnitrate suspension (in which the particles carry positive charge initially) and sulfamerazine suspension in which the drug (sulfamerazine) particles carry negative charge initially as in the figures shown above.

Surfactants

Flocculation have been brought about by using both ionic and non-ionic surfactants. However, the concentrations of these surfactants to achieve flocculation is critical because they act as wetting agents also to bring about dispersion of the powder particles in a dispersion medium.

Polymers

Polymers act as flocculating agents by forming a 'bridge' between particles. The sedimentation volume is higher in a suspension in which polymers have been used to bring about flocculation. eg Xanthumgum

Flocculation in structured vehicle

A suspension with controlled flocculation may look unsightly because the sediment volume will be lower than the total volume of the suspension. An ideal formulation would be a suspension with controlled flocculation supported in a structured vehicle.

To a suspension in which the particles have been flocculated to a desired degree, a polymer which is lyophilic is added to obtain a structured vehicle. Most of the pharmaceutical suspensions are prepared in aqueous medium and hence a hydrophilic polymer is used to form structured vehicle. Some examples of hydrophilic polymers are carboxy methyl cellulose, carbopol, veegum, tragacanth, bentonite etc.

These structured vehicle forming hydrophilic colloids are negatively charged and are compatible with suspensions which have been flocculated with anion of the electrolyte (For example PO_4^{-3} of monobasic potassium phosphate). That is, if the suspended particles carry a positive charge initially and are flocculated with monobasic potassium phosphate, a hydrophilic polymer may be added to form structured vehicle. Otherwise, to a suspension (with particles carrying negative charge) which has been flocculated with aluminium chloride, if a hydrophilic polymer is added, it results in an incompatible product. Under such conditions, the sign of the particle (negative charge) may be changed to positive sign and then a hydrophilic polymer may be added after flocculating the particles with the use of anion of an electrolyte. The change in sign (from negative to positive) may be brought about by using hydrophilic protective colloid. (This is similar in mechanism of protecting a hydrophobic colloid with hydrophilic colloid).

In general, a physically stable suspension may be produced

(a) by reducing the particle size by a suitable method

(b) by adding a suitable suspending agent to increase the viscosity of the medium to an optimum level and

(c) by the use of suitable quantity of proper electrolyte to cause flocculation to a desired level in a structured vehicle. The agents used to produce structured vehicle invariably act as suspending agents.

(d) Due to temperature fluctuations there may be change in particle size, distribution and polymorphic forms. They are destabilising processes. The growth in particle is termed "Oswald ripening" and this occurs during storage. This may alter absorption rate and in turn bioavailability of drugs. When temperature is raised, crystals of most drugs may dissolve and form supersaturated solution which favour crystal growth. This can be prevented by adding certain polymers or surfactants. Sulphathiazole and acetaminophen crystal growth can be prevented by the addition of high molecular weight polyvinyl pyrrolidone. The molecules of the polymer attach to the free space of drug crystal lattice and form a non-condensed net like film over the drug crystal. In addition the polymer is surrounded by a hydration shell. It is represented as follows in Fig. 119.

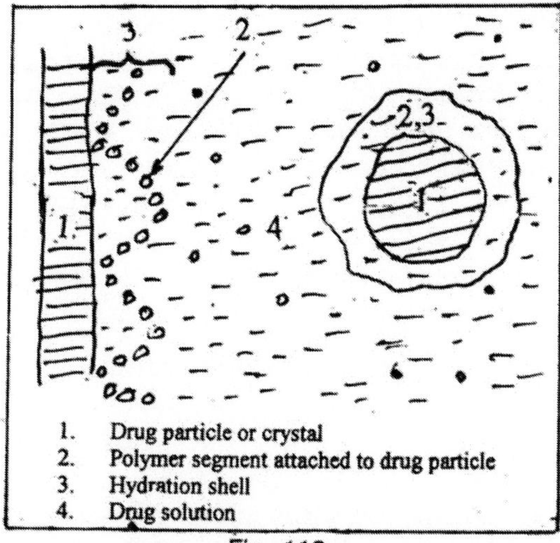

Fig. 119

(e) Stability of suspension may also decrease owing to interaction with excipients dissolved in the dispersion medium.

Example 1 In sulfamerazine suspension containing non-ionic surfactant as wetting agent, sorbitol is used as flocculating agent. The amount of sorbitol required depends upon the cloud point of surfactant. The lower the cloud point, the less sorbital is needed to induce flocculation.

Example 2 Charge on the preservative: Cetyl pyridinium chloride (a cationic surfactant) is used as preservative in suspensions. If more quantity is added, the positive charge on the preservative may reverse the charge of the dispersed particles (eg. Negatively charged zinc oxide may get reversed on the addition of cetyl pyridinium chloride). If the preservative molecules get adsorbed on the suspended particles, free fraction of preservatives in water get reduced and this also leads to lesser preservation.

Chemical stability

In suspensions, the suspended particles are practically insoluble in the liquid vehicle and hence the chances of chemical reaction are very less. But, many drugs in suspension have a finite solubility and so may be susceptible to degradation. However, it may be assumed that the dissolution is not rate-limiting on degradation.

Thus to get a stable suspension at the time of formulation as well as during storage all the above factors should be taken into account.

1.6. Rheologic properties of Suspensions

The principles of rheology are applicable to the flow properties of the suspensions. The flow property of a suspension becomes important as it is required to pour the suspension out of the container to withdraw a dose of the product. It is also important in the case of external preparations which are suspensions as they must spread properly over the affected area when applied.

The viscosity as well as change in flow properties of the suspension will affect the rheological properties of the suspension greatly. Ideally, a suspension should have a high viscosity at low shear rates and a low viscosity at high shear rates. In a suspension under storage, the only shear is due to settling of particles. At this low shear rate, the viscosity of the suspension must be high. During shaking of the bottle a high shear rate is produced and at this high shear rate, the viscosity should fall to a low value. Such a property may be derived from pseudo-plastic substances such as tragacanth, sodium alginate and sodium carboxy methyl cellulose which are used as suspending agents.

However, a suspending agent which is thixotropic as well as pseudoplastic may have the property of forming a gel on standing and becoming fluid when shaken. Thus a suspension containing such a combination of suspending agents may prove to be ideal one. Such a combination of property may be obtained from a mixture of bentonite (which is thixotropic) and carboxy methyl cellulose (which is pseudoplastic).

1.7. Pharmaceutical applications of suspensions

(a) *For oral use:* A suspension provides convenient means of administering an insoluble drug as compared to tablets or capsules as far as swallowing is concerned. For adsorptive or antacid properties, usually suspensions are fast acting because of more surface area. e.g. Kaolin, magnesium carbonate, calcium carbonate and magnesium trisilicate. Insoluble derivatives of drugs are often used to reduce the unpleasant taste. e.g. Chloramphenicol palmitate. Insoluble drugs which are susceptible to hydrolysis are dispensed as dry syrups and are reconstituted with water at the time of use. e.g. *Ampicillin dry syrup.*

(b) *For external use:* Number of lotions are of suspension type (e.g. calamine lotion for protective action on the skin). Semisolid suspensions are pastes (e.g. Magnesium sulfate paste, Zinc and salicyclic acid paste, Tooth paste etc). The performance and acceptability of these preparations depend upon the sedimentation and rheological properties.

(c) *For injections:* Insoluble drugs which are susceptible to hydrolysis are dispersed as sterile powders in vials. At the time of their use, they are reconstituted with sterile water for injection. e.g. *Penicillin injection.* Suspension injections provide for sustained action. e.g. *Streptomycin oily injections.*

2. EMULSIONS

An emulsion is a dispersion of a liquid as globules in another liquid, both the liquids being immiscible with each other. (Example: dispersion of oil in water or dispersion of water in oil). The diameters of the globules usually vary from 0.1 to 10 μm, although globule diameters as small as 0.01 μm and as large as 100 μm are possible in some emulsions. Emulsions having globules of mean diameter about 5 μm are called fine emulsions and emulsions with large globules are refered to as coarse emulsions. The emulsion is said to be thermodynamically unstable since the globules coalesce and the phases will ultimately separate. To stabilise an emulsion, a third substance called emulgent or-emulsifier or emulsifying agent is invariably added to the emulsion. The emulsion may be a dilute dispersion, a concentrated dispersion or semisolid. The liquid emulsions are opaque, milky white, and viscous. The semisolid emulsions are called creams

2.1. Types of emulsion

In an emulsion one liquid phase is essentially polar (aqueous) while the other liquid is relatively non polar (eg. oil).

(a) Oil in Water type emulision

(a) When the oil is distributed as globules throughout the aqueous- continuous phase, the emulsion is called oil in water (o/w) type emulsion (Fig.120) Medicinal emulsions for oral administrations are usually o/w type emulsions. It is prepared so to mask the unpleasant odour and taste of certain medicinal oils and also to increase the absorption. Absorption of shark liver oil is facilitated when given in the form of emulsion. The various emulsifying agents used for producing o/w type emulsions are acacia gum (has more of emulsifying property and less of viscosity building property and hence called primary emulsifying agent), tragacanth gum (has more of viscosity building property and less of emulsifying property and hence called secondary emulsifying agent), starch, methyl cellulose, sodium carboxy methyl cellulose, soluble salts of alginic acid and gelatin. Finely divided solids like aluminium hydroxide yield o/w type emulsions (*Liquid Paraffin Magnesium Hydroxide Emulsion*). Non-ionic surfactants such as tweens and natural emulsifying agents such as acacia, soidum carboxy methyl cellulose are used in oral emulsions.

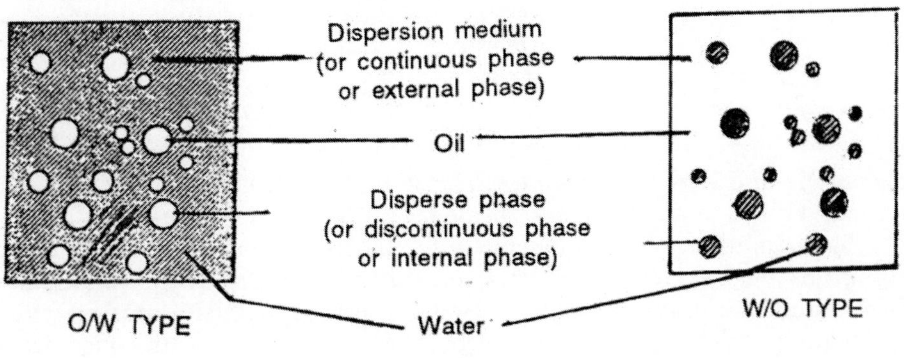

Fig. 120

O/w type emulsions may also be used externally Eg. *Turpentine Liniment and Vanishing Cream*. The various emulsifying agents are sodium lauryl sulphate, triethanolamine stearate, monovalent soaps like sodium oleate, glyceryl monostearete mixed with a monovalent soap or alkyl sulphate etc. Surfactants or mixture of surfactants having HLB values in the range 8-16 will yield o/w type emulsions.

(b) Water-in-oil type emulsion

When water is distributed as globule in oily continuous phase, the emulsion is called water in oil type emulsion (w/o emulsion). (Fig. 120) These emulsions are mainly for external use. Certain food such as butter and some salad dressings are w/o emulsions. The w/o emulsions used externally are Cold cream, Oily Calamine Lotion, Oily Zinc Cream etc. The various emulsifying agents used are polyvalent soaps like calcium palmitate, sorbitan esters (spans), cholesterol and wool fat. Surfactant or a mixture of surfactants whose HLB value is between 3 and 6 yields w/o type emulsions.

(c) Multiple emulsion or complex emulsions

In this oil globules surrounded by water layer are dispersed as complex globules in continuous oil medium (i.e. o/w/o) or water globules surrounded by oil layer are dispersed as complex globules in continuous water medium (w/o/w). It is only of theoritical importance.

In multiple emulsions both hyphophobic and hydrophilic emulsifiers are used. O/W/O emulsions are formed better by lipophilic non-ionic surfactant using gum acacia emulsified systems. W/O/W emulsions may be prepared first by forming W/O emulsion from isopropylmyristate (oil), sorbitan-mono-oleate (emulgent) and distilled water. this emulsion is added to a polyoxyethelene sorbitan mono oleate solution in water to produce finally W/O/W emulsion - a multiple emulsion. Such multiple emulsions may be used for prolonged action, taste masking, more effective dosage forms, parenteral preparations, protection of the drug against external environment and enzyme entrapment.

(d) Micro emulsions

These emulsions are clear transparent solutions. They appear to represent a state intermediate between thermodynamically stable solubilised solutions and thermodynamically unstable emulsions. They contain droplets of oil in water phase (o/w) or droplets of water in oil (w/o) with diameters of about 10 to 200 nm and the volume fraction of the dispersed phase varies from 0.2 to 0.8.

For making micro emulsion with a surfactant, a co-surfactant is also used. An anionic surfactant (sodium lauryl sulphate or potassium oleate) is dispersed in an organic liquid such as benzene and a small amount of water is added. The gradual addition of pentanol (lipophilic co-surfactant) to the above gives a clear solution at 30°C. The surfactants form an adsorbed film on the microemulsion particles to prevent coalescence. Thus the micro emulsion contains a large or swollen micelles containing the internal phase similar to solubilized solutions. The globule size of the internal phase may also be reduced by using sonication or ultra frequency waves. Usually the emulgent should be 20 to 30% of the weight of the oil used. In the preparation of W/O systems, oil is blended with the emulgent and the water is added to produce the emulsion. Micro emulsions are used for solubilisation of drugs in pharmaceutical systems, for making some cosmetics, also used in food industries, and for making wax polishing products.

Recently micro-emulsions are being studied as drug delivery systems. They may be used to increase bioavailability of drugs poorly soluble in water by incorporation of the drug in the internal phase. Micro emulsions have also been considered as topical drug delivery system and the experiments revealed that delivery of certain drugs from microemulsions was faster and showed deeper penetration into the skin. Several patents were made by scientists for topical delivery of certain antihypertensive and antiinflammatory drugs formulated in microemulsions.

2.2. Applications of emulsions

1. Medicinal agents which have objectionable taste and odour (for example, shark liver oil, castor oil, olive oil etc) may be formulated into o/w emulsions to mask the taste and to make palatable.
2. Oil soluble vitamins (A,D,E and K) are absorbed more completely when they are made into fine emulsions than when they are administered as oily solutions.
3. O/w type emulsions are used as a dosage form for intravenous administration of oils and fats with high calorific value to patients who can not ingest food by other means and the globules in this emulsion should be similar to the size of chylomicrons (nearly colloidal size). The choice of emulsifying agent for intravenous emulsions are restricted to gelatin, lecithins and some non-ionic surfactants. Only edible oils are used as oily phase
4. Radio-opaque emulsions are being used as diagnostic agents in X-ray examination.
5. Emulsions of both the types (o/w and w/o) are extensively used to prepare pharmaceutical preparation for external use and as cosmetic preparations. Such a product should be easily spreadable, water washable non-staining and more acceptable to the patients. Eg: Cold cream and vanishing cream
6. Emulsification is used in aerosol products to produce foams. The propellant that forms the dispersed liquid phase within the container vapourises when the emulsion is discharged from the container.
7. Emulsions afford protection to drugs susceplible to oxidation or hydrolysis.
8. Liquid paraffin is used as purgative when taken orally and is not absorbed. It should not be made into fine emulsion since fine globules may be absorbed.
9. Some enemas are made as emulsions either for local action (Eg. soap enemas) or to influence drug action.
10. Solid drugs which show poor solubility may be dissolved in the oil and emulsified. From this emulsion, the biovailabity is more (as compared to tablet or suspension. Eg. non-steroidal antifungal agents).

2.3. Identification of type of emulsions

Mainly the emulsions are either o/w type or w/o type. They may be identified by the following tests.

(a) Dilution test

Generally addition of the continuous phase to an emulsion will lead to dilution and the addition of internal phase to an emulsion will lead to separation of the added liquid.

Accordingly, addition of water to o/w type emulsion leads to dilution of emulsion without any separation of added water. However separation will occur with w/o type emulsion. Similarly, addition of oil to o/w type emulsion leads to separation of the added oil. However dilution occurs with w/o type emulsion by the addition of oil.

(b) Dye test

A small quantity of water soluble dye such as methylene blue or brilliant blue may be dusted on the surface of an emulsion. If the emulsion is of o/w type the dye will dissolve in the continuous phase and diffuse throughout the water. If the emulsion is of w/o type, the water soluble dye will lie in clumps on the surface.

Alternatively, a small quantity of oil soluble dye may be added to the emulsion and shaken. If a drop of the emulsion is examined under mircoscope, the external phase is stained indicating the emulsion is w/o. If the internal phase is stained (i.e. coloured spots may be seen), the emulsion is o/w type.

In a similar manner, the test can be carried out with water soluble dye.

(c) Electrical conductivity test

Water is a good conductor of electricity especially when it contains dissolved electrolytes whereas oil is a bad conductor of electricity. This fact is utlised to find out the type of emulsion.

An electrical circuit is shown in the Fig: 121. The emulsion is kept in a vessel with two electrodes dipped in. It is connected to a battery, switch and a bulb in series. The circuit is closed by switching on. If the bulb glows continuously, it indicates that the continuous phase in the emulsion is water and the emulsion is o/w type. If the bulb flickers (not glowing continuously) the emulsion is w/o type.

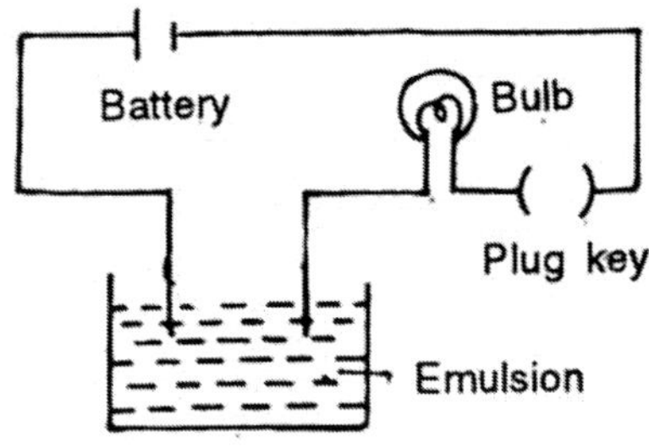

Fig.121. Electrical conductivity test

(d) By observing the creaming or sedementation pattern in emulsion

Creaming is the upward movement of the internal phase in an emulsion (i.e. positive creaming). Creaming occurs only in o/w emulsions. It is nothing but the separation of lower and higher density liquids. The liquid with lower density tends to move upwards. Sedimentation (negative creaming) is the downward movement of particles towards the bottom of the container. It occurs only in w/o type emulsion. It is also a process of separation of liquids with different densities. In this case the liquid globules with higher density (i.e water) settle at the bottom.

2.4. Theories of emulsification

Viscosity theory: As per this theory, an increase in viscosity of an emulsion will lead to an increase in stability. This theory failed to explain about the milk which shows considerable stability even though its viscosity is less.

Film theory or Adsorption theory: As per this theory, the added emulsifying agent forms a mechanical film by getting adsorbed at the interface of the liquids (i.e. at the interface between the dispersed globules and the dispersion medium) and offers stability to the emulsion. However, this theory could not explain the formation of type of emulsion.

Wedge theory: According to this theory, monovalent soaps like sodium stearate give o/w type emulsion and divalent soaps like calcium stearate give w/o type emulsion.

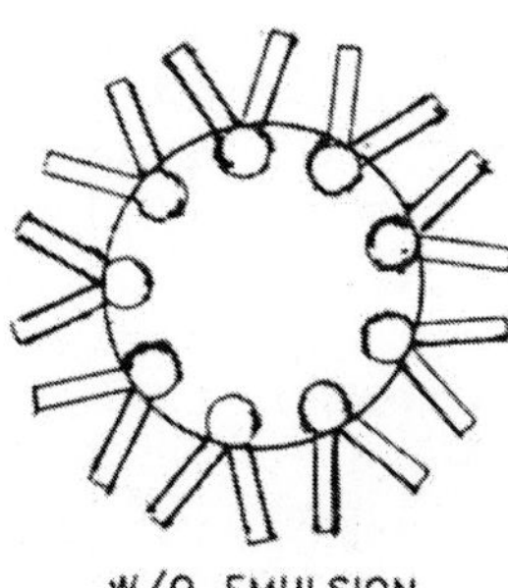

Fig. 122

This was explained by the successful accommodation of the soaps at the interface and subsequent possible orientation of the soap molecules to give the type of emulsion (Fig. 122).

For example, sodium stearate may be represented as follows.

$C_{17}H_{35}COONa$ or

and its accomodation is possible only in o/w type emulsion.

In the case of divalent soap, calcium stearate, the represertation may be presented as follows

$$\begin{matrix} C_{17}H_{35}COO \\ C_{17}H_{35}COO \end{matrix} \Big> Ca \quad \text{or}$$

Its acomodation is possible in w/o type emulsion.

This theory could not explain the stability of an emulsion. Another defect in this theory is that calcium stearate will ionise and will not exist as a wedge.

Interfacial tension theory In accordance with this theory, the added emulsifying agent reduces the interfacial tension between the oil and water phases and thus a stable emulsion is formed. This theory could not explain the formation of type of emulsion.

Thus there is no universal theory of emulsification. Any theory, to be meaningful, should be capable of explaining

(a) type of emulsion formed

(b) stability of emulsion

Modern approach:

The modern approach about the theory of emulsification is as follows.

When a liquid is shaken with another immiscible liquid, the liquid in small quantities disperse as fine droplets in another liquid which is in large quantity. Depending upon the agitation or the shear rate used, the size of the droplets vary. The higher shear rates produce smaller droplets. The time of agitation is also important. The mean size of the droplets decreases rapidly in the first few seconds. The limiting size range is generally reached within one to five minutes. Such a dispersion is thermodynamically instable and the two liquids separate rapidly into two clearly defined layers which are thermodynamically stable. It is due to the fact that cohesive forces between the molecules of each liquid is greater than adhesive forces between the molecules of the two liquids. The existence of an emulsion is the result of the two competing process – one is the dispersion of one liquid in the form of droplets throughout the other and the other is the combination of these droplets to reform initial bulk liquid. The first process increases the free energy and the second process results in decrease in free energy i.e. the process is spontaneous. Therefore, for a stable emulsion, it is necessary to promote dispersion by using a well operating machinery to produce fine droplets in a short period of time and to minimize the second process by using certain parameters to stabilize emulsion. The various parameters are

a) When one liquid is broken into small particles, the interfacial area of the globules is enormous as compared to surface area of the original liquid. For example if 1 cm^3 of mineral oil is dispersed into globules of a volume of 0.01 μ (10^{-6}cm) into 1 cm^3 of water, the surface area of the oil droplets becomes 600 sq. meters. The surface free energy associated with this area is about 34×10^7 erg or 8 calories. The total volume of the system ($2cm^2$) remains the same. Thus, the system becomes thermodynamically instable. Hence the droplets tend to flocculate (aggregation of droplets) and subsequently coalesce (fusing of the agglomerate into a larger drop) To prevent this, emulsifying agents are added to give stable coherent interfacial film surrounding each droplet and this results in the reduction of interfacial tension. The emulsifying agents may be divided into three groups.

a) *Surface active agents.* These are adsorbed at oil/water interface to form monomolecular films and thus reduce surface tension.

b) *Hydrophilic colloids.* These are adsorbed at oil-water interface to form multimolecular film.

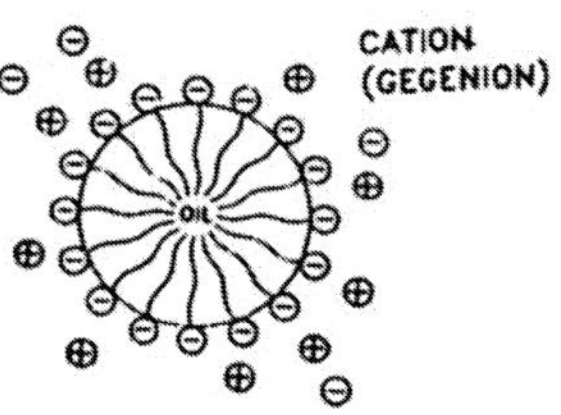

Fig. 123

c) ***Finely divided solids:*** These are adsorbed at the oil-water interface to form particulate layer.

(a) Monomolecular adsorption

Surface active agents or amphiphiles reduce interfacial tension because of their adsorption at the oil-water interface to form monomolecular layer. A good emulsifying agent will reduce the interfacial tension to 1 dyne/cm and thus the surface free energy of the system is reduced to one sixtieth of that calculated earlier. In addition to this the monomolecular layer prevent coalescence between droplets. Such a film should be flexible so that it is capable of reforming rapidly if broken. An additional effect promoting stability is the presence of a surface charge which will cause repulsion between adjacent particles.

The presence of charges on the surface of oil globules create an electrical double layer around each globule. (Fig: 123) Overlapping of these double layer gives rise to a repulsion which opposes the *van der waals* forces of attraction. The variation in net potential of interaction due to combined effects of repulsive and attractive forces between oil globules in an o/w emulsion is given as follows.

If the potential barrier is high, globules will bounce apart if the approaching globules are able to overcome the energy of barrier (due to thermal ef-

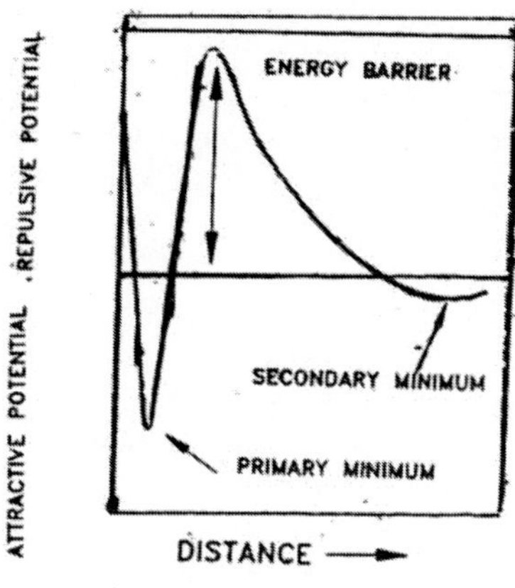

Fig. 124

fects, decomposition of surfactant, addition of oppositely charged electrolytes or surfactants) they pass into primary minimum and the emulsion may break which now depends upon the strength of the adsorbed film. Flocculation may occur in the secondary minimum but the globules are separated by a layer of continuous phase. Refer Fig.124 The aggregates can be separated by a mechanical agitation.

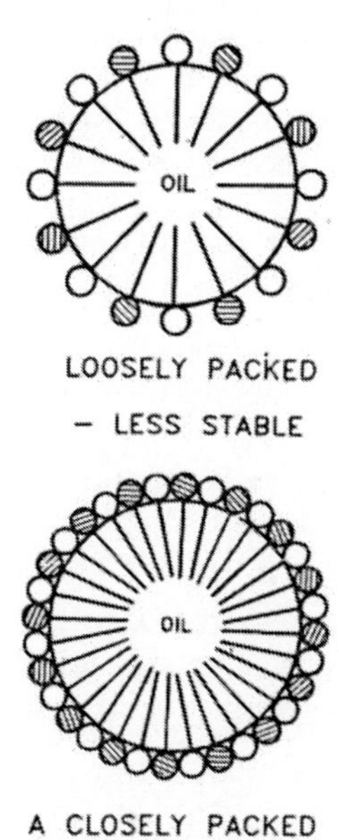

Fig. 125

Between the surfactant molecules adsorbed at the interface, repulsion may occur due to like charges. Hence to promote adsorption, lipophilic hydrocarbon chain of sufficient length must be present. That is why potassium stearate ($C_{17}H_{35}COOK$) has more emulsion stabilising ability than potassium laurate ($C_{11}H_{23}COOK$) Combination of emulsifiers is preferred to a single emulsifier to produce stable emulsions.

The adsorption of a water soluble surfactant at oil-water interface is also promoted by the presence of an oil soluble surfactant in the oily phase. The effect is mutual which leads to the formation of a closely packed film (Refer Fig.125) called complex condensed film which provides for more stability.

Example:

a) a combination of water soluble sodium lauryl sulphate (1 part) and oil soluble cetostearyl alcohol (9 parts) (It is called emulsifying wax)

b) a combination of water soluble cetrimide (1 part) and oil soluble cetostearyl alcohol (9 parts) (It is called cetrimide emulsifying wax)

The type of emulsion that is produced (o/w or w/o) depends upon the property of emulsifying agent. It is referred to as hydrophile lipophile balance (HLB) that is the balance between the polar and non polar nature of the emulsifier. The HLB values of surfactants have been discussed under Interfacial phenomena.

O/w emulsion are formed when the HLB value of the emulsifier is in the range of about 8 to 16 and w/o emulsions are formed when the range is 3 to 6. For example, span 60 having a HLB value of 4.7 will produce w/o emulsion and a blend of tween 20 and span 20 having a HLB value of 12 will yield o/w emulsion. Thus, the type of emulsion is a function of relative solubility of the surface active agent, the phase in which it is more soluble being the continuous phase. (It is called Bancroft rule). An emulsifying agent with high HLB value is soluble in water and it produces o/w emulsion and that with low HLB value is oil soluble producing w/o emulsion.

Davies has proposed that the type of emulsion formed depends on the coalescence kinetics of the two liquid phases when they are shaken together in the presence of an emulsifying agent. Say the coalescence rate of oil globules dispersed in water is rate 1 and the coalescence rate of water globules dispersed in oil is rate 2. When an emulsifying agent having a HLB value 7 is used, rate 1 will be less than rate 2 and therefore an o/w emulsion will result.

(b) Multi molecular adsorption

Hydrocolloids form multimolecular layer adsorbed at the interface. They are strong and resist coalescence. They do not cause appreciable lowering of interfacial tension. An auxiliary effect with these hydrocolloids is the significant increase in the viscosity of the medium. Since they are hydrophilic, they promote only o/w type emulsions. Their use is limited because of availability of large number of synthetic surfactants. The mechanical strength of gel barrier may be increased by increasing gelation which is more effective at iso-electric point. With anionic hydrocolloids such as carboxy methyl cellulose gelation is induced at low pH and the film formed is rigid.

(c) Solid particles adsorption

Finely divided solid particles that are wetted to some degree by both oil and water can act as emulsifying agents. They concentrate at the interface and produce a film around each droplet (particulate layer) and this effect prevents coalescence strongly because of the mechanical strength of the film. Those powders that are wetted preferentially by water form o/w emulsions and those that are wetted easily by oil tend to form w/o emulsion. An extremely rigid interfacial film of close packed particles can be produced by capillary force as shown in the diagram. (Fig.126)

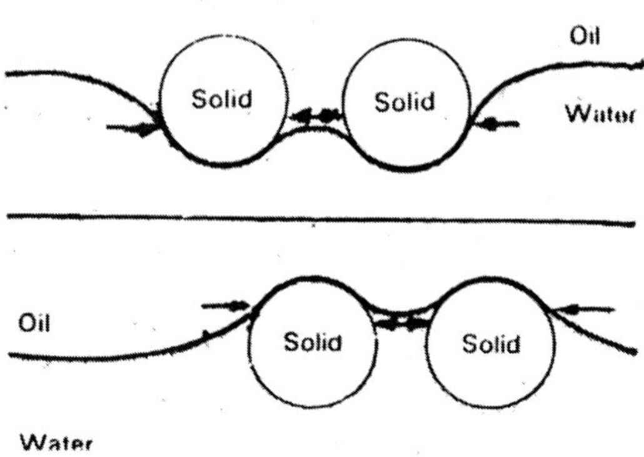

Fig. 126. Capillary forces cause similar particles cohere strongly

Other factors influencing stability of emulsions

In the case of w/o emulsion, ionisation of substances in oil is weak. However ***electrical double layer*** may be formed in the water globules dispersed in the oil. The diffuse part of such layers is thick. Hence potential energy barriers to flocculation is lower in w/o than in o/w emulsions. Flocculation occurs more easily in w/o type emulsion.

Solvation effects The hydrophilic groups of adsorbed emulsifier may have thick solvation sheaths which aid in the prevention of flocculation of oil globules. Another school of thought is that solvation sheath of short range do not contribute to stability of emulsion.

Stearic effects Hydrophilic group of many non-ionic emulsifying agents consists of extensive poly ethylene oxide chains. Oil globules carrying adsorbed molecules of this type behave in a manner that they are coated with a thick layer of hydrophilic colloid which prevents flocculation of oil globules.

2.5. Emulsifying agents

An emulsifying agent should have the following desirable properties.

(a) Should have effective surface active property and should reduce surface tension to below 10 dyne/cm.

(b) Should get adsorbed quickly around the droplets (or globules) as a condensed, non-adherent film which will prevent coalescence.

(c) Should impart the droplet an adequate electric potential so that mutual repulsion results

(d) Should increase the viscosity of the emulsion

(e) Should be effective in a reasonably low concentration

(f) Should be non toxic

(g) Should be odourless and tasteless and if there is taste and odour, they should be compatible with the product.

(h) Should have good chemical stability

(i) Should be compatible with the other ingredients in the emulsion.

Type	Type of film	Examples
Synthetic surfactants	monomolecular	**1. Anionic**
		Soaps: Potassium laureate and triethanolamine stearate.
		Sulphates: Sodium lauryl sulphate and alkyl poly oxyethylene sulphate
		Sulphonates: Dioctyle sodium sulphosuccinate
		2. Cationic: *Quaternary ammonium compounds* Cetyltrimethyl ammonium bromide
		3. Nonionic
		Polyoxyethylene fatty alcohol ethers
		Sorbitan fatty esters
		Poly oxyethylene sorbitan fatty acid esters.
Natural	Multimolecular	**Hydrophilic colloids** Acacia, gelatin
	Monomolecular	Cholesterol, Lecithin
Finely divided solids	solid particle (particulate layer)	**Colloidal clays** Bentonite veegum
		Metallic hydroxides magnesium hydroxide.

Auxiliary emulsifying agents

Name	Composition	Uses
Bentonite	Colloidal hydrated aluminium silicate	Hydrophilic thickening agents and stabiliser for o/w and w/o lotions and creams.
Cetyl alcohol	chiefly $C_{16}H_{33}OH$	Lipophilic thickening agent and stabiliser for o/w lotions and liniments.
Glyceryl mono stearate	$C_{17}H_{35}COOCH_2\,CHOH\,CH_2OH$	
Magnesium hydroxide	$Mg(OH)_2$	Hydrophilic stabiliser for o/w emulsions.
Methyl cellulose	Series of methyl esters of cellulose	Hydrophilic thickening agent and stabiliser for o/w emulsions. It is a weak o/w emulsifier.
Silice gel	Hydrous oxides of silica	Hydrophilic stabiliser in ointments,
Sodium alginate	Sodium salt of alginic acid, a purified carbohydrate extracted from giant kelp.	Hydrophilic thickening agent and stabiliser for o/w emulsion.
Sodium carboxy methyl cellulose	Sodium salt of carboxy methyl esters of cellulose	"
Stearic acid	A mixture of solid acids and fats, chiefly stearic and palmitic	
Stearyl alcohol	Chiefly $C_{18}H_{37}OH$	Lipophilic thickening agent and stabiliser for o/w lotions and ointments.
Tragacanth	Dried gummy exudate of the species Astragalus	Hydrophilic thickening agent and stabiliser for o/w emulsions. It is a weak o/w emulsifier.
Veegum	Colloidal magnesium aluminium silicate	Hydrophilic thickening agent and stabiliser for o/w lotion and creams.

Concentration of the emulsifier

The concentration of the emulsifier required to form a condensed film around the droplets of the dispersed phase to give a stable emulsion is calculated as follows.

Say 100 gm of an oil having a density of 1 is to be emulsified in 100 ml of water.

If the desired particle diameter (i.e. of droplet diameter) is 1 μ, then the particle diameter in terns of cm is 1×10^{-4} cm.

Volume of particle

$$= \frac{\pi d^3}{6} = 0.524 \times 10^{-12}\ \text{cm}^3$$

Total number of particles in 100 grams.

$$= \frac{100}{0.524 \times 10^{-12}} = 191.0 \times 10^{12}$$

surface area of each particle $= \pi d^2$

$$= 3.142 \times (1 \times 10^{-4})^2 \text{cm}^2$$

$$= 3.142 \times 10^{-8}\ \text{cm}^2$$

Total surface area

$$= 3.142 \times 10^{-8} \times 191.0 \times 10^{12}$$

$$= 600 \times 10^{4} \text{ cm}^2$$

If the area that each molecule occupies at the oil-water interface is 30×10^{-16} cm^2

we require $\dfrac{600 \times 10^4}{30 \times 10^{-16}} = 2 \times 10^{21}$ molecules.

suppose the molecular weight of the emulsifying agent is 1000, then the required weight is

$$\frac{1000 \times 2 \times 10^{21}}{6.023 \times 10^{23}} = 3.32 \text{ grams.}$$

This calculation may serve as a guide to determine the weight of emulsifying agent (approximately) needed for the preparation of an emulsion.

Selection of emulsifying agent

Selection of an emulsifying agent depends on the use to which the emulsion is required. For example, it may be required for an emulsion meant for internal, external or parenteral use. The desirable properties expected must be satisfied. Selection based on HLB for an emulsion which may be o/w or w/o may be given as follows.

First method

To produce emulsions of o/w type emulsifiers in the HLB range of 8-18 are tried and for w/o type emulsifiers in the range of HLB 3-16 are tried.

Second method

Griffin evolved a series of required HLB values for a particular material to be emulsified.

Substance	HLB value for O/W	HLB value for W/O
Cotton seed oil	6-7	-
Petrolatum	8	-
Bees wax	9-11	5
Paraffin wax	10	4
Mineral oil	10-12	5-6
Methyl silicone	11	-
Lanolin, anydrous	12-14	-
Lauryl alcohol	14	-
Castor oil	14	-
Kerosene	12-14	-
Cetyl alcohol	13-16	-
Stearyl alcohol	15-16	-
Carbon tetrachloride	16	-
Lauric acid	16	-
Oleic acid	17	-
Stearic acid	17	-

The HLB values are algebraically additive. By taking emulsifiers with low HLB value and high HLB value proportions of the emulsifiers required to produce the required HLB value may be worked out. If we use two emulsifiers of HLB values 3 and 18, to get a HLB value of 10, the required proportions can be obtained as follows by a method called allegation method.

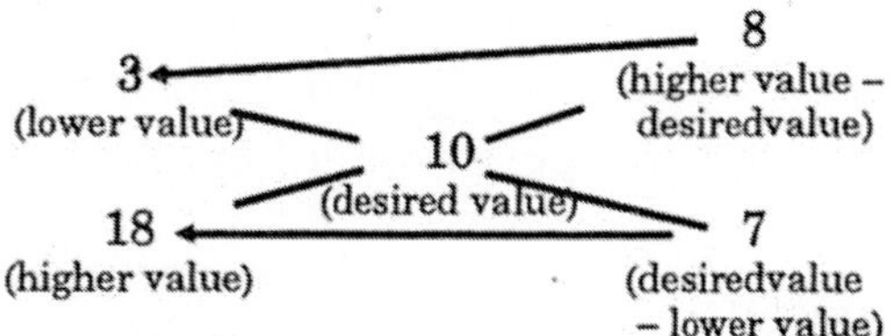

2 parts of the emulsifier with HLB value 3 and 7 parts of the emulsifier with HLB value 18 will give a blend with HLB value 10.

Third method

If the HLB value of an emulsifier to emulsify an oil is not known, it may be necessary to determine this value. For this, determination, various blends of emulsifiers are prepared to give a wide range of mixtures with different HLB values and then the emulsions are prepared. The physical stability of the emulsions are assessed. The blend which gives better stability is the required HLB value for the emulsifier.

Normally mixtures of emulsifiers give a better emulsion due to a) production of required HLB value for the emulsifier mixture 2) formation of mixed interfacial film (complex condensed film) with more stability and cohesiveness and 3) provide better consistency and feel for the product.

2.6 Stability of emulsions

Stability of emulsions is characterised by

(a) absence of coalescence of internal phase

(b) absence of creaming

(c) maintenance of elegance with respect to color, odour and other physical properties.

The various instabilities of the emulsions are

(a) flocculation and creaming

(b) coalescence and breaking

(c) phase inversion.

(a) Flocculation and Creaming

Creaming results from flocculation and concentration of globules of the internal phase. If the disperse phase is less dense than the continuous phase (o/w type emulsion) a creamy layer (containing concentrated globules of the internal phase) collects at the top of the emulsion since the velocity of sedimentation becomes negative. It is called upward creaming. In the case of w/o type emulsion, creaming occurs in a downward direction since the velocity of sedimentation is positive i.e. sedimentation of the dispersed globules takes place. Creaming occurs as a result of density difference between the dispersed phase and the dispersion medium. Creaming is not a serious problem since it is reversible and redistribution (or redispersion) of the internal phase occurs on shaking the container.

The rate of sedimentation of a droplet particle is governed by ***Stoke's law***. According to this law, the rate of creaming may be decreased by increasing the viscosity of the dispersion medium. Using viscosity improvers or thickening agent such as methyl cellulose, tragacanth, and sodium alginate. The particle size of the globules may be reduced by homogenisation. If the average particle size of the emulsion is reduced, the rate of creaming is reduced considerably when the globules are reduced to a diameter below 2 to 5 μ, Brownian movements set in at room temperature Creaming is prevented by Borwnian movement. Adjusting the density difference between oil and water also increases the stability but this method is not suitable for pharmaceutical preparations. Creaming of emulsion is also called sedimentation pattern of emulsions.

b) Coalescence and breaking

The coalescence (aggregated globules merge into larger drops) of the dispersed particles lead to complete separation of oil and water. It is a serious problem since simple shaking fails to resuspend the globules uniformly throughout the medium.

Factors causing breaking

a) A substance which is incompatible with the emulsifier, destroys the emulsifier ability.

Example: effect of large anions on cationic emulsifier, effect of calcium and magnesium ions on monovalent soaps, effect of phenolic substances on cetomacrogol.

b) On increasing the temperature the number of collisions between globules will increase leading to cracking or breaking of the emulsion. This is because the energy barrier between the globules is overcome by thermal effects. It is made use of in accelerated stability tests on the stability of emulsion.

c) Increased temperature may coagulate certain type of macro molecular emulsifying agents.

d) Freezing of aqueous phase will produce ice crystals which exert pressure on globules.

e) Attempt to incorporate excessive amounts of disperse phase may cause breaking of emulsion.

Critical point cracking It is defined as the concentration of the internal phase above which the emulsifying agent cannot produce a stable emulsion. In some emulsions, the value may be as high as 74%. Instability results from the irregular shape and size of the globules. Generally a phase volume ratio of 50/50 results in about the most stable emulsion. Attempts to incorporate more than about 74% of oil in o/w emulsion leads to cracking.

(c) Phase inversion

In o/w emulsion stabilised with sodium stearate can be inverted to w/o type by adding calcium chloride to form calcium stearate

Inversion may also be produced by alterations in phase volume ratio. For example, an o/w emulsifier is mixed with oil and a little quantity of water, a w/o type emulsion is produced by agitation. Since water volume is less, it forms w/o emulsion. But when more water is added slowly, phase inversion occurs and o/w type emulsion is produced. Inversion has also been observed when an emulsion which has been prepared by heating and mixing the two phases, is cooled. It is due to the temperature dependent changes in the solubilities of the emulsifying agents. Phase inversion can be prevented by choosing proper emulsifying agent in suitable concentration. Wherever possible, it is better to see the internal phase does not exceed 50% of total volume of the emulsion.

Phase inversion technique is sometimes used to produce emulsions with fine droplet sizes.

Preservation of emulsions

Some antimicrobial agents are added for preservation of emulsions to protect against microbial attack Frequently a preservative exhibits a lower antimicrobial activity in an emulsion than in a solution. It is because of the 'partitioning effect' of the agent between the oil and water. This effect causes a lowering of the effective concentration of the antimicrobial agent in water. Hence sufficient additional amount of antimicrobial agent should be added to make amends for the amount partitioned into the oily phase so as to get the 'effective concentration' of the antimicrobial agent in the aqueous phase. The chemical stability of the various components of emulsion is also important since some materials may be more prone to degradation in the emulsified state than they are in the bulk solution.

Assessment of stability of emulsions

Assessment of stability of emulsions may be undertaken by observing the rate of separation of the disperse phase as a distinct layer (degree of creaming) from emulsion. This method is suitable only for unstable emulsions that exhibit creaming quickly. For ac-

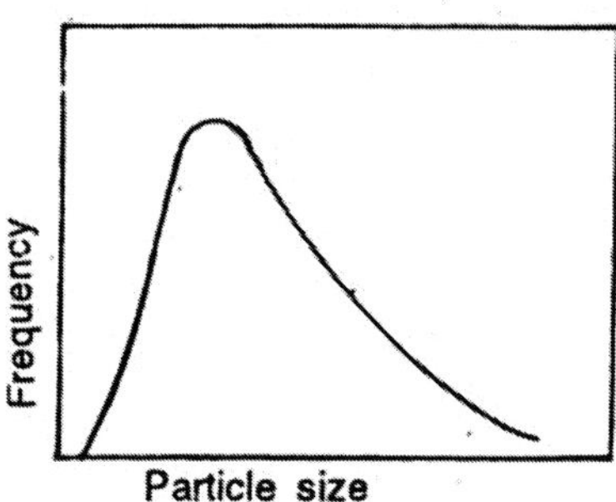

Fig. 127. Globule size distribution in an emulsion

celerated study, the rate of creaming may be increased by centrifugation.

A precise assessment can be made by studying the changes in size distribution of globules in an emulsion with time. Measurement of globule size can be undertaken using a microscope. In this method, initially the particle diameters are measured and a size frequency distribution of particles is obtained as a graph (Refer Fig.127). The size distribution study is carried out at different time intervals. The changes in the shape of the curve shown indicate instability Stability can be assessed in terms of the rate at which such changes occur.

A more reliable result can be obtained by calculating changes in the number of globule per mililiter

Other methods such as coulter counting, turbidimetric analysis and temperature tests have also been used to evaluate new emulsifying agents and to determine the stability of emulsion.

Semi solid emulsions (or creams)

Creams find variety of uses in cosmetics as emollient, protective or as bases to prepare medicinal creams One such example is cold cream.

Phase equilibria and formulation

The student is advised to refer the phase diagram discussed under phase equilibria to understand emulsion formulation based on phase equilibria

A ternary phase diagram is given in Fig:128 as an example to understand the various phases that may exist in different regions within the triangular diagram

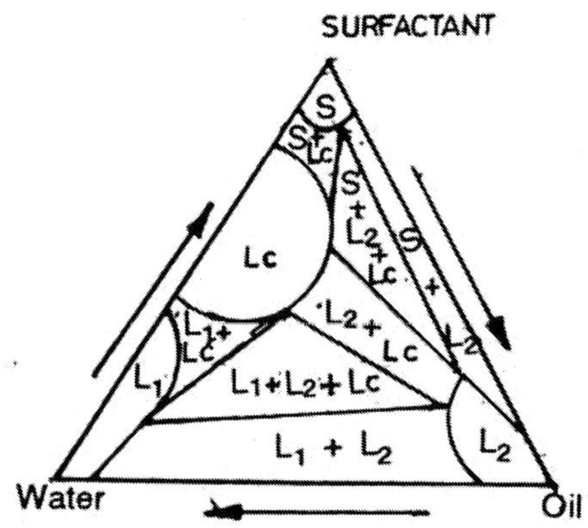

Fig. 128. Phase diagram of surfactant-oil-water system

The compositions at different regions are represented in the diagram. L_1 and L_2 represent aqueous and oily phases respectively. Each corner represents the higher concentrations of surfactant, water or oil. Refer the diagram where each corner has been represented as surfactant, water or oil.

Near the corner represented as surfactant, we find solid surfactant phase (which may be disregarded for our discussion). Below this, we find solubilised systems i.e. micelles exist in which oil and water are solubilized. LC represents a liquid crystalline phase with lamellar structure which may be represented by the figure shown.

As we move down, i.e. as the concentration of surfactant is being

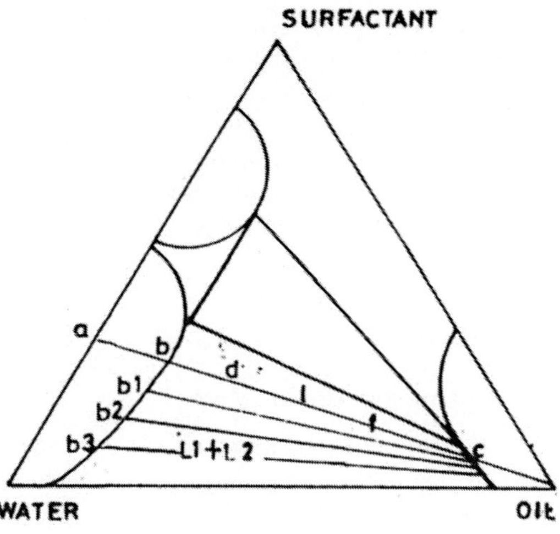

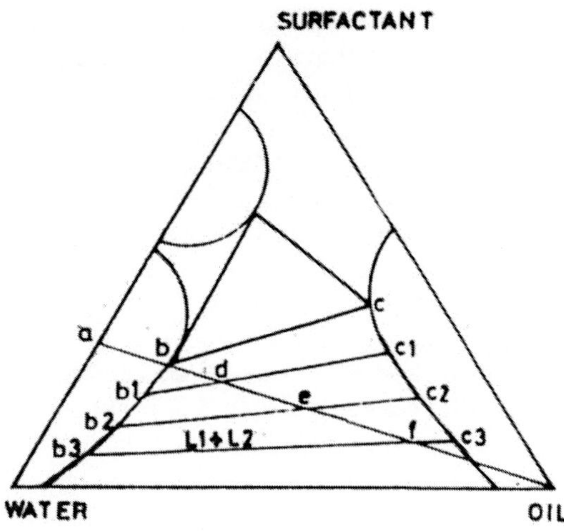

Fig. 129

reduced, we find the phases $S + L_2 + LC, L_2 + Lc, L_1 + L_c$ and $L_1 + L_2 + L_c$.

In the case of $L_2 + L_c$ and $L_1 + L_c$, it may be considered that L_2 is dispersed in L_c and L_1 is dispersed in L_C. As regards $L_1 + L_2 + L_c$ this region may be considered as an emulsified system and either the L_1, L_2 or L_c can be continuous phase for the other two i.e. L_2 and L_c or L_1 and L_2 or L_1 and L_c can be dispersed phase.

$L_1 + L_2$ represents the conventional emulsion. This occurs at a low concentration of surfactant. The student may be aware of the fact that for emulsification purpose only a low concentration of surfactant i.e. emulsifying agent is used.

Therefore, with such a diagram, it is possible to know how the changes in concentration of oil, water and surfactant have an effect in the preparation of solubilised or emulsion systems. It may be ascertained that various concentrations of the ingredients needed for a stable emulsion leading to a successful formulation of an emulsion which is relatively stable. Batch to batch variations may also minimised.

One must be aware of the fact that the areas of regions of various phases represented in the diagram varies for different surfactant and oil used.

This ternary diagram approach has been used to demonstrate the effect of phase volume ratio also. It was found that an o/w emulsion was produced when 45% and more of water was used and less than this amount resulted in w/o emulsions.

The phase diagram has also been used for

1. Viscosity dependence on phase volume ratio

2. rheologic properties dependence on phase volume ratio and type of emulsions.

It may be expected that these properties change on the location of the system within the triangular ternary diagram. (Fig: 129)

It is also possible to study the effects produced as one of the components is varied or effects produced on adding a different component. For example, effect of addition of oil to the system containing 30% of surfactant can be explained. Two situations can occur. In the first case consider a line drawn at 30% of surfactant concentration to the corner of the oil. As this line is parallel to other the lines, it is also considered as one of the tie lines. In the tie line shown, we find two conjugate phases corresponding to the concentrations at b and c occur between b and c. The compositions of the two conjugate phases L_1 and L_2 depend on the direction of the tie line running across the $L_1 + L_2$ phase region. In the first situation, the continual addition of oil brings about no change in the compositions of the two phases b and c but only the relative amounts vary as shown by d, e, and f. Addition of oil produces a charge in phase volume ratio and hence the effect of phase volume on stability, viscosity emulsion type etc may be investigated.

In contrast to the first situation, continual addition of oil to the system may produce a change in the direction of tie lines thereby indicating a change in the composition at points d,e and f If a line is drawn at 30% surfactant concentration to the corner of the oil, we find the line cut the tie lines i.e. it is not parallel. In this case, the composition of the two conjugate liquids L_1 and L_2 at point d is given by b_1 and c_1; the composition at e by b_2 and c_2 and at f by b_3 and c_3. In this case we study the effect of varying concentration of oil as well as the effect of varying composition of the two conjugate phases themselves.

2.7 Preparation of emulsions

Small scale method: Mortar and pestle method

It is used for emulsions which are stabilized by a multimolecular film at the interface. Consequently the emulgents used are acacia, tragacanth, agar, chondrous, cellulose derivatives, ect. There are two basic methods (wet gum method and dry gum method) for the preparation of such emulsions. The emulsions produced show polydisperse globules with wide range of sizes.

Wet gum method

In this the emulgent is placed in the mortar and dispersed in water to form a mucilage. The oil is added in small amounts with continuous trituration, each portion of the oil is emulsified before adding the next increment. The optimum ratio of fixed oil; water and acacia is 4:2:1 to prepare initial emulsion called primary emulsion. The ratio of volatile oil, water and gum is 3:2:1. The ratio varies with emulgents.

The primary emulsion should be triturated at least for five minutes. Then sufficient water is added to produce the final volume.

Dry gun method

In this, the gum is added to the oil and dispersed in a mortar and pestle. The water is added in little quantities at a time with trituration to produce the primary emulsion.

Preparations of emulsions by wet gum method and dry gum method may be carried out by shaking or agitation in bottles rather than in a mortar and pestle.

Large scale methods

The selection of emulsion making machines depends on

1. the amount of emulsion to be processed
2. flow characteristics

3. need to blend ingredients such as powders
4. the temperature involved.
5. the desired rate of cooling if elevated temperature is used for the preparation.

When an emulsion is prepared, nergy must be spent to form an inter-ace (i.e. extensive interface by the reduction in size of the globules of the internal phase) between the oily and aqueous phases. The emulsion making machines may be agitators, colloid mill, homogenisers and ultrasonic devices.

Agitators

Small electric mixers are used to prepare an emulsion at the prescription counter. In this, the oil, emulgent and water are mixed and transferred to the mixer. The beater within the mixer is operated electrically to induce shearing stress to get a stable emulsion.

Waring blenders (Fig. 130) disperse the internal phase efficiently. The shearing action is produced by rapidly rotating blades operated electrically. This mixer transfers large amount of energy to get an emulsion from the crude mixture of oil, water and the gum. It is most suitable for preparing fluid emulsions.

Production size agitators Fig. 131 include rapidly rotating blade with baffles and scrapper. It is the most suitable one to prepare creams. This instrument has a rapidly rotating blade operated by a motor. The stator (holder of the contents of the emulsion) is provided with two baffles to induce proper mixing and agitation. A scrapper is made to operate nearer to the inner surface of the vessel to avoid dead spots during mixing. The vessel is jacketed to facilitate heating or cooling during the processing.

Colloid mills

A colloid mill Fig. 132 consists usually a stator and a rotor which revolves at a greater speed. A crude emulsion is passed between the stator and the high speed rotor revolving at a speed of 2000-18000 rpm. The clearance (the gap) between the rotor and stator is adjustable usually from 0.001 inch upward.

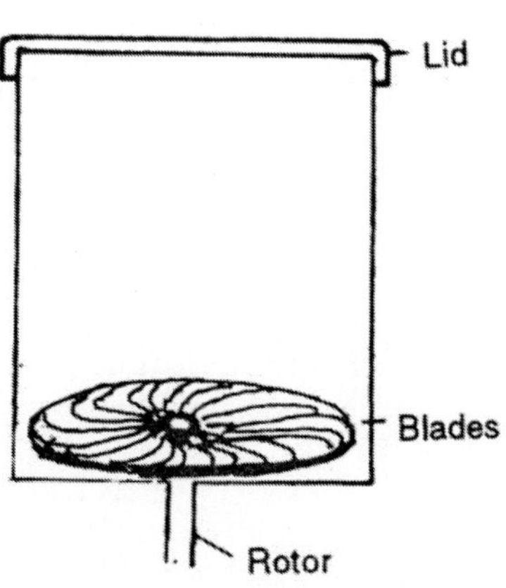

Fig. 130 Warring blendor

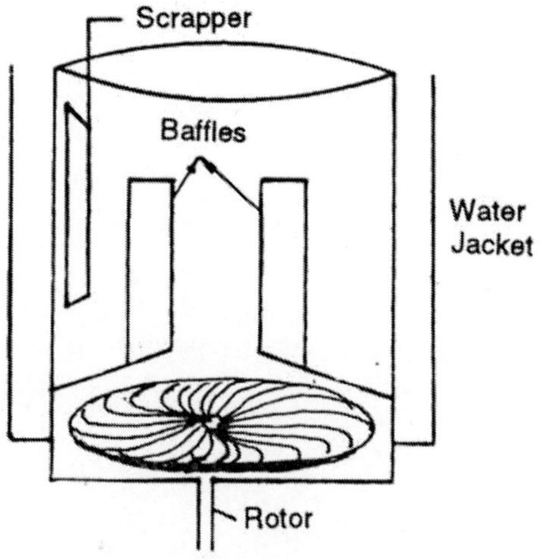

Fig. 131. Production size agitator

The emulsion mixture is subjected to a tremendous shearing stress which effects a fine emulsion. During operation, temperature of the emulsion increases and hence it is necessary to cool the equipment by circulating cold water when the emulsion is being formed.

Homogenisers and viscolizers

In these, the mixed phases are passed between a finely ground valve and a seat under high pressure of the order of 1000-5000 lb/sq. inch. This high pressure produces an atomization which is enhanced by the impact received by the atomized mixture as it strikes the valve head.

Homogenisation is done in two ways – either the ingredients of the emulsions are mixed and passed through the homogeniser to produce a fine emulsion or an emulsion prepared by some other means may be passed through a homogenizer.

Silverson mixer homogeniser

Models are available for batch processes Fig: 133 as well as for continuous type to process a few milliliters to several liters. The machine consists of a head under which turbine blades are attached to a motor through a rod. When operated the rod as well as the turbine blades rotate at a high speed. During operation this head is immersed in the coarse emulsion taken in a vessel. The emulsion is sucked in and thrown through the mesh cover by the rotating blades. Due to large shearing and impaction, a fine emulsion is produced. The disadvantage in this method is that the emulsion show increased creaming tendencies.

Gaulin two stage homogeniser

To avoid the above disadvantage, a two stage homogeniser may be used. One such homogeniser is the Gaulin two stage homogeniser. Fig. 134 In this the coarse emulsion is passed through the first valve at a high pressure of 3000-5000 lb/sq. inch and then through a second valve at a reduced pressure of 1000 lb/sq. inch. This breaks down any clusters formed in the first stage.

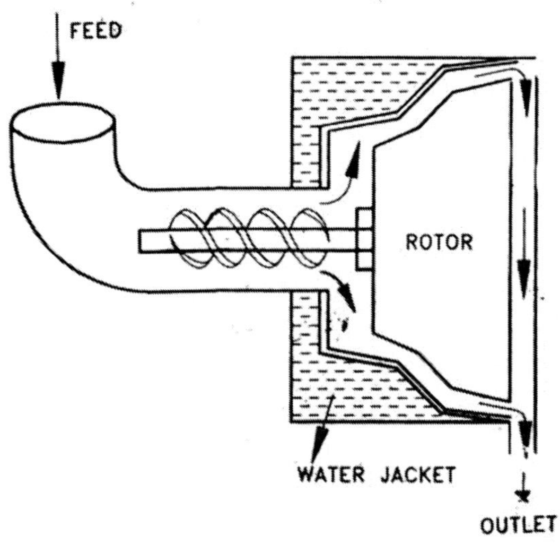

Fig. 132. A colloid mill

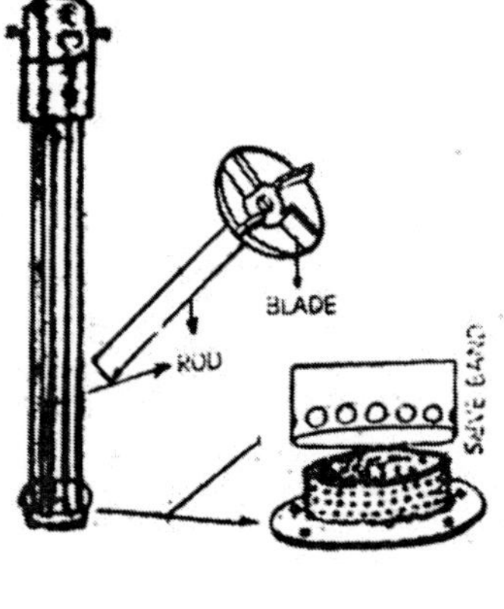

Fig. 133. Silversion mixer emulsifier

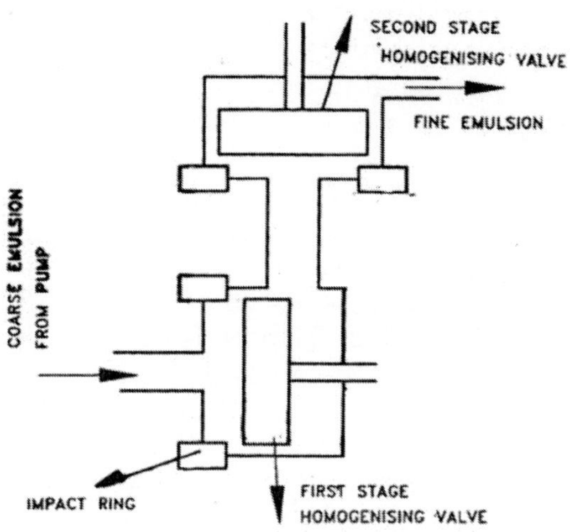

Fig. 134. Gaulin two-stage homogeniser

A homogeniser does not incorporate air in the final product. Insufficient emulsifying agent may spoil the emulsion since homogenisation produce more surface area. The temperature rise also is not large during homogenisation.

Ultrasonic devices (Rapisonic homogeniser)

Ultrasonic vibration of high frequency (100,000–500,000/sec) is produced by a suitable technique. A tube containing crude mix of the emulsion is exposed to this vibrations. The liquid develops regions of compressions and rarefaction. Cavities are formed in the regions of rarefaction and these collapse with great force which produces emulsification. This method will produce stable emulsions only with liquids of low viscosity. It is not applicable for large scale production. Fig.135.

2.8. Rheologic properties of emulsions

Various factors which decide the rheological properties of emulsions are phase volume ratio, particle size dis-

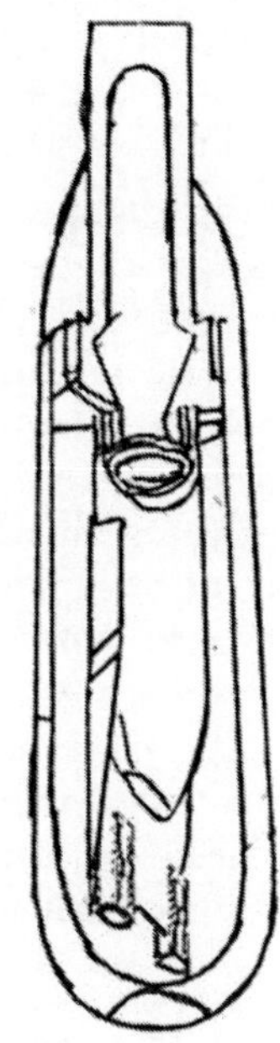

Fig. 135. Rapisonic homogeniser

tribution and the viscosity of the internal phase. When the volume concentration of the dispersed phase is as low as less than 0.05, the system exhibits Newtonian flow. As the volume concentration is increased, the system becomes resistant to flow and exhibits pseudoplastic flow. At sufficiently higher concentrations, plastic flow occurs. When the fraction of volume concentration approaches 0.74, phase inversions may occur with sizable change in viscosity. Reduction in mean globule size increases the viscosity.

The viscosity of thin liquid film, say 100 to 200 Å thickness is several times the viscosity of the bulk liquid. In concentrated emulsions, when the thickness of the continuous phase between adjacent droplets approaches the above said dimensions, higher viscosities are observed. Thus the continuous phase can affect the flow properties of the emulsion by its own viscosity. By increasing the shear on the emulsions, reduction in viscosity occurs which is due to decrease in viscosity of the continuous phase as the distance of separation of the globules are increased.

The third component that influences the viscosity of the emulsion is the emulsifying agent which will affect the particle flocculation and interparticle attractions and in turn will modify the flow. The greater the concentration of the emulsifying agent, the higher will be the viscosity of the product. The physical and electrical properties of the films also affect the viscosity. It has also been found that for a given amount of oil soluble component, water soluble ionic surfactants produce stiffer creams than equal molar concentration of a non-ionic surfactants.

Although the emulsified products are subjected to a wide variety of shear stresses during their preparation, the viscosities of the final products decide their flow properties, performance, spreadability (in the case of dermatologic and cosmetic products), syringeability through hypodermic needle (in the case of parenteral emulsions) and removability (from a bottle or tube).

FOAMS

A foam is a coarse dispersion of a gas or air in a liquid (i.e. solution) which is present as thin films of colloidal dimensions.

Foams have high interfacial area and hence are unstable in thermodynamic sense. The stability of foams may be affected by two factors:

1. the tendency of the liquid film to become thinner due to drainage of liquid.

2. the tendency to rupture as a result of disturbances such as vibration, heat and diffusion of gas from small bubbles to large bubbles. The diffusion of gas from small bubbles to large bubbles is facilitated due to the fact that small bubbles exert more internal pressure than large bubbles.

Solutions of short chain acids and alcohols form transient or unstable foams. Persistent foams are formed by solutions of surfactants and hence are more stable. This stability can be attributed to electrical double layer repulsion or stearic stabilisation. Stearic stabilisation occurs with lyophobic colloidal particles whose surface has an absorbed layer of non-ionic polymeric material such as gums, non-ionic surface active agents and methyl cellulose. The stearic interaction results when the polymeric layers of two approaching particles overlap.

Foams find application in pharmaceutical products as aqueous and non-aqueous spray preparations for topical, rectal and vaginal medication and for burn dressings and in cosmetics. (eg. shaving cream)

Anti-foaming agents find greater application in pharmacy because there is a need for the destruction of foams in some pharmaceutical processing. They are used to prevent foam in liquid preparations and in fermentation process where foaming is a nuisance. Foam inhibitors are used in the treatment of flatulence, in the elimination of gas, air or foam from the gastrointestinal tract prior to radiography and for the relief of abdominal distension and dyspepsia.

Anti foaming agents are of two types. They are foam breakers such as n-octanol, ether and foam inhibitors such as polyamides and silicones.

Suggestions for Practicals

1. *Determination of the most suitable suspending agent from among the given suspending agents for a indiffusible substance.*

Preparc a series of each of 100 ml of **5% zinc oxide** suspensions in water containing **one gram** of the suspending agents **(given) - bentonite**, acacia, gelatin, sodium carboxymethyl cellulose and tragacanth. To prepare the suspension, take the zinc oxide and the suspending agent in a mortar. Triturate with a small volume of water to make a paste. Add water slowly with continuous trituration to produce three fourth of the final volume and to get a suspension in which the particles are uniformly distributed. Transfer each of the suspensions separately into separate measuirng cylinders. Make up the volume of each suspension to 100 ml. Shake well and leave he measuring cylinders undisturbed. Note down the volume of sediment in each of the measuring cylinders at definite intervals of time say 10, 20, 30, 40, 50 and 60 minutes. Keep a control which is a suspension of zinc oxide in water without the suspending agent.

Tabulate the results as shown

Time in minutes	Volume of sediment V_u	Sedimentation volume $F = \frac{V_u}{V_o}\left(\text{or } \frac{V_u}{100}\right)$

(Sedimentation volume 'F' is the ratio of final volume (V_u) to the original volume of the suspension (V_o). In this case V_o is 100 ml).

Draw a graph by plotting time (in minutes) on x-axis versus 'F', the sedimentation volume on 'y' axis.

An ideal suspension will show 'F' value equal to 1 indicating sedimentation has occurred and the caking tendency is absent. Compare the 'F' values of the suspensions prepared with different suspending agents and report the suspending abilities of the suspending agents in terms of sedimentation volume in the decreasing order.

2. *Determination of Degree of Flocculation induced by a flocculating agent in a suspension.*

Prepare five separate suspensions each of 100 ml of 5% W/v of zinc oxide in water containing 0% (control), 1%, 1.5%, 2% and 2.5% w/v of aluminium chloride as the flocculating agent. Transfer each suspension separately into 100 ml measuring cylinders. Shake well all the cylinders and leave them undisturbed. As in the previous experiment, read the volume of sediment at different intervals say 0, 10, 20, 30, 40, 50 and 60 minutes in each of the measuring cylinders. Note down the final volume (i.e ultimate volume) which is constant for a considerable period of time. Calculate the sedimentation volume (F) for each of the suspension including the control. Consider the control as the suspension which is deflocculated. The sedimentation volume of deflocculated is represented as F_x.

Tabulate the results as follows:

For suspensions containing flocculating agent (Aluminium Chloride)

Time in minutes	Volume of sediment V_u	Sedimentation Volume $\left(F = \frac{V_u}{100}\right)$

For control (deflocculated suspension)

Time in minutes	Volume of sediment V_u	Sedimentation Volume F_x $\left(F_x = \frac{V_u}{100}\right)$

Then, the degree of flocculation (*beta*) is given by

$$\beta = \frac{F}{F_x} = \frac{\text{ultimate sedimentation volume of the flocculated suspension}}{\text{ultimate sedimentation volume of the deflocculated suspension}}$$

Compare the β (degree of flocculation) of suspension containing different concentrations of deflocculating agent and report. Likewise different flocculating (monovalent and divalent) may be used and compared.

3. *Effect of viscosity on sedimentation*

Prepare five zinc oxide suspensions in water (10% w/v) each of 100 ml containing 0% (control), 5%, 10%, 20% and 30% w/v of glycerin. Transfer them in 5 separate measuring cylinders. Shake well and leave them undisturbed. Read out the sediment volume in each of the cylinders at different time intervals. Read the sediment volume when it remains constant for a considerable period of time. Report the effect of viscosity on the sedimentation rate and sedimentation volume (viscosity of each of the solution of glycerin in water can be determined separately using Oswald's viscometer).

4. *Study of combined of flocculating agent and structured vehicle on the physical stability of suspensions.*

Prepare four suspensions each of 100 ml as directed below.

1. 5% w/v of bismuth subnitrate in water (control)
2. 5% w/v of bismuth subnitrate and 2% w/v of sodium carboxy methyl cellulose in water.
3. 5% w/v of bismuth subnitrate in water with 50 millimoles of KH_2PO_4 (flocculating agent)
4. 5% w/v of bismuth subnitrate and 2% w/v of sodium methyl cellulose in water + 50 millimoles of KH_2PO_4.

Perform the experiment and read the ultimate sediment volume. Calculate the sedimentation volume (F) and report on the physical stability of the suspensions.

5. *Determination of the type of emulsion and study of some parameters.*

Prepare an emulsion as directed below with the ingredients and quantities shown.

Liquid paraffin	-	50 ml
Acacia gum	-	17 g
Purified water	-	100 ml

Take 34 ml of water in a mortar. Disperse the gum acacia in water by trituration to get a mucilage. Add liquid paraffin a little at a time to the muscilage with constant trituration until all the oil is added. Obtain an uniform emulsion with further trituration. Make up the volume to 100 ml with water. Perform the following:

1. find out the type of emulsion by dilution with water. Perform the dye test also (refer the text)
2. Find the effect of addition of oil to the emulsion.
3. Keep the emulsion undisturbed to observe for any creaming.
4. heat the emulsion and find out the effect on creaming and observe any cracking.
5. Cool the emulsion in a refrigerator and observe for any cracking.
6. Study the globulze size using a microscope and assess the stability of emulsion by measuring the size distribution of globules at different time intervals during storage.

XI. KINETICS AND CATALYSIS

1. Chemical kinetics concerns with the study of rates of chemical reactions. A number of principles and related rate processes involved in the study of chemical kinetics are of immense help in the proper formulation and stabilisation of pharmaceutical products.

Instability in formulations is mainly due to decomposition. The speed of decomposition follows the rate process. Dissolution as well as diffusion from solid dosage forms follows rate processes. The rate processes are also applicable to the study of absorption, distribution and elimination of drugs.

For a manufacturer, the principles of kinetics are of immense help in the performance of stability studies. Accelerated stability studies are undertaken to predict the stability of a product within a short period of time i.e. in determining the shelf-life of a product.

Thus, the principles studied under chemical kinetics provide a considerable advantage in the development of stable dosage forms. The manufacturer also gains considerable economic advantage in marketing a new product after formulation because of this approach. It is also possible to select the best formulation which will be stable for a long time from among a series of formulations.

2. Order of Reaction

The rate of a reaction refers to a change in concentration of the reactant with time. The order of a reaction refers to the way or manner in which the rate of the reaction changes with concentration of the reactants. It expresses the experimentally determined dependence of the reaction rate upon the concentration of the reactants.

2.1. First order reaction

When the rate of reaction is proportional to the first power of the concentration of a single reactant, the reaction is said to be first order with respect to the single reactant.

In this order of reaction, a single reactant decomposes directly into one or more products and may be represented as follows

$$A \longrightarrow \text{products}$$

$$\frac{d[A]}{dt} \quad \ldots (1)$$

Then the rate of reaction, is directly proportional to the concentration of the reacting substance $[A]$. Expressing this mathematically at any time t after replacing $[A]$ by C

The equation (1) can be written as

$$-\frac{dC}{dt} = kC^n \quad \ldots (2)$$

or, $-\dfrac{dC}{dt} = kC^1$ for first order reaction

Separating the variables, we can write equation (2) as

$$-\frac{dC}{C} = k\,dt$$

in which C is the concentration of reactant remaining unreacted (or undecomposed) at time t, and k is the first order rate constant. Fig. 136-A.

Integrating the equation (3) between the limits when $C = C_0$ (initial concentration) at $t = 0$ and $C = C$ at $t = t$

$$-\int_{C_0}^{C} \frac{dC}{C} = k \int_{0}^{t} dt$$

$$-(\ln C - \ln C_0) = k(t - 0)$$

$$-\ln C + \ln C_0 = kt$$

Multiplying both sides by minus (–) we obtain

$$\ln C - \ln C_0 = -kt$$

$$\text{or, } \ln C = \ln C_0 - kt \qquad \text{... (4)}$$

Converting the natural logarithm into common logarithm, we can write, equation (4) as

$$2.303 \log C = 2.303 \log C_0 - kt$$

Dividing both sides of equation with the factor 2.303 yields,

$$\log C = \log C_0 - \frac{kt}{2.303} \qquad \text{... (5)}$$

This equation describes the first order kinetics as a function of logarithm of concentration, time and reaction rate constant.

The value of k for the reaction is calculated from the slope obtained by plotting $\ln C$ or $\log C$ against time using the linear form of equation (4) or (5). The slope is equal to $-k$ if equation (4) is used for plotting and it is $-k/2.303$ if equation (5) is used for plotting. The rate constant, k, for first order reaction has units of reciprocal time (time^{-1})

The straight line (Fig. 136-B) produced by plotting $\ln C$ or $\log C$ against t is an identifying characteristic of first order reaction in which the rate of reaction is proportional to the concentration of a single reactant.

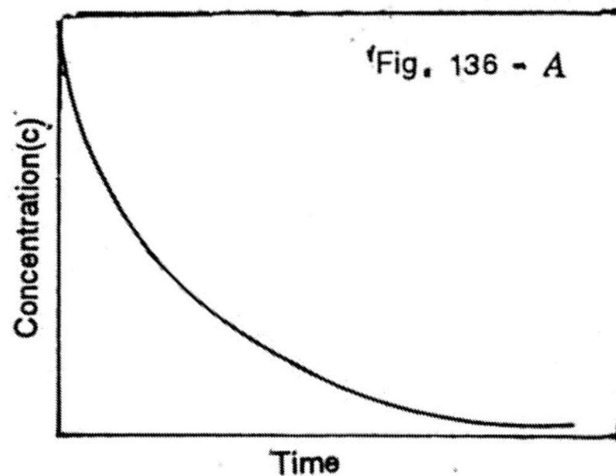

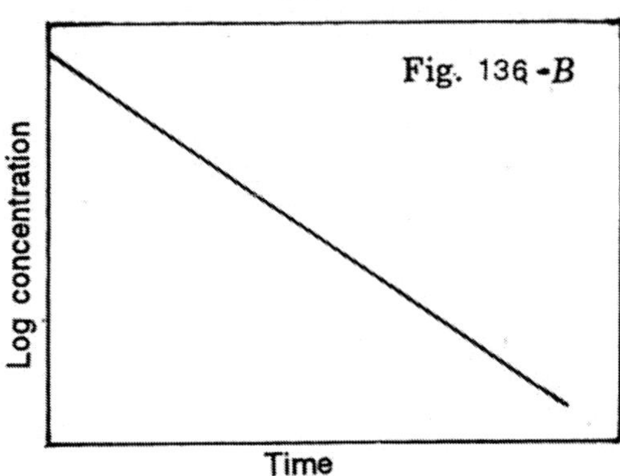

Fig. 136

The equation (5) can be rearranged to obtain

$$k = \frac{2.303}{t} \log \frac{C_0}{C} \qquad (6)$$

A modification of this equation is one in which C_0, the initial concentration is replaced by a and C by $(a - x)$ where x is the concentration reacted at time t. It is given as

$$k = \frac{2.303}{t} \log \frac{a}{a - x} \qquad \text{... (7)}$$

Sometimes, C_0 either is not known or is not a suitable reference concentration. In such cases, the equation (3) may be integrated between the limits $C = C_1$ at $t = t_1$ and $C = C_2$ at $t = t_2$.

$$-\int_{C_1}^{C_2} \frac{dC}{C} = -k \int_{t_1}^{t_2} dt$$

$$-(\ln C_2 - \ln C_1) = k(t_2 - t_1)$$

$$-\ln C_2 + \ln C_1 = k(t_2 - t_1)$$

$$k = \frac{\ln C_1 - \ln C_2}{t_2 - t_1} \quad \ldots (8)$$

$$\text{or, } k = \frac{\ln C_2 - \ln C_1}{t_1 - t_2} \quad \ldots (9)$$

The equation (7) may be written in logarithmic form as

$$k = \frac{2.303}{t_2 - t_1} \log \frac{C_1}{C_2} \quad \ldots (10)$$

The concentration terms in the first order kinetics express the fact that the concentration decreases exponentially with time. This can be understood by referring to a graph (Fig. 136-B) obtained by plotting concentration against time. Equation of first order kinetics can, then, be written in an exponential form as follows

$$\ln C = \ln C_0 - kt$$

$$\ln \frac{C}{C_0} = -kt$$

Taking inverse logarithms on both sides of equation, we can write

$$\frac{C}{C_0} = e^{-kt}$$

Which can be simplified to

$$C = C_0 \cdot e^{-kt} \quad \ldots (11)$$

$$\text{or } C_0 = C \cdot e^{kt} \quad \ldots (12)$$

Some examples of first order reaction are

(a) *Inversion of cane sugar*

In this active mass of water does not change appreciably in dilute solutions. The rate of chemical reaction depends upon concentration of sucrose only. In the stoichiometric equation, only one molecule of sucrose is involved hence it is considered to follow first order kinetics.

(b) *Hydrolysis of methyl acetate*

$$CH_3COOCH_3 + H_2O \rightleftharpoons CH_3COOH + CH_3OH$$

In this water is taken in larger quantity and hence active mass of water is not changed appreciably. Although two molecules (in the stoichiometric equation) react in the equation, only one molecule is considered to be involved in the reaction with change in concentration and therefore it is called pseudo first order kinetic reaction.

(c) *Decomposition of procaine hydrochloride in ammonium hydroxide-hydrochloric acid buffer, pH 9.7, at* 50°C. It follows pseudo first order kinetic.

(d) *Decomposition of hydrogen peroxide in aqueous solution in the presence of finely divided platinum*

$$H_2O_2 \longrightarrow H_2O + O$$

(e) *Radioactive disintegration*

(f) *Decomposition of nitrogen peroxide*

$$N_2O_5 \longrightarrow 2NO_2 + (O)$$

2.2. Half life

By observing the figure (136A), one can understand that theoretically first order reaction takes infinite period of time for the completion of the reaction (i.e. for all the reactant to undergo reaction). Hence a statement of time needed for complete decomposition would be meaningless. Actually the rate subsides ordinarily in a finite period of time at which the reaction may be considered to be almost complete. Hence it is quite satisfactory to calculate what is called half-life rather than the time required for a substance to decompose completely.

Half-life of a reactant may be indicated by symbols such as $t_{1/2}$, $t_{0.5}$ or $t_{50\%}$. It is defined as the time required for the initial concentration of a reactant to get reduced to half its initial value in a reaction. Simply, it is the time required for the reactant to reach 50% concentration of its initial value because of decomposition. It may also be defined as the time required for half of the reactant to undergo reaction. Suppose a product contained an initial concentration of 10 mg/5 ml of a drug then the time required for half of the drug to get decomposed would be the half-life i.e. the time required for the product to get reduced to 5 mg/5 ml of the drug would be the half-life of the product. If a first order reaction is followed through 10 half-lives, less than 0.1% of initial concentration of a reactant will remain unreacted. However in practice, it is often enough to follow through two or three half-life periods.

The half-life may be obtained as follows for the first order reaction.

$$t = \frac{2.303}{k} \log \frac{C_0}{C}$$

$$t_{1/2} = \frac{2.303}{k} \log \frac{C_0}{1/2\, C_0}$$

$$= \frac{2.303}{k} \log 2$$

$$t_{1/2} = \frac{0.693}{k} \quad \text{... (13)}$$

In pharmaceutical field, the time for the drug to decompose by 10% is an important value to know. It is also important to note that $t_{1/2}$ or $t_{10\%}$ does not depend on concentration. That is, it takes the same time for the concentration of the drug to go from 0.5 mole to 0.25 mole as it would take to go from 0.01 mole to 0.005 mole.

2.3. Second order reaction

A second order reaction refers to a reaction in which the experimentally determined rate of reaction is proportional either to second power of the concentration of a single reactant or to the first power of the concentrations of two reactants.

If two reactants A and B react at a rate proportional to the concentration of each i.e. $[A]$ and $[B]$, we can write

$$-\frac{d[A]}{dt} = -\frac{d[B]}{dt} = k\,[A][B]$$

If a and b represent the initial concentrations of A and B respectively and x is the amount of each of A and B reacting in time t, the reaction rate $\frac{dx}{dt}$ is given as

$$\frac{dx}{dt} = k(a-x)(b-x) \quad \text{... (14)}$$

Where $(a-x)$ and $(b-x)$ represent the concentration of A and B remaining unreacted at time t.

For a simple case, if the initial concentration of A and B are equal (i.e. $a = b$) the above equation (14) can be written as

$$\frac{dx}{dt} = k(a-x)^2 \quad \text{... (15)}$$

On integration between the limits $x = 0$ at $t = 0$ and $x = x$ at $t = t$.

$$\int_0^x \frac{dx}{(a-x)^2} = k \int_0^t dt$$

$$\left(\frac{1}{a-x}\right) - \left(\frac{1}{a-0}\right) = kt$$

$$\frac{x}{a(a-x)} = kt \quad \text{... (16)}$$

$$\text{or } \frac{1}{a} \cdot \frac{x}{(a-x)} = kt$$

$$\text{or } \frac{1}{at} \cdot \frac{x}{(a-x)} = k \quad \text{... (17)}$$

If the initial concentrations of A and B are not equal (i.e. $a \neq b$), integration of the equation (14) yields.

$$\frac{2.303}{(a-b)} \log \frac{b(a-x)}{a(b-x)} = kt \quad \text{... (17a)}$$

If $x/a(a-x)$ is plotted against t with reference to equation (16), it will yield a straight line. The slope of the line gives the value of k.

If the initial concentrations of A and B are not equal, the equation (17a) is used for plotting. That is, if $\log b(a-x)/a(b-x)$ is plotted against t, it will yield a straight line. Then the slope of the line is given by $(a-b)\, k/2.303$

The rate constant k for a second order reaction has units of liter $mole^{-1}$ sec^{-1}

The half-life for a second order reaction is obtained as follows

Consider the equation (16)

$$k = \frac{1}{at}\frac{x}{a-x}$$

$$\text{At } t = t_{1/2}, x = \frac{1}{2}a$$

Substituting these values in the equation

$$k = \frac{1}{at_{1/2}} \frac{1/2\,a}{a - 1/2\,a}$$

$$k = \frac{1}{at_{1/2}} \frac{\frac{1}{2}a}{1/2\,a}$$

$$k = \frac{1}{at_{1/2}}$$

On rearrangement,

$$t_{1/2} = \frac{1}{ak} \text{ or } t_{1/2} \propto \frac{1}{a} \quad \text{... (18)}$$

In second order reactions $t_{1/2}$ is significant only when a single reactant or when two reactants of same initial concentrations are involved.

The most common rate processes encountered in the consideration of drug stability are the first and second order reactions. When a reaction happens to be of higher order, it is always convenient to adjust the experimental conditions in such a way that except the concentration of one reactant, all the other concentrations of reactants are made to remain constant throughout the experiment. For example, the saponification of an ester by hydroxide (NaOH or KOH) is second order reaction. This second order reaction can be made to follow first order kinetics provided the hydroxide is taken in great excess or the hydroxide ion is maintained constant by using a buffer system. The actual rate constant k is then obtained by dividing the experimentally determined apparent first order rate constant by the concentration of hydroxide ion maintained constant throughout the experiment. Thus a *pseudo* or *apparent* first order reaction can be defined as a second order reaction or bimolecular reaction that is made to behave like a first order reaction. In such a reaction, the rate is determined by one of the reactants even though two reactants are present since the second reactant does not show significant changes in concentration. Hydrolysis of an ester in presence of large excess of water is an example of *pseudo* first order reaction whereas the hydrolysis of an ester by using alkali is the second order reaction.

Examples of second order reactions are

(a) Decomposition of ozone into oxygen

$$2O_3 \longrightarrow 3O_2$$

(b) Conversion of benzaldehyde to benzoin

$$2C_6H_5CHO \longrightarrow 2C_6H_5CH(OH)COC_6H_5$$

(c) Hydrolysis of an ester by an alkali

$$CH_3COOC_2H_5 + NaOH \rightleftharpoons CH_3COONa + C_2H_5OH$$

Ethyl acetate is mixed with an equal quantity of sodium hydroxide solution and the reaction mixture is kept at a constant temperature. In the stoichiometric equation two species of molecules are involved in the reaction and both undergo appreciable change in their concentration and hence it is called second order kinetic reaction.

(d) Decomposition of chlorbutol in sodium hydroxide solution at 25°C follows second order kinetic reaction.

(e) Thermal decomposition of acetaldehyde follows second order reaction.

$$2CH_3CHO \longrightarrow 2CH_4 + 2CO$$

2.4. Third order reaction

A third order reaction refers to a reaction in which the experimentally determined reaction rate is proportional to

1. the first power concentration of each of the three reactants or
2. the first power concentration of one of the two reactants and to the second power of the second reactant or
3. the third power of the concentration of a single reactant.

It may be represented as

$A + B + C \rightarrow$ products or

$2A + B \rightarrow$ products or

$A + 2B \longrightarrow$ products or

$3A \longrightarrow$ products

For the reaction

$A + B + C \longrightarrow$ products, the rate law is:

$$-\frac{d[A]}{dt} = -\frac{d[B]}{dt} = k[A][B][C]$$

If a, b and c represent the concentrations of A, B and C respectively and when $a = b = c$,

$$\frac{dx}{dt} = k(a-x)^3$$

On integration, the equation will yield

$$k = \frac{1}{2t}\left[\frac{1}{(a-x)^2} - \frac{1}{a^2}\right] \quad \text{... (19)}$$

When $k = k_{1/2}$, $x = 0.5a$ or $1/2a$ and on substitution in equation (19)

$$t_{1/2} = \frac{1}{a^2} \times \frac{1.5}{k} \text{ and } t_{1/2} \propto \frac{1}{a^2} \quad \text{... (20)}$$

Examples of third order reactions are

(a) Formation of nitrogen peroxide

$$O_3 + 2NO \longrightarrow 2NO_2$$

(b) Reduction of ferric chloride by stannous chloride

$$2FeCl_3 + SnCl_2 \longrightarrow 2FeCl_2 + SnCl_4$$

2.5. Zero order reactions

In certain reactions, the rate of chemical reaction is independent of the concentration of the reactant molecules and is known as zero order reaction. It is mathematically expressed as

$$-\frac{d[A]}{dt} = k_0 \cdot [A]^0 \quad \text{... (21)}$$

Replacing $[A]^o$ by C^o, the equation is given by.

$$-\frac{dc}{dt} = k_0 C^0 \quad \text{... (22)}$$

Where $k_0 =$ rate constant for zero order reaction. Since $C^0 = 1$, the equation is written as

$$-\frac{dc}{dt} = k_0 \quad \text{... (23)}$$

The above equation shows that the rate of reaction in zero order kinetics is independent of concentration of the reactant but it proceeds at a fixed rate. The fixed rate is K, the rate constant. That is, the concentration decreases at a fixed rate irrespective of the initial concentration of the reactant.

Thus, if a drug in a product degrades at the rate of 1.0 mg per day, the rate of degradation will be 1.0 mg/day irrespective of initial concentration of the drug in the product. Suppose the initial concentration of the drug in the product was 100 mg, then the drug would be completely degraded in 100 days.

The above equation (23) may be written as

$$-dC = k_0 dt \qquad \text{... (24)}$$

Integrating the equation between the limits when $C = C_1$ at $t = t_1$ and $C = C_2$ at $t = t_2$, (where $C_1 > C_2$ and $t_1 > t_2$)

$$-\int_{C_1}^{C_2} dC = k_0 \int_{t_1}^{t_2} dt$$

$$-(C_2 - C_1) = k_0(t_2 - t_1)$$

Rearranging the above equation, we obtain

$$k_0 = -\left(\frac{C_2 - C_1}{t_2 - t_1}\right) = \frac{C_1 - C_2}{t_2 - t_1} \text{ or } \frac{C_2 - C_1}{t_1 - t_2} \qquad \text{... (25)}$$

The equation (24) may also be integrated between the limits $C = C_0$ at $t = 0$ and $C = C_t$ at $t = t$.

$$-\int_{C_0}^{C_t} dC = k_0 \int_0^t$$

$$-(C_t - C_0) = k_0(t - 0)$$

$$\text{or, } C_0 - C_t = k_0 t \qquad \text{... (26)}$$

(Sometimes $C_0 - C_t$ is replaced by x, the concentration reacted in time t and the equation becomes $x = kt$)

$$\text{or, } C_0 = C_t + k_0 t \qquad \text{... (27)}$$

$$\text{or, } C_t = C_0 - k_0 t \qquad \text{... (28)}$$

The equation indicates that concentration in a zero order reaction at any time t is equal to the initial concentration minus the product of reaction rate constant and time.

In multisulfa product, the velocity of colour fading is found to be constant and is independent of concentration of the colourant used. That is, colour fading follows zero order kinetics. Then, the equation is given by

$$A_t = A_0 - k_0 t \qquad \text{... (29)}$$

where A_t = absorbance at $t = t$

A_0 = absorbance at $t = 0$

k_0 = zero order rate constant

In some pharmaceutical preparations such as suspensions, degradation follows zero-order kinetics. In suspensions, the concentration of a drug in solution depends on the drugs equilibrium solubility. As the drug in solution decomposes, more drug goes into solution from the suspended drug particles so that concentration remains constant. It is to be understood that the drug's concentration in solution remains constant despite its degradation with time because the solid drug acts as reservoir of drug.

The equation for the degradation of that drug in solution is the same for an ordinary solution of the drug with no reservoir of drug to replace that depleted or decomposed. That is, the degradation follows first order kinetics and is given by

$$-\frac{dC}{dt} = kC$$

where C is the concentration of drug remaining undecomposed at time 't' and k is known as the first order rate constant. When C is rendered constant (as in suspension) the equation is given as

$$kC = k_0 C^0$$

The above first order equation then becomes

$$-\frac{dC}{dt} = k_0$$

where k_0 is rate constant for zero order reaction and the equation is apparent zero order equation. It should also be understood that once all the suspended particles have gone into solution, the reaction changes to first order kinetics.

Half-life of zero order

The half-life of a zero-order can be obtained from the equation

$$C_t = C_0 - k_0 t$$

The half-life ($t_{1/2}$) is the time when C_t is equal to $\frac{1}{2} C_0$. Substituting these values in the above equation, we get

$$\frac{1}{2} C_0 = C_0 - k_0 \, t_{1/2}$$

On rearranging, it gives

$$t_{1/2} = \frac{C_0 - \frac{1}{2} C_0}{k_0} = \frac{\frac{1}{2} C_0}{k_0}$$

$$t_{1/2} = \frac{C_0}{2k_0} \quad \text{... (30)}$$

The initial concentration corresponding to C_0 is ordinarily written as 'a' and hence $t_{1/2}$ can also be written as

$$t_{1/2} = \frac{a}{2k_0} \quad \text{... (31)}$$

Examples of zero order reactions are

(a) Decomposition of hydrogen iodide at the surface of gold. At sufficiently higher pressure, the catalyst surface is covered by HI molecules and thus the concentration of the reactant remains constant throughout the reaction.

(b) In hydrogen iodide formation concentrations of hydrogen and iodine, have no effect on the reaction, but exposure to sunlight will induce the reaction spontaneously between hydrogen and iodine to yield hydrogen iodide. This photochemical reaction follows zero order kinetics.

(c) Decomposition of sparingly soluble drugs in aqueous solution follow zero order kinetics (the apparent zero order) since the amount of drug decomposed in the solution is replaced by the dissolution of some of the suspended drug and thus the concentration of the drug in the solution remains constant e.g. suspension of asprin.

(d) Colour fading in multisulfa formulation.

Reactions of higher order

Tetramolecular and higher order reactions are very rare since chance of simultaneous collisions of more molecules at a time is not possible as per kinetic molecular theory.

3. Methods to determine the Order of Reaction

3.1. Substitution method

The most obvious method is the one in which the quantities a, x and t are determined experimentally and the values are substituted in the respective order of reaction. The equation that yields a constant value of k for a series of time intervals, indicates the order of reaction.

3.2. Graphical method

This is a simple method. In this, instead of substituting the values in the respective equations of the order of reaction, the values are used to plot a graph.

If a straight line is obtained by plotting the concentration (a) against time (t), it indicates a zero-order reaction. If $\log(a-x)$ versus t yields a straight line it is first order. For a second order a plot of $\frac{1}{(a-x)}$ versus t yields a straight line provided the initial concentration of the two reactants involved in the reaction are same. The reaction is of third order when a plot of $\frac{1}{(a-x)^2}$ versus t results in a straight line with all the three reactants at the same initial concentrations.

3.3. Half-life method

A general expression for the time to complete half the reaction i.e. half life, $(t_{1/2})$, is given by

$$t_{1/2} \propto \frac{1}{a^{n-1}}$$ where $n =$ order of the reaction.

Starting with two different initial concentrations a_1 and a_2 for the same reaction, the half-lives $(t_{1/2})_1$ and $(t_{1/2})_2$ are determined respectively

$$\therefore (t_{1/2})_1 \propto \frac{1}{a_1^{n-1}} \text{ and } (t_{1/2})_2 \propto \frac{1}{a_2^{n-1}}$$

Dividing one by another, we obtain,

$$\frac{(t_{1/2})_1}{(t_{1/2})_2} = \frac{\frac{1}{a_1^{n-1}}}{\frac{1}{a_2^{n-1}}} \text{ or } \frac{a_2^{n-1}}{a_1^{n-1}} = \left(\frac{a_2}{a_1}\right)^{n-1}$$

In logarithmic form

$$\log(t_{1/2})_1 - \log(t_{1/2})_2 = n - 1(\log a_2 - \log a_1)$$

$$\text{or } \frac{\log(t_{1/2})_1 - \log(t_{1/2})_2}{\log a_2 - \log a_1} + 1 = n$$

where $n =$ order of the reaction.

The half-lives can be determined by plotting a versus t at two different concentrations a_1 and a_2. Then the half time at $\frac{1}{2}a_1$ and $\frac{1}{2}a_2$ are read from the graph. The values obtained are substituted in the above equation and n is arrived at and that gives the order of reaction.

If $(t_{1/2})_1 = (t_{1/2})_2$, it is first order reaction since in a first order $t_{1/2}$ is independent of concentration 'a'. For a zero-order $t_{1/2}$ is proportional to the initial concentration a. For a second order in which $a = b$ (i.e. in which the concentration of the reactant A is equal to the concentration of the reactant B) $t_{1/2}$ is proportional to $\frac{1}{a}$ and for third order in which $a = b = c$, $t_{1/2}$ is proportional to $\frac{1}{a^2}$.

4. Complex Reactions

Reactions are not as simple as the stoichiometric equation would show. Hence it is not possible to express many reactions by simple zero, first, second or third-order.

Very often two or more reactions take place at the same time. Accordingly they are called complex reactions. They may be

1. Reversible reaction (or opposing reactions)

   $$A + B \rightleftharpoons C + D$$

2. Parallel or side reactions (or simultaneous reaction)

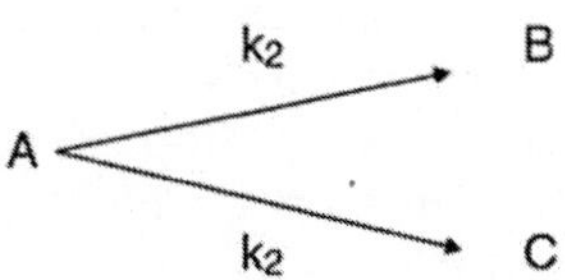

e.g. General acid base catalysed reactions.

3. Series or consecutive reactions.

$$A \xrightarrow{k_1} B \xrightarrow{k_2} C$$

e.g. Depletion ot glucose in acid solution and degradation of hydrocortisone semisuccinate at 70°C over a narrow pH range.

Decomposition of chlorthiazide gives a final product which is produced by a series of consecutive first order kinetics.

Theoretically, all reactions are reversible. In most of the cases, the reverse reaction may be disregarded as it does not alter the concentration very much. If the reverse reaction cannot be ignored, the equilibrium constant must be taken into account in the evaluation of specific reaction rate constant.

For the kinetic study of chemical reactions in the case of consecutive reactions, the reaction which proceeds at a slower rate may be considered. If a number of steps are involved in a reaction, the slowest of the steps is the rate determining step for the overall reaction.

Parallel reactions are quite common particularly in organic compounds. In the kinetic study, the one which predominates over all the other is selected.

Experiments may show a reaction order which is non-integral or fractional for complex reactions. Inspite of that, the order of reaction with respect to each reactant can be determined by controlling the concentrations of other reactants. In this way the integral reaction order with respect to each component can be arrived at.

Steady state approximation: Michaelis Menton Equation

The rate laws of a number of kinetic processes cannot be integrated exactly. It is better to postulate a reasonable reaction sequence and then the rate law may be derived.

The steady state approximation may be employed to derive the rate law. This may be illustrated by deriving the Michaelis Menton equation

Michaelis and Menton assumed the interaction between a drug (or substrate) D with an enzyme E to yield product P.

The sequence of reaction may be represented as follows

$$E + D \underset{k_2}{\overset{k_1}{\rightleftharpoons}} (E.D) \xrightarrow{k_3} P$$

Where $(E.D)$ is a complex which ultimately yields the product 'P'.

Then, the rate of product formation is given by

$$\frac{dp}{dt} = k_3[\text{E.D}] \quad \ldots (32)$$

There is no easy method by which the concentration of the complex (E.D) can be obtained. However D, P, and E_t, the total concentration of enzyme can be measured.

The rate of formation of $(E.D)$ is

$$\frac{d[E.D]}{dt} = k_1[E][D] - k_2[E.D] - k_3[E.D] \quad \ldots (33)$$

$$\text{or, } \frac{d[E.D]}{dt} = k_1[E][D] - [E.D](k_2 + k_3) \quad \ldots (34)$$

The concentration of $E.D$ is always much less than the concentration of D and P and is also constant throughout most of the reaction. Then, it may be written as

$$\frac{d[E.D]}{dt} = 0 \quad \ldots (35)$$

$$\text{i.e., } k_1[E][D] - [E.D](k_2 + k_3) = 0$$

or,

$$[E.D]_{SS} = \frac{k_1[E][D]}{(k_2 + k_3)} \quad \ldots (36)$$

The subscript 'SS' is to refer the concentration of $E.D$ at steady state.

$$\text{But } E_t = E + [E.D]_{SS} \quad \ldots (37)$$

$$\text{or, } E = E_t - [E.D]_{SS}$$

Substituting for E in the above equation

$$[E.D]_{SS} = \frac{k_1 D(E_t - [E.D]_{SS})}{k_2 + k_3} \quad \ldots (38)$$

$$= [E.D]_{SS}(k_2 + k_3) = k_1 D E_t - k_1 D[E.D]_{SS}$$

$$= [E.D]_{SS}(k_2+k_3) + k_1D[E.D]_{SS} = k_1DE_t$$

$$= [E.D]_{SS} = \frac{k_1DE_t}{(k_2+k_3)+k_1D} \quad \ldots (39)$$

$$\text{or, } [E.D]_{SS} = \frac{DE_t}{k_m + D} \quad \ldots (40)$$

$$\text{where } k_m = \frac{k_2+k_3}{k_1}$$

The rate of product formation is already given as (refer equation 32)

$$\frac{dp}{dt} = k_3[E.D]$$

Under steady state, the equation (32) may be written as

$$\frac{dp}{dt} = k_3[E.D]_{SS} \quad \ldots (41)$$

Substituting this into equation (40)

$$\frac{dp}{dt} = \frac{k_3DE_t}{k_m + D} \quad \ldots (42)$$

Where k_m is Michaelis-Menton constant

When D is present in very large excess, all the enzyme E_t is present as $E.D$. In otherwords, all the enzyme is combined with the drug and reaction proceeds at maximum velocity i.e. $\left(\frac{dp}{dt}\right)_{max}$

Replacing $\left(\frac{dp}{dt}\right)_{max}$ by V and k_3E_t by V_m and since $[E.D]$ is equivalent to E_t, the equation (42) becomes

$$V = \frac{V_mD}{k_m + D} \quad \ldots (43)$$

The equation (43) may be inverted to obtain the linear form of equation which is known as Lineweaver-Bunk equation as follows

$$\frac{1}{V} = \frac{k_m + D}{V_mD}$$

$$= \frac{1}{V} = \frac{k_m}{V_mD} + \frac{D}{V_mD}$$

$$\frac{1}{V} = \frac{k_m}{V_mD} + \frac{1}{V_m}$$

$$\text{or, } \frac{1}{V} = \frac{k_m}{V_m} \cdot \frac{1}{D} + \frac{1}{V_m} \quad \ldots (44)$$

A plot of $\frac{1}{V}$ versus $\frac{1}{D}$ gives a straight line with an intercept $\frac{1}{V_m}$ in the ordinate. The slope is k_m/V_m.

It is possible to calculate k_m; the Michaeles-Menton constant from the values of V_m and k_m/V_m.

The kinetics of capacity limited of saturable processes can best be described by Michaeles-Menton equation.

5. Factors Influencing Reaction Rates

Many factors affect the rate of reaction other than concentration. They are:

5.1. Temperature

In general, the rate of degradation increases with rise in temperature. Usually it increases by a factor of between two and three fold for every 10°C rise in temperature.

The influence of temperature on the reaction velocity (k) is given quantitatively by *Arrhenius* equation. The equation in the exponential form is

$$k = Ae^{-Ea/RT} \quad \ldots (45)$$

where k = specific rate of degradation (i.e. reaction velocity constant)

A = frequency factor (Arrhenius factor)

E_a = energy of activation

R = gas constant

T = absolute temperature

The frequency factor is a measure of frequency of collisions that may be expected between the reacting molecules.

Energy of activation (or heat of activation) refers to the energy required for effective collision to cause a reaction between molecules.

Expressing the equation in logarithmic form

$$\ln k = -\frac{Ea}{RT} + \ln A \quad \text{... (46)}$$

Converting to common logarithmic form:

$$\log k = \frac{-Ea}{2.303R} \cdot \frac{1}{T} + \log A \quad \text{... (47)}$$

where $\log A$ is a constant

If log of k values is plotted against the reciprocal of temperature ($1/T$), it yields a straight line (Fig. 137). Then the slope is given by $-\Delta Ea/2.303R$. From this value, the heat of reaction can be calculated.

It is also possible to obtain the value of Ea by plotting $\log t_{1/2}$ against $\frac{1}{T}$ (Fig. 138)

$$t_{1/2} = \frac{0.693}{k}$$

$$\text{or } \log k = \log 0.693 - \log t_{1/2} \quad \text{... (48)}$$

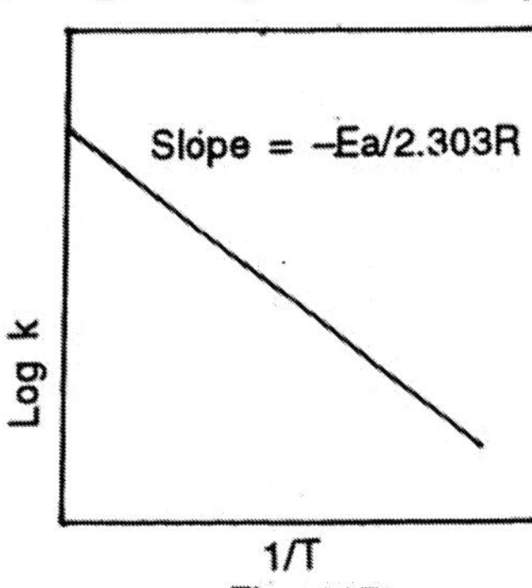

Fig. 137

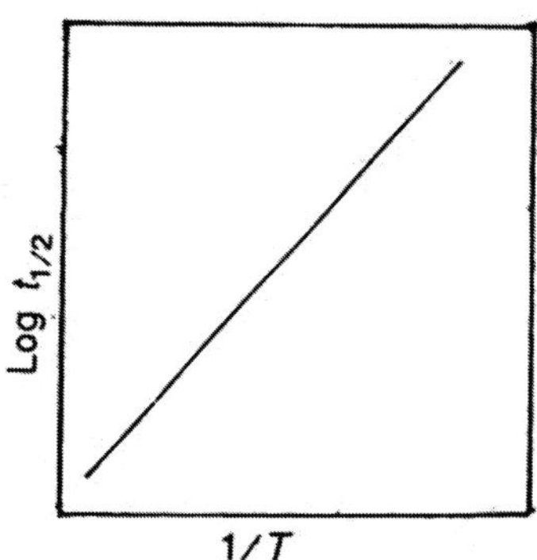

Fig. 138

Thus, on substitution in equation (47) yields

$$\log t_{1/2} = \log 0.693 - \log A + \frac{Ea}{2.303R} \cdot \frac{1}{T}$$

$$\text{or, } \log t_{1/2} = \frac{Ea}{2.303R} \cdot \frac{1}{T} + \text{constant} \quad \text{... (49)}$$

where constant $= (\log 0.693 - \log A)$

A straight line is obtained by plotting $\log t_{1/2}$ against $1/T$. The slope of the line is equal to $Ea/2.303R$ and from this Ea can be calculated.

Ea may be also obtained by writing equation 47 for two different temperatures and substracting as follows

At a temperature t_2, the equation (47) is given as

$$\log k_2 = -\frac{Ea}{2.303R} \cdot \frac{1}{T_2} + \log A \quad \text{... (50)}$$

At a temperature t_1, the equation 47 is given as

$$\log k_1 = -\frac{Ea}{2.303R} \cdot \frac{1}{T_1} + \log A \quad \text{... (51)}$$

where $t_2 > t_1$

Substraction equation (51) from (52) we obtain

$$\log \frac{k_2}{k_1} = \frac{E_a}{2.303R}\left(\frac{T_2 - T_1}{T_2 T_1}\right) \quad \text{... (52)}$$

This temperature dependency relationship is useful when the heat of activation (energy of activation) is in the range of 10 to 30 k.cal/mole (*solvolytic process*). If Ea is only 2 to 3 k.cal/mole (*diffusion* or *photolysis*) little advantage is gained. In the same way if the heat of activation is 50 to 70 k.cal/mole (*pyrolysis of polyhydroxylic substances*), the rate of degradation is so fast that it becomes difficult to make use of this relationship.

Arrhenius equation is only an empiric relation and it gives the effect of temperature on an observed rate constant. The temperature dependence especially of uni- and bi-molecular reactions appears to reflect a fundamental physical requirement that must be satisfied for the occurence of a reaction.

The physical requirement is given by collision state theory or simply collision theory. According to this theory a collision must occur (at a particular temperature) between molecules for a reaction to take place. Further, the collision must be effective i.e. a reaction between molecules does not take place unless the molecules are of certain energy. Thus, the rate of reaction can be considered proportional to the number of molecules of a reactant having sufficient energy. From this it may be understood that all collisions will not lead to reaction and only those collisions with sufficient energy are effective leading to a reaction. If 'Z' is the collision number (it is the number of collisions per second per cubic centimeter) and P, the probability factor (it takes into account that not every collision between molecules does lead to reaction), then, combining the both gives the Arrhenius factor 'A' (i.e. $Z + P = A$) and is termed the frequency factor and it refers to the frequency of collisions between molecules. E_a is the minimum kinetic energy a molecule must possess to undergo a reaction.

Transition state theory: It is an alternative to the collision theory. According to this theory, there is an equilibrium between the normal reactant molecules and the activated complex of these reacting molecules. Decomposition of this activated complex yields the product. But in this, the amount of energy required for a reaction may be less. For an elementary bimolecular process the reaction may be written as

$A + B$	$[A....B]^*$	$\longrightarrow P$
Normal reactant molecules	Activated complex (i.e. activated reactant molecules in transition state)	Product molecule

5.2. Ionic strength

Ionic strength of a solution may influence the rate of degradation in accordance with the equation.

$$\log k = \log k_0 + 1.02\, Z_A\, Z_B \sqrt{\mu} \quad ... (53)$$

Z_A and Z_B = charges carried by the reactants A and B in solution respectively

k = the rate constant of degradation

k_0 = the rate constant at infinite dilution.

μ is the ionic strength which is defined as half the sum of the terms obtained by multiplying the concentration of each of the ionic species Z_A and Z_B present in solution by square of its valence and may be given as

$$\mu = \frac{1}{2} \Sigma\, C_A\, Z_A^2 \text{ and } \mu = \frac{1}{2} \Sigma\, C_B \cdot Z_B^2 \quad ... (54)$$

If $\log k$ is plotted against μ, the following curves may be obtained. (Fig.139) Three possibilities are there for an increase in the ionic strength. When the reactant is positively charged[1] and is undergoing hydrogen ion catalysis, an increase in ionic strength (by the addition of electrolytes such as sodium chloride) produces an increase in the rate of reaction (i.e. k is increased). If one of the reactants is a neutral molecule[2] an increase in ionic strength does not affect the rate of reaction and hence it is independent of ionic strength. The third possibility is that an

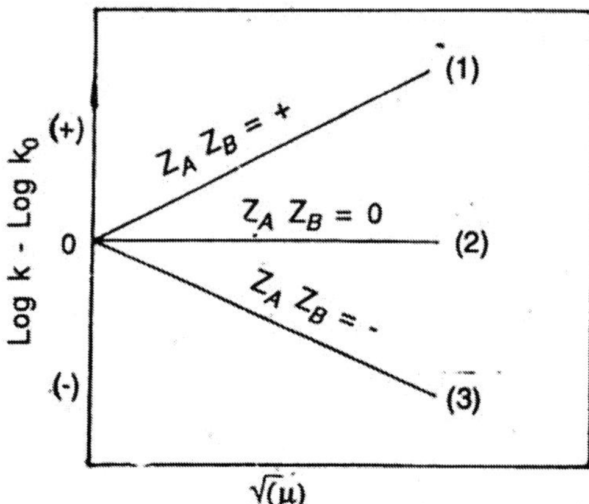

Fig. 139

increase in ionic strength decreases the rate of reaction when positively charged reactant undergoes hydroxyl ion catalysis[3].

5.3. Solvent effect

Hydrolysis is due to reaction with water. Therefore replacement of water with non-aqueous solvents such as alcohol, propylene glycol has often been used. This replacement of a part or all of the water is undertaken to reduce decomposition by hydrolysis. For example, elixir of phenobarbitone contains glycerin and alcohol. Hydrolysis of aspirin is reduced in alcohol-propylene glycol. However, there may be hydrolysis even in the presence of non-aqueous solvents such as alcohol. For example, cyclamic acid degrades at a faster rate in non-aqueous vehicle than in aqueous vehicle.

It may be said that degradation depends on the relative solubilities of the reactants and the degradation products in a given solvent system, dielectric constant of the solvent system and the chemical nature of the reactant species.

The quantitative relationship between the reaction velocity constant of degradation and the solubility is given by the equation considering a reaction.

$$A + B \longrightarrow \underset{\text{(activated complex)}}{(A....B)*} \longrightarrow \text{products}$$

as $$\log k = \log k_0 + \frac{V}{2.303R} \cdot \frac{1}{T} (\Delta\delta_A + \Delta\delta_B - \Delta\delta^*) \quad ...(55)$$

where k = observed reaction velocity constant

k_0 = reaction velocity constant in an infinitely dilute solution exhibiting ideal behaviour.

V = an approximation for the molar volumes of the reactants A and B and the activated complex formed during the reaction and prior to the formation of the products.

δ_A, δ_B and δ^* = the solubility parameters of the reactants A, B and the activated complex respectively

It is assumed that the properties of the activated complex and the products are similar and therefore $\Delta\delta^*$ may be taken as the difference in polar characteristics between the solvent and the products. The $\delta^* = 0$ indicates similar polar characteristics between the solvent and the products and the δ_A and $\delta_B = 0$ indicates similar polar characteristics between the solvent and the reactants. If $\Delta\delta^* = 0$, and $\Delta\delta_A + \Delta\delta_B > 0$, (i.e. polar characteristics are dissimilar), the term $\frac{V}{2.303RT}(\delta_A + \delta_B - \delta^*)$ will be positive. Then the reaction velocity (k) will be greater than that in an ideal solution. On the other hand, if $\delta_A + \delta_B = 0$, and $\delta^* > 0$, then the term $\frac{V}{2.303RT}(\delta_A + \delta_B - \delta^*)$ will have a **negative value** indicating lower reaction **velocity (k)** than in the case of an ideal **solution.**

In general, it may be said that the solvents which are highly polar will accelerate the reactions that yield products with greater polar characteristics than the reactants (i.e. yield products with higher solubility than that of the reactants). If the products formed have less polar characteristics than that of the reactants (i.e. if the reactants are more soluble than the products) then, the reaction rate will be retarded.

5.4. Dielectric constant

It has been already mentioned that the dielectric constant has an influence on the reaction rates. Dielectric constant is a property of liquids and therefore the dielectric constant of the solvents affect the rate of hydrolytic reaction and the effect depends on the presence or the absence of an electric charge on the reactant molecule. If the hydrolytic degradation involves a charged reactant molecule as well another ionic species (H^+ or OH^-) in the system, then the quantitative expression explaining the effect of dielectric constant on reaction rate may be given as

$$\ln k = \ln k_{\varepsilon = \infty} - \frac{NZ_AZ_Be^2}{RTr^*}\frac{1}{\varepsilon} \quad \text{... (56)}$$

where k = observed reaction rate in a solvent of dielectric constant ϵ.

$k_{\epsilon = \infty}$ = reaction rate constant in a solvent of infinite dielectric constant.

N = Avagodro's number.

Z_A and Z_B = charges on the two ionic species (the charged reactant and H^+ or OH^- species).

e = value of charge (i.e. the unit of electric charge)

r^* = distance between the ionic species in the activated complex.

If $\ln k$ is plotted against $\frac{1}{\epsilon}$, it yields a straight line. If Z_A and Z_B carry similar charges, the slope of the line will be negative and hence a decrease in dielectric constant of the solvent will result in a decrease in the rate of hydrolytic degradation. A decrease in dielectric constant can be caused by the addition of a non-aqueous solvent such as ethyl alcohol or propylene glycol or by the replacement of aqueous solvent with non aqueous solvent in part or in whole.

If Z_A and Z_B carry opposite charges, the straight line obtained by plotting $\ln k$ against $\frac{1}{\epsilon}$ will be positive. In this instance, a decrease in dielectric constant will result in an increase in the hydrolytic degradation.

If the reactant (drug) is a dipole carrying no charge and is involved in a reaction with an ion, the relationship between dielectric constant and the reaction velocity constant is given by

$$\ln k = \ln k_{\epsilon=\infty} + \frac{NZ_A^2 e^2}{2RT}\left(\frac{1}{r_a} - \frac{1}{r^*}\right)\frac{1}{\epsilon} \quad \ldots (57)$$

where Z_A = the charge on the ionic hydrolytic species

r_a = the radius of the ionic species

r^* = the radius of the activated complex.

As before, if ln k is plotted against $\frac{1}{\epsilon}$, a straight line is produced. r^* being the radius of activated complex (i.e. combined radius of the dipole and the ion) is always larger than r_a and hence the slope of the line will always be positive. Therefore ln k will increase on increasing $\frac{1}{\epsilon}$. That means a decrease in the dielectric constant of the solvent system will only increase the rate of reaction.

For example, degradation of the antibiotic, chloramphenicol catalysed by hydrogen ion (H^+) in water-propylene glycol was found to increase on decreasing the dielectric constant of the solvent system by increasing the concentration of propylene glycol. However, the replacement of water by other solvents is frequently employed in pharmacy to stabilise drugs against possible hydrolysis though there is a small increase in degradation rate which may be outweighed by enhancement of solubility of the drug in the solvent of lower dielectric constant.

5.5. Specific Acid-base catalysis

Hydrolytic degradation is catalysed by hydrogen (H^+) or hydroxyl (OH^-) ions. The magnitude of the rate of degradation is dependent on pH. Hydrogen ion catalysis dominates at lower pH ranges (i.e. at higher concentrations of hydrogen ion) whereas hydroxyl ion catalysis predominates at higher pH range (i.e. at higher concentration of hydroxyl ions). The degradation rate can be independent of pH at intermediate pH range. Thus, the degradation reaction is said to occur by acid-base catalysis when the rate law for such an accelerated degradation is found to contain a term that involves the concentration of hydrogen ions [H^+] or the concentration of hydroxyl ions [OH^-].

The rate of degradation product formation, $\frac{dp}{dt}$ dependent on specific acid-base catalysis, may be given for an ester in terms of the general rate law as below.

$$\frac{dp}{dt} = (k_0 + k_1 [H^+] + k_2 [OH^-]) [S] \quad (58)$$

where k_0 = rate constant for solvent catalytic effect

k_1 = rate constant for specific hydrogen ion effect

k_2 = rate constant for specific hydroxyl ion effect

$[S]$ = solvent concontration.

For this, the observed reaction rate constant (k_{obs}) is given by

$$k_{obs} = k_0 + k_1 [H^+] + k_2 [OH^-] \quad \ldots (59)$$

At low pH, the hydrogen ion concentration is high and hence $k_1 [H^+]$ is greater than k_0 or $k_2 [OH^-]$. Then the observed reaction rate constant is given by

$$k_{obs} = k_1 [H^+] \quad \ldots (60)$$

and in this case specific hydrogen ion catalysis is observed.

At high pH, the hydroxyl ion concentration is high and hence $k_2 [OH^-]$ is greater than k_0 or k_1 [H$^+$]. The equation is then written as

$$k_{obs} = k_2 [OH^-] \quad ... (61)$$

and in this case, specific hydroxyl ion catalysis is observed.

At intermediate pH, or if the products of $k_1 [H^+]$ and $k_2 [OH^-]$ are small in value, the equation is written as

$$k_{obs} = k_0 \quad ... (62)$$

and in this case, the reaction is solvent catalysed.

If the reaction medium is slightly acidic, both the solvent and the specific hydrogen ion (acid) catalysis are involved. On the other hand, if the reaction medium is slightly alkaline, both the solvent and the specific hydroxyl ion (base) catalysis are involved in the degradation process.

The influence of pH on degradation can be determined by measuring the degradation at several hydrogen ion concentrations and obtaining a plot of log of rate constant (log k) versus pH The point of inflection of such a plot represents the pH of optimum stability.

5.6. General Acid-base catalysis

Buffers are commonly employed in the formulation of pharmaceutical liquids to maintain the pH of the solution. Though the pH is maintained constant at an optimum level, one or more of the components of the buffer can catalyse the degradation and the reaction is said to be subject to general acid-base catalysis. If the catalytic component is acidic, it is general acid catalysis and if the catalytic component is basic, it is general base catalysis. Common buffer salts which have been found to have catalytic effects are acetates, phosphates and borates.

In order to determine whether a particular pharmaceutical liquid product is catalysed by the buffer system employed, the ionic strength and the ratio of the buffer components (to keep the pH constant) are kept constant while the concentration of the buffer component is altered. If degradation occurs at different concentrations (instead of maintenance of the pH constant) of the buffer components, the reaction is said to be subject to general acid base catalysis. In that case, keeping the ratio of buffer components constant, the concentration of buffer components should be kept as low as possible to minimise the catalytic effect of the buffer components.

5.7. Catalysis

Often chemical reactions are catalysed by catalysts as already mentioned. A catalyst is a substance which alters the speed of a reaction without itself being altered chemically. A catalyst does not alter the equilibrium of a reversible reaction but speeds up the reaction to attain equilibrium at a shorter time. A catalyst remains unaltered chemically at the end of a reaction.

A catalyst is considered to combine with the reactant and form an activated intermediate complex which then decomposes to regenerate the catalyst and yields the product. Catalysis is also considered to occur at the surface of the catalyst in the case of heterogeneous catalysis (Refer under catalysis for further details).

5.8. Light

Light induces chemical reactions. Radiations of proper frequency must be absorbed to cause a chemical reaction (degradation). Photochemical decompositions do not depend on temperature for activation of the molecules. These reactions are usually complex and proceed by a series of steps.

Pharmaceutical compounds which undergo photochemical decomposition are riboflavin, phenothiazines, nifidipine, chlordiazepoxide, etc (Refer under Photochemistry for further details).

6. Stability Problems and Testing

Pharmaceutical preparations or products often may exhibit physical or chemical reactions and that may end in instability. Due to such instability, the preparation gets deteriorated. This deterioration may lead to

(a) reduction in the activity of a preparation

(b) formation of toxic products

(c) an inelegant product.

Apart from these effects, microbial contamination also may cause deterioration of the product. Ultimately the product becomes unacceptable.

Hence it is necessary to perform stability testing to find out the extent of deterioration or degradation and to ensure the degradation has not exceeded an acceptable level assuring.

1. the safety of the patient and
2. the activity of the product

Decomposition or degradation of active ingredients (drug substances) in pharmaceutical preparations may occur by hydrolysis, oxidation-reduction, racemisation, decarboxylation, ring clevage, photolysis, isomerisation and epimerisation.

Physical degradation of pharmaceutical products may be due to loss of water, loss of volatile constituents, absorption of water, crystal growth, polymorphic changes, and colour changes.

However the degradative reactions leading to chemical instability in pharmaceutical products are mainly the hydrolysis and oxidation-reduction.

6.1. Hydrolysis

Many pharmaceutical preparations contain esters or amide functional groups that undergo hydrolysis in solution. Hydrolysis is a reaction of an ester or amide with water. Though hydrolysis can occur with pure water the presence of a catalyst which supplies hydrogen (H^+) ions or hydroxyl ions (OH^-), is needed to promote the reaction.

The ester hydrolysis whether acid catalysed or alkali catalysed can in general, be represented as follows:

$$\underset{\text{ester}}{R'-\overset{\overset{\Large O}{\|}}{C}-OR} + H_2O \qquad \underset{\text{acid}}{R'-\overset{\overset{\Large O}{\|}}{C}-OH} + \underset{\text{alcohol}}{HOR}$$

This reaction denotes second order reaction. However, it is possible to treat this as *pseudo*-first order reaction by keeping H^+ or OH^- at a considerably higher concentration or by keeping H^+ or OH^- concentrations essentially constant by the use of buffers.

In the study of degradation of drugs by ester hydrolysis, first order kinetic expressions have been employed whenever possible.

The drugs which undergo ester hydrolysis may be procaine, atropine, aspirin etc.

Amide hydrolysis is similar to ester hydrolysis but it forms an amine instead of an alcohol. It may be represented as follows:

$$\underset{\text{amide}}{R-\overset{\overset{\Large O}{\|}}{C}-\overset{\overset{\Large H}{|}}{N}-R'} + H_2O$$

$$R-\overset{\overset{\Large O}{\|}}{C}-OH + \underset{\text{amine}}{H_2 \cdot N-R'}$$

Examples of amides that undergo amide hydrolysis are niacinamide, phenethicillin, chloramphenicol, barbiturates, penicillins etc.

Amides have in general greater stability than the structurally similar esters.

Ring alteration: Hydrolytic reactions may also proceed by ring cleavage with subsequent attack by H^+ or OH^- ions. Examples of drugs which undergo hydrolysis by ring alteration are hydrochlorothiazide, pilocarpine and reserpine.

6.2. Protection against Hydrolysis

Pharmaceutical liquid preparations containing water are the most susceptible to hydrolysis, e.g. solutions, suspensions and emulsions. Solid dosage forms such as tablets and granules may also undergo hydrolysis because of entry of water vapour from the atmosphere or because of water of crystallisation in other ingredients.

Hydrolysis of drug products such as powders, granules, tablets and capsules may be prevented by avoiding contact with water vapour. It involves the control of atmospheric humidity during preparation, purification, and packaging. Extra protection can be achieved by way of including porous envelops containing 'esiccants (like silica gels) in the conainers.

In the case of liquid dosage forms, he method of protection is by reducing he rate of hydrolysis. This may be chieved by adjusting the pH to an opimum level at which the catalytic effect of H^+ or OH^- ions (specific acid base catalysis) are at a minimum by the inlusion of proper buffer solutions.

If the hydrolytic degradation is general acid-base catalysed i.e. by the acid and basic species (i.e. acid and its conjugate base) of the buffer solution in addition to H^+ or OH^-, the buffer concentration should be kept at a minimum.

Hydrolytic reactions may in general be minimized by partial or full replacement of water (i.e. by a reduction in dielectric constant) with a solvent of lower dielectric constants such as alcohol, glycol, glucose and mannitol solutions.

Complexation is also a method by which hydrolytic reactions may be inhibited. For example, benzocaine is protected against hydrolysis by forming a molecular complex of benzocaine with caffeine.

By modification of chemical structure by increasing the length of or by branching the acyl or alkyl-groups, the rate of hydrolysis of an ester may be decreased owing to stearic hinderance.

Hydrolysis is a solvolytic reaction and hence the degradation by hydrolysis depends on solubility of the drug. Hence, by reducing the solubility of the drug by forming less soluble salt or ester of the drug, hydrolysis can be decreased. For example, insoluble chlorthiazide (may be formulated as suspension) is less prone to hydrolysis than its soluble sodium salt. Solvolysis can be reduced by preparing difficultly soluble esters and other derivatives. For example chloramphenicol palmitate is difficultly soluble ester which can be formulated as suspension.

Erythromycin is an antibiotic. It gets degraded in the acidic environment as found in stomach. To protect the drug, erythromycin is converted into an ester. The ester remains inactive until the drug is released from the ester by enzymatic hydrolysis in the body (prodrug concept).

Sterile dry powders (penicillin powder) or dry syrups (ampicillin syrup) are prepared and dispensed to exclude water till it is used and at the time of usage, they are reconstituted with water for injection or purified water respectively. This is to avoid hydrolytic decomposition.

6.3. Oxidation - reduction

The instability of a considerable number of pharmaceutical preparations are due to oxidative decomposition of active ingredients. Oxidation involves the addition of oxygen or the removal of hydrogen. Oxidation and reduction occur simultaneously. A substance is said to be oxidized if one or more electrons are removed from it. The simplest type of oxidation involves the removal of an electron. For example, ferrous ion is oxidised to ferric ion by the elimination of an electron.

$$Fe^{++} \longrightarrow Fe^{+++} + 1e$$

Autoxidation is the most common form of oxidative decomposition that occurs in many of the pharmaceutical preparations and it involves a free radial chain process. The rancidity occurring in fixed oils is due to autoxidation during storage.

Autoxidation is a reaction of a substance with molecular oxygen (present in air) and it involves free radical chain process. The autoxidation of an organic substance may be simply represented as follows:

Chain initiation: Induced by benzoyl peroxide or ultra violet light or heat in which free radicals are produced.

$$RH \xrightarrow[hv]{} R^0 + (H) \quad \text{free radical}$$

Chain propagation:

$$R^0 + O_2 \longrightarrow RO_2^0$$

$$RO_2^0 + RH \longrightarrow RO^0 + OH^0 + R^0$$

Chain termination:

$$R^0 + HI \longrightarrow RH + I^0 \quad \text{(stable free radical)}$$

$$RO_2^0 + X \longrightarrow \text{inactive products (termination by inhibitor)}$$

where HI and *X* are chain inhibitors.

$$\left.\begin{array}{l} R^0 + R^0 \\ RO_2^0 + RO_2^0 \\ RO_2^0 + R^0 \end{array}\right\} \longrightarrow \text{inactive products (self termination)} \quad \begin{array}{l} R-R \\ RO_2 - RO_2 \\ RO_2 - R \end{array}$$

In an autoxidative degradation, only a small amount of oxygen is needed to initiate the reaction and thereafter oxygen concentration is relatively unimportant.

Heavy metals such as copper, ion, cobalt, and nickel catalyse the oxidative degradation (For e.g. oxidation of ascorbic acid is catalysed by copper ions).

Many oxidative degradations are catalysed by hydrogen and hydroxyl ions.

Some solvents other than water may have a catalysing effect on oxidations. For example, aldehydes, ethers, and ketones may cause free radical reactions.

The kinetics of overall oxidative degradation processes are influenced by heat and light. The degradation of pharmaceutical substances by oxidative degradation follows first order or second order kinetic expressions.

Some drugs that undergo oxidative decomposition are ergometrine, epinephrine, heparin, paraldehyde, tetracyclines, vitamin D, K, C etc.

6.4. Protection against oxidation

Most oxidative degradation of pharmaceutical compounds are probably autoxidative and hence antioxidants that are effective against atmospheric oxygen are often used to provide protection against autoxidation. They may be ultraviolet absorbers such as phenyl salicylate and 2-hydroxy benzophenone; hydroperoxide destroyers such as organic compounds of sulphur and phosphorous; metal deactivators (by complexation) such as chelating agents like citric acid, ethylene diamine tetra acetic acid (EDTA) and 8 hydroxy quinone; and chain terminating agents (antioxidants) such as butyl hydroxy anisole (BHA), nor-dihydroxyguariaretic acid (NDGA) and gallic acid esters such as propyl and *n*-butyl gallates.

The effectiveness of antioxidants can be increased through the use of synergists such as chelating agents and it also depends on the concentrations used, the solution pH and packaging.

When oxidation is catalysed by hydrogen and hydroxyl ion, the pH of optimum stability must be ensured.

Water soluble antioxidants act by undergoing oxidation in preference to the drug. Oil soluble antioxidants prevent free radical chain processes.

Antioxidants commonly used for aqueous systems are sodium bisulphite, sodium sulphite, sodium metabisulphate, ascorbic acid, thioglycerol etc.

Antioxidants commonly used for oil systems are ascorbyl palmitate, hydroquinone, propyl gallate butylated hydroxy anisole (BHA), α-tocopherol and butylated hydroxy toulene (BHT).

Oxidation of fats and oils may be retarded by hydrogenation. Drugs which are attacked by atmospheric oxygen may be protected by replacing the air in the container with an inert gas. For example ergometrine injection is protected against oxidation by replacing the air with inert gas nitrogen in the ampoules.

An effective antioxidation (preservation against oxidation) can be obtained by taking into account some or four factors. For example, drug substances such as ascorbic acid and epinephrine (adrenaline) may be stabilised by excluding oxygen, buffering the solutions to a favourable pH, using metal-free solvents, adding chain inhibitors, excluding light and storing at a low temperature.

6.5. Photolysis

Degradation in pharmaceutical substances occur when they are exposed to light. Exposure to light may produce oxidation-reduction, ring rearrangement or modification and polymerisation. The shorter the wave length of light, the greater is the effect of light in initiating the chemical reaction because of higher energy.

A photochemical reaction may be accompanied by a thermal reaction. However, this thermal reaction is entirely different in character from that of ordinary thermal reaction. The thermal reaction once induced by light may continue after the light source has been withdrawn. The energy available in photochemical reaction is much greater than in a normal thermal reaction. For details refer under photochemistry.

The possible orders of photochemical reactions are second order, first order and zero-order. Few drugs which are affected by light are Nifedipine, chlordiazepoxide, and fursemide.

Photochemical reactions can be reduced by storing the product in darkness. Amber-coloured bottles are used to minimize these reactions. Packaging the bottled liquid in cartons also act as a physical barrier to light.

DL-methionine was found to have photostabilising effect on ascorbic acid solution buffered by phosphate and not by citrate at pH 4.5. Uric acid was found to produce a photoprotective effect in buffered and unbuffered solution of sulphathiazole sodium.

British Pharmaceutical Codex defines a light resistant container is one that does not transmit more than 15% of radiation between 290 and 450 nm.

7. Accelerated Stability Testing

If pharmaceutical preparations or new formulations are stored under normal conditions, their instabilities are detectable only after long storage periods. Such a method is time consuming and uneconomical. In an attempt to reduce the time required to obtain information in instabilities, various tests are undertaken. These tests involve storage of the preparations under conditions that will accelerate decomposition at a faster rate. As there is rapid deterioration when stored under conditions that place a higher stress or challenge to the preparations, the instability becomes detectable at a short period.

The most common stresses often used is the temperature (i.e. elevated temperatures). The other stresses may be humidity and light or any other stress related to a particular preparation.

The objectives of accelerated stability testing may be

1. the best formulation from a series of different initial formulations may be selected because rapid detection of decomposition is made possible.
2. it is useful to predict the shelf-life of a product (i.e. to predict the expiry date).
3. it provides for a rapid means of quality control.

7.1. Prediction of shelf-life

Shelf-life is the period during which a dosage form keeps its qualities. The predication of shelf-life is based on applying the Arrhenius equation which gives the effect of temperature on rate constant, k of a chemical reaction.

Fortunately, it is not required for the purpose of stability prediction to determine the mechanism of degradation. The stability of any active component in a pharmaceutical preparation can be evaluated by determining some property of the degradation (such as colour disappearance, concentration) under accelerated storage conditions as a function of time. If this function can be linearised with any of the chemical kinetic reaction orders (i.e. it refers to the determination of the order of reaction), temperature dependency of the degradation can be obtained with the help of Arrhenius equation. Then it is possible to determine the chemical stability of the active ingredient for an extended shelf-storage period under normal conditions of storage. In otherwords, the period during which the preparation will remain stable under normal conditions of storage can be determined.

Consider a multisulphanomide preparation whose instability is measured in terms of colour disap-

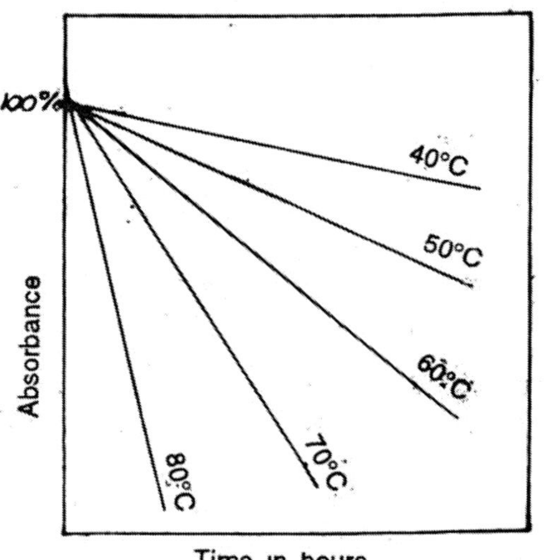

Fig. 140

pearance. The preparation is subjected to different elevated temperatures say 40°C, 50°C, 60°C, 70°C and 80°C to accelerate the degradation (measured in terms of colour intensity decrease). Plots of changes in absorbance at 500 nm (measured by the use of photocolorimeter) for each elevated temperatures against time are obtained (Fig. 140). Such a plot shows that changes in absorbance versus time is linear as shown in the figure.

The linear curves obtained for different elevated temperatures show that colour loss is following zero order kinetics in accordance with the equation.

$$A_t = A_0 - kt$$

where A_t = absorbance at time t

A_0 = absorbance at time zero i.e. initial absorbance

k = rate constant.

The slopes of the lines represent the rate of change in colour with time for different temperatures and the value of k, for each temperature can be obtained from the respective slope. The k value becomes greater and greater as the temperature is increased.

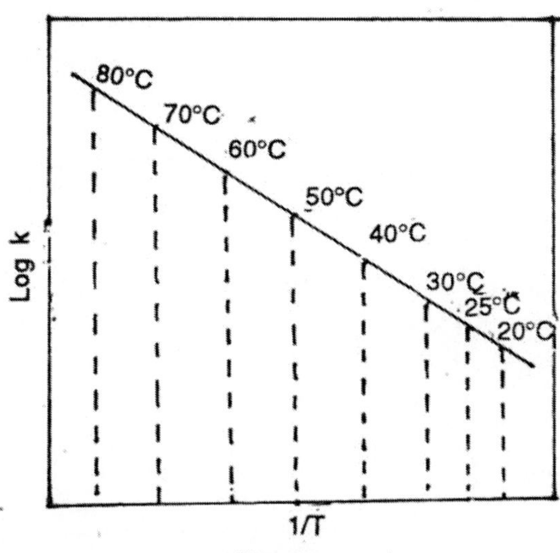

Fig. 141

Then, an Arrhenius plot of log k values versus the reciprocal of the absolute temperature (T) is obtained. Such a plot may be shown in Fig. 141.

Since the plot is linear, the stability of the preparation may be predicted at ordinary room temperature by extrapolating the curve to the lower temperature say 25°C. The k value is then read out for the lower temperature (say 25°C) and from this value, the shelf life period may be calculated using zero-order kinetic equation, $A_t = A_0 - kt$

For example, in order to predict the time for the absorbance to fall from 0.470 (A_0) at time zero to 0.225 (A_t) at time t, representing the potency of the preparation has fallen below the desired level for use, the zero order reaction is used. Assume at 25°C, the rate constant is $2.09 \times 10^{-5}\ hr^{-1}$.

Using zero order equation,

$$A_t = A_0 - kt$$

$$kt = -A_t + A_0$$

$$t = \frac{-A_t + A_0}{k}$$

and substituting the values at t (25°C), the shelf-life period is given as

$$t = \frac{(-0.225 + 0.470)}{2.09 \times 10^{-5}}$$

$$\doteq 11722 \text{ hours or } 488 \text{ days.}$$

The shelf-life period is nearly 1 year 4 months.

Suppose the concentration is measured as a function of time at different elevated temperatures and the degradation (shown by a decrease in concentration) follows first order kinetics, the shelf life period can be calculated as shown in the example that follows.

Suppose the initial concentration is 90 units/ml and the specific decomposition rate k is obtained by using Arrhenius plot is $3.63 \times 10^{-5}\ hr^{-1}$ at room temperature 25°C.

Suppose the concentration falls below 40 units/ml, it is not potent for use. Then the expiration date can be predicted considering the date of manufacture as 1.8.94.

The initial concentration (c_0) at time zero is 90 units/ml.

The final concentration (c) at time 't' is 40 units/ml.

k at 25°C = 3.63×10^{-5} per hour.

Using the first order kinetic equation,

$$t = \frac{2.303}{k} \cdot \log \frac{c_0}{c}$$

and substituting the values

$$t = \frac{2.303}{3.63 \times 10^{-5}} \log \frac{90}{40}$$

= 22344 hrs or 2 years6 months

The various steps involved in the prediction of shelf-life may be summarised as follows:

1. The preparation for which the stability is to be determined is divided into 5 or 6 portions and each portion is stored at different temperatures say 40°, 50°, 60°, 70° and 80° in order to accelerate the degradation.
2. Samples from each portion are withdrawn at different intervals of time and determined from the remaining concentrations.
3. The order of reaction (whether zero, first or second order) is determined by plotting the appropriate function of the concentration (whether a, $\log (a - x)$ or $1/(a - x)$) against time and the linearship relation is determined (This one is graphical method. Other methods such as half life method or substitution method also can be used).
4. From the slopes of the lines, the reaction velocity constant k for the degradation at each of the elevated temperatures is calculated.
5. Employing the Arrhenius relationship, the reaction velocity constant k for the degradation at room temperature (generally 25°C) is determined. This may be obtained from the linear plot of the logarithm of the k values for various elevated temperatures against the reciprocals of absolute temperatures and then extrapolating the curve to 25°C and reading off the k value at 25°C.
6. The k value obtained for 25°C is then substituted in the appropriate rate equation (already determined order of reaction) and an estimate is obtained for the time during which the product will remain potent (i.e. shelf-life period).
7. Appropriate calculation is carried out to find out the amount of drug to be added in excess (overage) to compensate for the loss during the shelf-life period to assure. 100% concentration in the product during use within its shelf-life period especially for vitamin formulations.

A similar method with some modifications has been suggested. In this method, a plot of log percent of

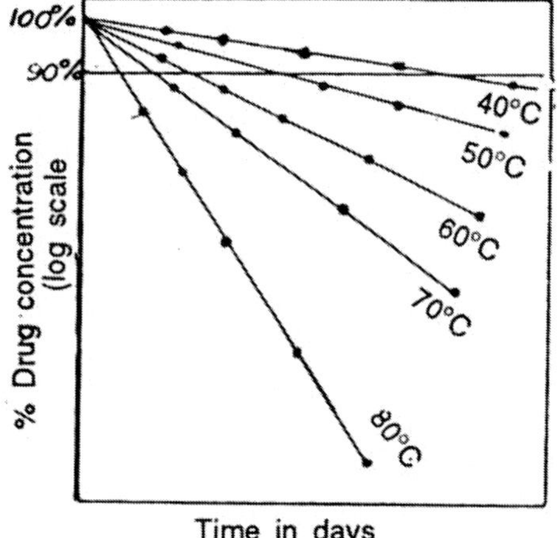

Fig. 142

drug remaining versus time in days is obtained as shown in Fig. 142.

From the above graph, (Fig. 142) the time for the potency to fall to 90% of the original value which normally means expiry date is read. Then the log time to 90% versus the reciprocal of either the Celsius or Kelvin scale is plotted as shown in Fig. 143.

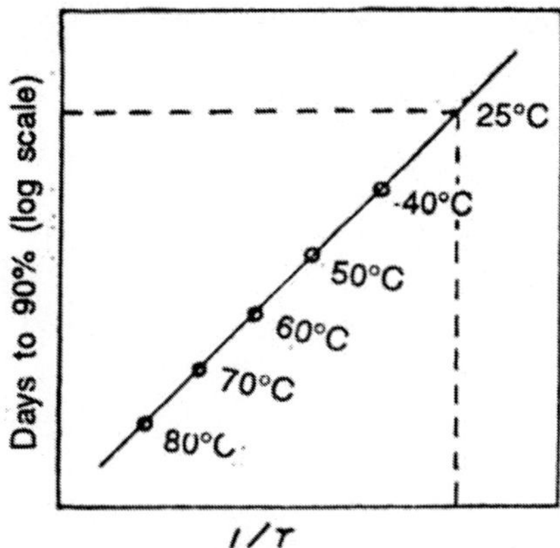

Fig. 143

The straight line of the curve is extrapolated to lower temperature and from this the number of days (which is the shelf-life period) at 25° is read directly.

An improved technique to evaluate stability by isothermal kinetics has been suggested by Rogers et al. In this technique the energy of activation and reaction velocity constant and the stability prediction are obtained in a single experiment. It involves raising the temperature of a product under test by programming the temperature to change at predetermined rate. Samples are withdrawn and analysed at suitable time intervals.

Temperature and time are related by

$$\frac{1}{T} = \frac{1}{T_0} + at \quad \text{... (63)}$$

$$\text{or } \frac{1}{T} - \frac{1}{T_0} = at \quad \text{... (64)}$$

where T_0 is the initial temperature and 'a' is the reciprocal heating rate constant and at any time during the run, the Arrhenius equation at time zero and at any time 't' may be given

$$\ln k_t = \ln k_0 - \frac{Ea}{R}\left(\frac{1}{T} - \frac{1}{T_0}\right) \quad \text{... (65)}$$

Substituting for $\frac{1}{T} - \frac{1}{T_0}$, the equation is

$$\ln k_t = \ln k_0 - \frac{Ea}{R} at \quad \text{... (66)}$$

Temperature being a function of time t, a measure of stability k_t is directly obtained over a range of temperature.

Overages:

Once the shelf-life has been determined, excess quantity of drug (overage) must be added in an unstable preparation (for e.g. vitamin preparations) to maintain 100% of the labelled amount of the drug during the shelf-life of the product. This can be easily calculated and added to the preparation at the time of manufacture so that 100% of the drug claimed on the label is assured throughout the shelf-life period.

This is not applicable to highly potent drugs. Overages, added in the formulations, should be within the limits compatible with therapeutic requirements and for shelf life period.

Many vitamins degrade at a finite rate when stored under ambient room temperature. To compensate for this finite rate of degradation, it is necessary to add overages during the formulation. Hence manufactures include excess quantities (i.e. overages) at the time of manufacture. The Organisation of the Pharmaceutical Products of India (OPPI)

VITAMIN	OPPI			FIP		
	Oral liquids in %	Tablets in %	Parenteral products in %	Oral liquids in %	Oral solids in %	Soft capsules in %
Vitamin A	100	75	50	60	60	75
Vitamin B_1	175	100	100	80	50	175
Vitamin B_2	150	100	100	80	80	100
Folic acid	100	-	100	50	80	-
Pantothenic acid	100	75	100	80	50	75
Vitamin C	175	-	-	50	-	100
Vitamin D	75	100	80	80	80	60

and Federation International Pharmaceutique (FIP) have recommended the overages shown in the Table. for various vitamins.

It may be noticed from the table, the OPPI overages are in general higher than FIP overages perhaps due to climate conditions.

7.2. Limitations of Accelerated Stability Testing

Stability predictions based on Arrhenius equation are valid only when the decomposition is a thermal phenomenon with an activation energy of about 10 to 30 k cal/mole.

The prediction may be invalid because at higher temperatures solvent produces unequal moisture concentration. There may be less humidity and oxygen solubility at higher temperatures whereas at room temperatures, there may be more moisture and oxygen content.

There is also a possibility of change in the order of reaction during the period of study. For example a zero order reaction may subsequently become a first order, second order and the activation energy may also change if the decomposition process is a complex process. Thus, there is a possibility that the application of higher stresses may cause reactions that would not take place at lower stresses (actual storage conditions).

During normal storage conditions, formulations are exposed to a variety of weather conditions and temperatures except a few which are stored at a particular temperature in a refrigerator or in a cold room. But in our experiments, the natural weather conditions are not simulated. The test would be more meaningful if it is performed in normal storage conditions.

In the case of disperse systems (emulsions and suspensions) when temperature is elevated, viscosity is decreased as a result of alterations in physical characteristics and this may introduce large errors in the prediction of stability.

7.3. Advantages of Accelerated stability testing

Even with all these difficulties, the accelerated stability testing is acceptable since the predicted shelf lives are sufficiently accurate when the data are analysed statistically as compared to shelf lives of the product stored under normal conditions.

8. Determination of the causes of decomposition

The causes of decomposition may be dependent upon

(a) chemical structures of drug substances

(b) chemical structures of decomposition products

(c) the properties of additives used, impurities present if any and the material of the container and

(d) storage conditions

The decomposition may be indicated by the appearance and odour of the preparation. A knowledge of the behaviour of similar compounds may also indicate the possible route of decomposition.

However a series of tests may be conducted to rule out the causes or to find out the causes of decompositions. A simple demonstration may help to understand clearly.

Consider a drug solution in water sealed in ampoules divided into six groups, three of which contain inert nitrogen gas in the space above the solution within the ampoules and the remaining consist of oxygen (or air) in the space above the solution within the ampoules. Now the ampoules are exposed to different conditions as shown below:

	Ampoules containing O_2 above the solution	Ampoule mark
1.	Exposed to light	A_1
2.	Exposed to heat	A_2
3.	Stored in dark	A_3

	Ampoules containing nitrogen gas above the solution	Ampoule mark
1.	Exposed to light	B_1
2.	Exposed to heat	B_2
3.	Stored in dark	B_3

The contents of ampoules are analysed, drawn at different time intervals.

The results may be summarised as follows:

(a) Decomposition in all the ampoules irrespective of the ampoules having oxygen or nitrogen above the solution indicates hydrolytic decomposition.

(b) Degradation by oxidation is indicated by the decomposition in only three groups of ampoules (A_1, A_2 and A_3) containing oxygen irrespective of exposure to light, heat or darkness.

(c) A photochemical reaction is indicated by the decomposition only in ampoules A_1 and B_1 groups exposed to light.

(d) Thermal decomposition is indicated by the decomposition only in A_2 and B_2 and not in all the other ampoules.

In a similar way, the effect of pH on decomposition of drug solutions can be carried out.

9. Accelerated Tests for Photochemical stability

Accelerated tests for photochemical stability can be done by inducing rapid decomposition by means of artificial light source of varying intensities simulating the effects of sunlight or room illumination. The relationship between the intensities of light and rate of photodegradation is a unique function of the formulation under test. In this method, photochemical decomposition is measured quantitatively. Extrapolation of the results to predict the effects of normal storage conditions is often difficult and thus warrants a development of a rational approach. However to overcome the problem of photodegradation, it is necessary to pack the formulation in amber coloured containers (bottles) and to store away from light. An extra protection from light is provided by placing the container in a carton box.

10. Accelerated tests for physical stability

Physical instabilities are many and are due to varied causes. Hence it is not possible to design a single universal test. However a general rule can be followed that if the formulations are stable under higher stresses, it will be stable under normal conditions.

(a) **Accelerated tests for moisture absorption** In this method, products are placed in an environment of high relative humidity and controlled temperatures. It is achieved by using a number of small cabinets each containing a different saturated salt solution that produces the desired humidity conditions. Now-a-days sophisticated environmental chambers are available to create required humidities and temperatures. The formulation (tablets, capsules etc) are kept both in packed forms and unpacked forms in the chambers and their physical and chemical stabilities are assessed. The results will indicate whether the product is susceptible to moisture and also whether the container needs to provide a high degree of protection.

(b) **Accelerated tests for emulsion stability** An emulsion is prepared in large quantities Small quantities are filled in a number of containers with closures and stored in a range of temperatures from 45° to 70°C. Temperature increases the thermal agitation and decreases viscosity of the continuous phase which leads to increased collisions of dispersed phase. If the emulsion withstand this higher stresses, it may be assumed that the emulsion will be stable under normal conditions of storage. The method is not applicable to emulsions containing drugs and emulsifying agents which undergo decomposition at higher temperatures since the conclusion will be erroneous. An alternate and best method is by centrifugation which accelerates rate of creaming in emulsions. The rate of creaming is directly proportional to the speed of ultracentrifuges upto 60,000 r.p.m. It is possible to predict sufficiently accurately about the creaming problems of majority of emulsions at normal storage conditions.

(c) **Accelerated tests for suspension stability** The stability problems with the suspension are setting of solid phase (dispersed phase) and formation of a solid cake and both are undesirable. Both the problems may be accelerated by centrifugation. High speed centrifugation is not preferable since it produces a close packed sediment. Low speed centrifugation equivalent to four times the gravitational force is preferred to study the physical stability.

Another stability problem with the suspension is crystal growth. For this study, temperature fluctuations under normal storage conditions are to be simulated. It is done by exposing suspensions between 23° and 33°C using a cycling time of 16 minutes. The cycling is normally repeated hundred times and crystal growth is observed. The crystal growth depends upon the particle concentration, the bulk particle solubility, temperature fluctuation range and the frequency of fluctuation.

11. Kinetics of drug decomposition in solid state

The breakdown of drugs in the solid state also occurs which is very important to decide the expiry date of solid dosage forms. Single component solid dosage forms degrade either by zero order or by first order reaction. The decomposition of multi drugs in solid dosage forms is more complex than single component and the decomposition may be zero or first order and sometimes it is difficult to differentiate between the two.

In tablets and other solid dosage forms, there is a possibility of solid-solid interaction which may be between drugs or between drugs and additives. This may be found out by running thin layer chromatography with the drug alone and drug-additive mixture. Any change in the R_f value of the drug indicates drug interaction. The interaction may also be studied by using diffuse reflectance spectroscopy.

Factors like temperature, hydrolysis, oxidation etc affecting liquid dosage forms also affect solid dosage forms. To protect from these factors, the dosage forms are packed suitably e.g. packing with metal foils, strip packing, putting in amber coloured bottles. Fading of color in tablets on exposure to light (photolysis reaction) in solid dosage forms is another problem. This photolysis was found to be a surface phenomenon. Other problems associated with the solid dosage forms are polymorphic transitions, sublimation and dehydration.

Various experimental methods used in solid state kinetics are reflectance spectroscopy, X-ray diffraction, thermal analysis, microscopy, dilatometry and gas pressure-volume analysis.

12. ICH, WHO, FDA guidelines on stability testing and shelf-life for International Registration of Pharmaceuticals.

To eliminate redundant and duplicate requirements for registration in individual countries, minimum acceptable standards are evolved by "International Conference on Harmonisation" (ICH) by selective countries (European countries, USA and Japan) for Worldwide marketing applications keeping in view globalisation and global trade. World Health Organisation (WHO) has advocated these standards to all its members representing 191 countries. The benefits in terms of saving time, cost and resources. ICH covered only New drug substances and product only. Hence WHO developed separate guidelines for stability testing of established drugs in conventional dosage forms. Food and Drugs Administration (FDA) of USA came out with still more strict guidelines. India has to follow these guidelines to promote its export potential.

World nations are divided into four climatic zones depending upon temperature and relative humidity prevailing in those countries.

Distribution of World nations into different zones

Region	Zone I and II countries	Zone III and IV countries
Europe	All countries	
America	Argentina, Bolivia, Chile, Canada, Mexico, Peru, Uruguay, **USA**	Barbados, Beliza, Costa Rica, Dominican Republic, Ecuador, El Salvador, Guatemala, Guyuna, Haiti, Honduras, Jamaica, Columbia, Cuba, Nicaragua, Dutch Antilles, Panama, Paraguay, Puerto Rico, Venezuela, All of these countries are assigned CZ IV
Asia	Afghanistan, Armenia, Azerbaijan, China, Georgia, Iran, Israel, **Japan**, Kazakstan, Kirighizia, Korea, Labanon, Nepal, Syria, Tadzhikistan, Turkey, Turkmenia, Uzbekistan	Behrain, Bangladesh, Hongkong, **India**, Indonesia, Irag(III), Jordan(III), Kampuchea, Qatar, Kuwait, Laos, Malaysia, Maldives Islands, Myanmar, Oman, Pakistan, Philippines, Saudi Arabia, Singapore, Sri Lanka, Taiwan, Thailand, United Arab Emirates, Vietnam, Yemen
Africa	Egypt, Algeria, Tunisia, Libya, Morocco, Namibia, Rwanda, South Africa, Zambia, Zimbabwe	Angola, Ethiopia, Benin, Botswana(III), Burkina Faso, Barundi, Djibouti, Ivory Coast, Gabon, Gambia, Ghana, Guinea, Cameroon, Kenya, Longo, Liberia, Madagascar, Malawi, Mali, Mauritania, Mozambique, Niger, Nigeria, Senegal, Sierra Leone, Somalia, Sudan, Tanzania, Togo, Chad(III), Uganda, Zaire, Central African Republic
Australian/ Oceanic	Australia, Newzealand	Fiji, Society Islands, Marshould Islands, New Caledonia, Papua-New Guinea, Samoa, Tonga

Zone 1:	Temperate;	temp;	20°C;	Relative Humidity	42%
Zone II:	Subtropical;	temp';	22°C;	Relative Humidity	52%
Zone III:	Hot/dry;	temp';	27.9°C;	Relative Humidity	35%
Zone IV	Hot/humid;	temp';	27.4°C;	Relative Humidity	76%

STABILITY DATA GENERATION: Protocol (8 steps)

1. Type, Size and No. of Batches

Drug Substances	Drug Products (Clinical Formulation)
At least 3 batches (minimum of pilot scales: Synthetic route, method of manufacture simulating final manufacture)	At least 3 batches preferably 3 different batch of drug substance (one may be from smaller: 25,000 to 50,000 tablet or capsule) (two should be at least pilot scale)
Quality is same as that to be used in clinical study (any stability in lab scale may be used as supporting data)	Quality same as that for marketing (Lab data not acceptable data on associated formulation or packaging may be used as supporting data)

2. Type, Size and source of container and closures

Drug substances : In proposed bulk container and closure

Drug product : In proposed dosage from container and closure proposed for storage and distribution meant for marketing

3. Storage Orientation for Full Interaction

Example: Vial in inverted position

4. Test Parameters (ICH Q6)

Drug assay, Analysis of Degradation products, Physical, Chemical Microbiological, Quality Attributes (Example Tablet: Dissolution test etc.), Loss of preservative, Release specification, Preservative Efficacy testing. etc.

USFDA gives elaborate guidelines: Assay and Degradation put together be 100% of initial value (Meet Adequacy of mass balance)

5. Test Methods: (ICH Q6)

"STP" be developed for analysis: Validated for specificity, accuracy, precision linearity: Limits for detection and quantification prescribed. (Replication if necessary)

6. Acceptance Criteria:

Derived from material used in pre and clinical studies and bioavailability studies is fixed as numerical limits.

Example: Moisture pickup, Viscosity, Particle size, assay, degradation products, impurities (individual and total upper limits)

7. Sampling time points: (Testing Frequency)

(a) Real time testing: (ICH) on samples (Long term)

Frequency of 3 month in first year (minimum period for initial submission)

Frequency of 6 month in second year & then annually (retest period submitted during assessment upto proposed shelf life)

(b) Accelerated conditions: (3 Points)

ICH	:	0, 3, 6 months if required. Additional samples at final time or a fourth time point.
USFDA	:	0, 2, 4 and 6 months
WHO	:	0, 1, 2, 3 appropriate, 6 months

(c) Intermediate conditions: (If failure occur at accelerated)

Four test points 0, 6, 9, 12 months

8. Test Storage Conditions

Current Practice

(a) Isothermal condition and

(b) Controlled humidity

Both a and b (For stability studies) mandatory

Instead of multi temperature testing, single accelerated testing is accepted (ICH, WHO and USFDA)

A. General Case: (For Drug substance and drug products)

Storage conditions for long term testing

Zone I and II Zone III & IV (ICH)	25° ± 2° C : 60% R.H ± 5% R.H
Zone III and IV (WHO)	30° ± 2° C 60% R.H ± 5% R.H

- Minimum time period at initial submission: 12 month continued for sufficient restest period for assessment.

Storage conditions for accelerated testing (ICH & WHO)

40°C ± 2°C; 75% R.H ± 5% R.H: minimum time period at initial submission: 6 months (Data submitted as impact study about short term excursion simulating shipping)

If the product is unstable in the above during 6 months Intermediate conditions performed

30°C ± 2°C ; 60% R.H ± 5% R.H; Minimum time period for initial submission at least 6 months out of 12 months

(a) Acceptance: Results within significant change otherwise not meeting specification.

Definition

1. Failure to meet acceptance criteria like appearance, colour, phase separation, resuspendability, caking, hardness, delivery, per actuation and as appropriate to product type
2. pH exceeding
3. Dissolution exceeding for 12 dosage units
4. Specific degradation exceeding
5. A 5% potency change from initial assay

B. To be stored in refrigerator (For drug substance and drug product)

Long term	:	5° ± 3°C minimum 12 months for initial submission
Accelerated	:	25° ± 2°C ; minimum 6 months

If significant change occur in accelerated

(a) Within 3 months, test not be continued but stress test data to be submitted (outside label condition) to cover shipping condition.

(b) Between 3 and 6 months any retest period (fourth) based on real time testing.

C. To be stored in a freezer (For drug substance and drug products)

Long term: 20° ± 5°C, ambient humidity; minimum 12 months at initial submission. Retest period depend on stability in long term.

Accelerated	:	5° ± 3°C; 60% ± 5%R.H	On a single batch to cover outside label condition (Shipping)
Stress testing	:	25° ± 2°C	

D. To be stored in deep freezer below – 20°C (For DS & DP) treated case by case basis

E. Drug product packed in impermeable container (ICH/USFDA)

- Semi solids in sealed aluminium collapsible tubes, injections in sealed glass ampoules
- No moisture or solvent entry or loss (Permanent barriers)
- Therefore conditions as above (General refrigerator, Freezer at any relative humidity).

F. DP packed in semi permeable containers: (Plastic Bag, Low density of polyethylene pouch for LVP, Ampoules and vials)

(i) Aqueous based products:

Evaluated for water loss under low RH

Study	Condition	Minimum time period at submission
Long	25° ± 2°C; 40% R.H ± 5% R.H	12 months
Intermediate	30° ± 2°C ; 60% ; R.H ± 5% R.H½	6 months
Accelerated	40° ± 2°C ; 60 % NMT 25% R.H	6 months (water loss after 3 months)

Significant change: Water loss of > 5%

After 3 months storage at accelerated

Required: Throughout the proposed shelf it should be within acceptance criteria.

(ii) Non Aqueous based product:

Any comparable approach may be followed

Stability Commitment: For DS and DP

- Long term study data on primary batches:

(a) If not covered proposed shelf life at time of approval, study to be continued to establish shelf life as well as for post approval

(b) If covered proposed shelf life post approval commitment not necessary

Evaluation for DS and DP

(i) Should be systematic approach

(ii) If data show little variation, (Apparent by looking): No for mal statistical analysis

(c) Accelerated stability data show more stable, shelf life may be extended at approval time (Limited cases)

(d) Stability of drug product after reconstitution or dilution to be provided as supportive information.

For Stability testing 3 types of equipments

(a) Humidity cum thermostatic chambers

(b) Refrigerators (5° ± 3°C : 15° ± 5°C)

(c) Thermostatic chambers with ambient humidity (25°C, 30°C, 40°C) Eg. for products in impermeable containers, ampoule, vial, etc. Available in standard companies (Ref. Table 7)

Some salient points are

1. Expiry date begins from quality control release of the batch. The date of release is not to exceed 30 days from production date irrespective of packaging date.
2. Expiry date is upto the last day of month.
3. ICH developed guidelines for photostability testing also. Samples are exposed to overall illumination of not less than 1.2 million hours and an integrated near K.V light of not less than 200 watt hours squaremeter is used. Fluorescent lamp or Xenon or metal halide lamp is used as light source.

   Drug substances or products are exposed both directly as well as in the proposed pack to establish the photoprotection ability of the package.
4. Storage condition necessary during shelf life should be mentioned on the label. ICH prescribes temperature specific range based on National/Regional requirements (vague terms like ambient temperature or room temperature should not be mentioned).

   WHO prescribes storage conditions as
   - Store at 2–8°C (under refrigeration, no freezing).
   - Store below 8°C (under refrigeration).
   - Store below – 5° to – 20°C (in freezer).
   - Store below – 18°C (deep freezer).
   - Store under normal conditions (it means store in dry, well ventilated premise of 15°C to 25°C upto 30°C. Extraneous odor, contamination, intense light should be excluded).
   - Storage conditions at the country of use also.

While clearing drugs from stores, one has to follow F.I.F.O system (First in First out system).

Stress testing for DS and DP: (Data outside labeled condition)

- Single batch of material
- Effect of accelerated temperature (EG. 50°, 60° ...) Humidity (75% RH or above), Oxidization, Photolysis, hydrolysis over different pH with solution or suspension

To establish intrinsic stability by studying degradation pathways and mechanisms, degradation products and to establish suitable analytical procedure and its validation (therefore stress testing will not predict physical changes). Since it may occur during shipping.

Although products of higher stresses unlikely in storage condition, (result from integral part of submissions).

13. Kinetics of Drug Transport in *vivo*

Drugs are administered into the body in various dosage forms (solution, suspension, powder, tablets, capsules, suppositories or injections) through various routes (oral, rectal or parenteral). The drugs are absorbed into the body and reach the site of action through blood (which transports the drug to various parts of the body) and exert a particular therapeutic response. The number of molecules that reach the site of action and the rate at which these molecules arrive depend upon various physico-chemical and biological factors. The absorbed molecules are distributed to various parts of the body, metabolised and excreted. The drug absorption, distribution, metabolism, and excretion can be quantified by kinetics and may be illustrated by a diagram in Fig. 144.

The drug in solution form either from gastrointestinal tract (G.I. tract) or from tissues enter the blood system. The drug binds with the plasma proteins. The free drug is distributed to receptor sites and in various other tissues. The free forms of the drug are also subject

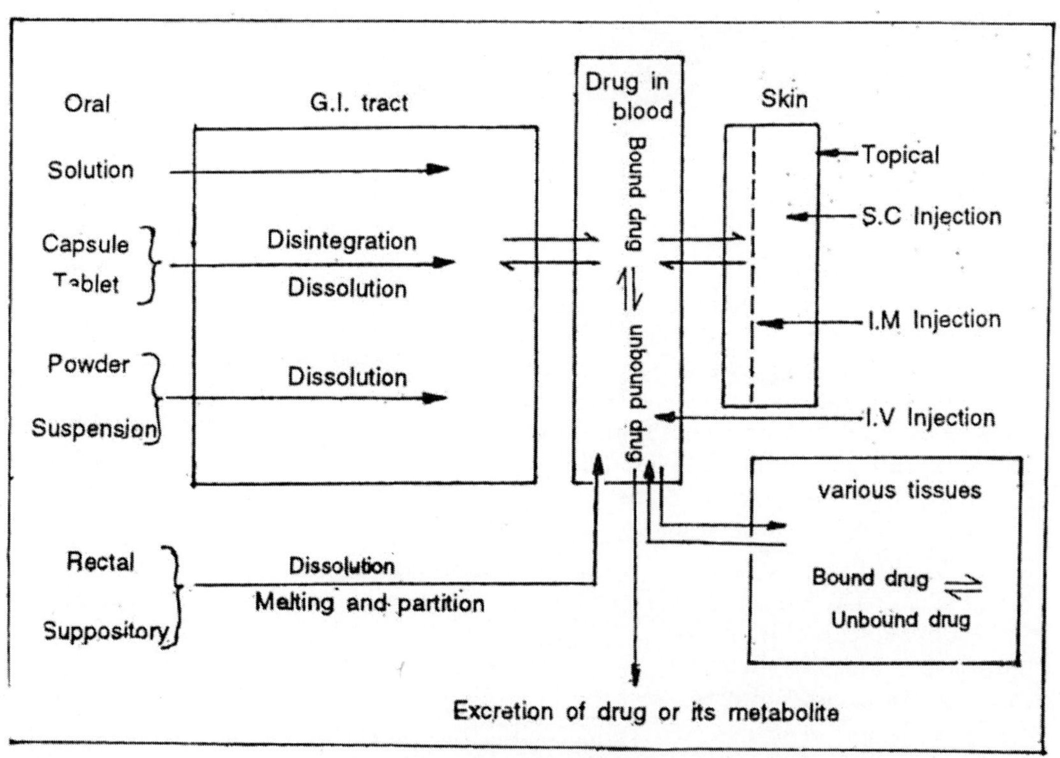

Fig. 144 Distribution of drugs in the body

to metabolism and excretion. To replace the lost drug, drug is released from the bound drug. The drug concentration in the plasma reflects the drug concentration in other tissues since the drug distribution in the body maintains a dynamic equilibrium. The drug concentrations in the plasma against different time intervals may be depicted as given below in Fig. 145.

The curve at the portion (1) indicates that the rate of absorption is more than the rate of elimination from the

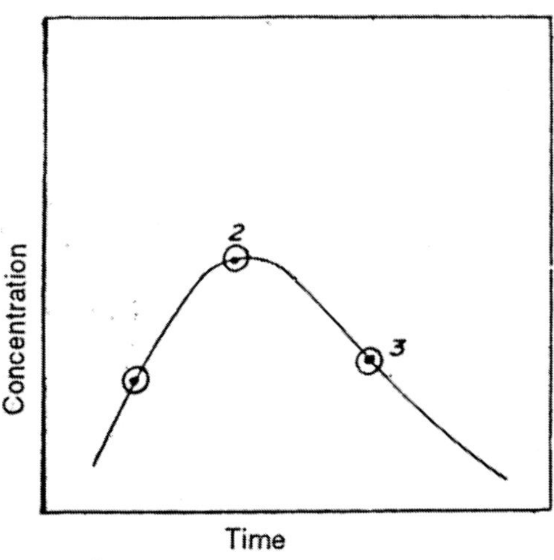

Fig. 145

body since more amount of drug is available at the absorption site. The curve at portion (2) indicates that the rate of absorption is equal to the rate of elimination. The curve at portion (3) indicates that the rate of elimination of the drug is greater than the rate of absorption of the drug since the absorption is ceasing.

From kinetics point of view, the drug absorption follows first order kinetics and the drug elimination also follows first order kinetics. In short, it is called 'first order in' and 'first order out'.

Another way of expressing the rate of change is biological half-life. It is the time required for the concentration to get reduced to half its initial value in the body fluids. The decrease in the drug concentration at the absorption site is expressed as biological half-life for absorption and is given by

$$(t_{1/2})_a = \frac{0.693}{k_a}$$

where $(t_{1/2})_a$ = biological half life for absorption

k_a = absorption rate constant derived from first order kinetic equation

Similarly the elimination of drug from the body is also expressed as biological half life for elimination $(t_{1/2})_{el}$ which is given by

$$(t_{1/2})_{el} = \frac{0.693}{k_{el}}$$

where $(t_{1/2})_{el}$ = biological half life for elimination

k_{el} = elimination rate constant derived from first order kinetic equation.

The elimination rate is more easily obtained in terms of the time taken to eliminate half the drug (biological half life for elimination) originally present in the blood from the inspection of the graph as given in Fig. 146.

The straight line portion of the elimination curve is extrapolated to cut the y axis which gives the original concentration C_0 at time zero. Then drawing a line (dotted line) from $\frac{1}{2} C_0$ to cut the x axis gives the biological half life for elimination.

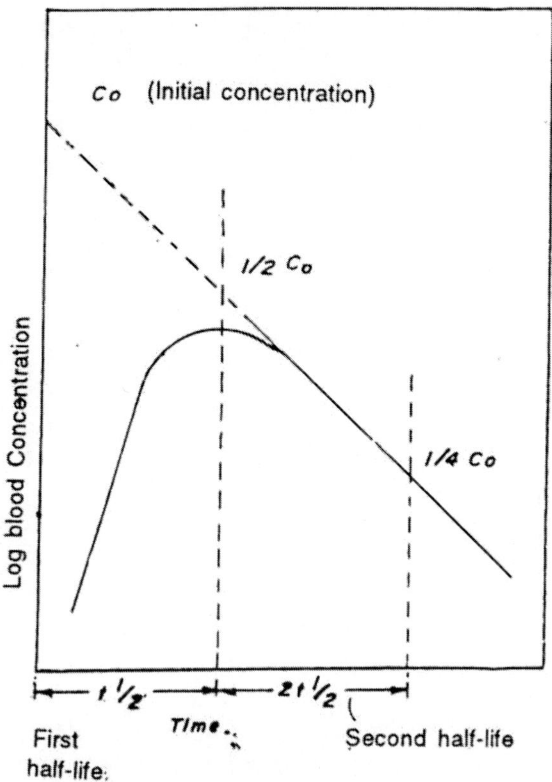

Fig. 146

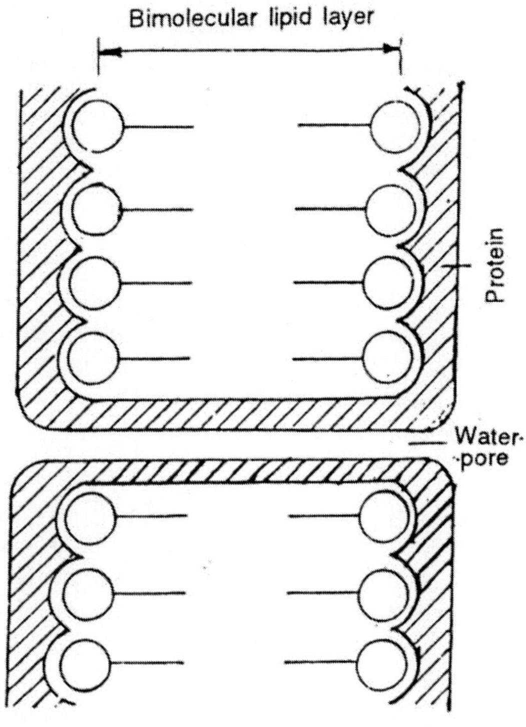

Fig. 147. Cell membrane

The distribution and metabolism of drugs can also be treated mathematically using kinetic equation.

Transport of drugs (for absorption or distribution or for elimination) has to occur through a barrier called biological membrane which may be represented by the following diagram.

Bi-molecular lipid layer A cell membrane (Fig. 147) is regarded as having two layers of lipoidal molecules (lecithin, cephalin, cholesterol, sphingomyelin etc) orientated with their polar groups facing outwards (polar groups of one layer facing other cells and polar groups of the second layer facing interior of cells) and the non-polar portion of both layers constituting core of the cell membrane. The bimolecular layer is stabilised by a layer of unfolded protein molecules both inside and outside the cell membrane. Thus the membrane is a lipid barrier (central portion of the cell membrane) which separates the aqueous intra and extra cellular fluids. The thickness of the membrane is about 75×10^{-7} mm and the structure is perforated by water filled pores having a radius of the order of 4×10^{-7} mm. The drug crosses the biological membrane in the following ways (i.e. the **mechanism of transport of drug** through the membrane).

13.1. Passive diffusion through lipid barrier

For any drug molecules to get partitioned into the cells, they have to undergo the following steps as shown in the diagram.

Aqueous phase (Extracellular)	Lipid phase (membrane)	Aqueous phase (Intracellular)
k_1 ⇌ $-k_1$	k_2 ⇌ $-k_2$	k_3 ⇌ $-k_3$
Partition	diffusion	partition

The first step is the partitioning of a drug between aqueous phase of the extracellular liquid and lipid phase of the membrane. The second step is the diffusion of the drug across the lipophilic portion of the membrane.

The third step is the partitioning of the drug from the lipid membrane into the intracellular liquid. The overall transport of the drug is affected by factors which influence these consecutive steps. The k values indicated in the diagram (as forward rate constants k_1, k_2 and k_3 and the reversible rate constants as $-k_1$, $-k_2$ and $-k_3$ respectively) refer to the rate constants of the processes. The rate determining step is the step which is the slowest. For example, for water soluble drugs, the first step is the rate determining step. Conversely for a lipid soluble drug, the third step is the rate determining step. For compounds (i.e. drugs) with intermediate characteristics, the second process becomes the rate limiting step.

Most of the drugs are weak electrolytes and exist in aqueous solution as a mixture of ionised and unionised forms. The unionised forms are less polar and more soluble in the lipid phase. Hence the body membranes are preferentially permeable to unionised forms of the drug molecules than to the ionised forms of the same molecule. In other words k_1 is extremely low for ions but much more for the corresponding unionised molecule.

In the gastro intestinal tract, the stomach is acidic and the intestine is alkaline. Weakly acidic drugs show more unionised forms than ionised forms in the stomach than in the intestine and hence are more absorbed from stomach than from the intestine. Weakly basic drugs show more unionised forms of the drug than ionised forms of the drug in the intestine and hence are more absorbed from the intestine than from the stomach. However, the surface area of the intestine (due to villi) is many times more than the surface area of the stomach and the transit time of the drug is also extended in the intestine. Because of these two factors, drugs are generally more absorbed from the intestine than from the stomach.

The diffusion of lipid soluble drugs occur via the membrane by passive diffusion. The rate of diffusion depends upon the concentration gradient (Refer Fick's Law of Diffusion).

13.2. Active transport of drugs across the membrane

Some substances are too large to pass through the pores in the cell membranes and too lipid insoluble to be transported by passive diffusion. But still they are transported across the membrane for which a special mechanism is proposed. The drug molecules form a complex with a carrier substance at one surface of the membrane (extra cellular), the complex moves across the membrane, it liberates the molecule (drug) at the other side (intra cellular), and the carrier returns to its original position. In this way, the substrate (i.e. drug molecule) moves across the membrane against a concentration gradient and thus the energy is spent in the transfer. Therefore this process is termed active transport.

The rate of transference in the special type of transport will depend upon the number of carrier molecules and a maximum rate is obtained when all the carrier molecules are involved in the process. Since the carrier molecules show some degree of specificity for substrates, some compounds with similar structure may compete with the normal substrate molecules and hence their transport is hindered.

13.3. Diffusion through water pores

The pores in the cell membranes are filled with water. Some anions may pass through the positively charged pores whereas cations may be hindered by electrostatic repulsion. The pore size is about 4×10^{-7} mm and any drug molecule having greater than this size cannot enter. The transport through the pores are due to diffusion, osmosis and filtration mechanisms.

Certain body membranes consist of sheets of epithelial cells and the pores between these cells may be as large as 4×10^{-6} mm (Eg. in the glomeruli of the kidney and in the epithelium of capillaries).

The kinetics of drug absorption through the membranes of gastrointestinal tract or from the tissue is influenced by a variety of physical, chemical, biological factors and additives present in the dosage forms.

13.4. Facilitated diffusion and ionic or electrochemical diffusion

A cell membrane carries positive charges on its outer surface and negative charges on its inner surface. Because of this, there is a potential difference or electrical gradient across the membrane. When a cationic drug approaches the cell membrane, it is repelled and only those molecules with high kinetic energy pass through ionic barrier. but once inside the cell, it is attracted by the interior of the cell. Of the ionic forms the anionic solutes permeate faster than the cationic forms.

For ionic drugs, transport across the membrane depends upon concentration gradient as well as electrical gradient. It is called electrochemical gradient which is the sum of the influences of the electric potential and the concentration differential across the membrane.

Once inside the cell, cations will be kept inside by the attractive negative charge of the interior of cell; intracellular concentration increases until the outward diffusion rate equals inward diffusion rate. It is called electrochemical equilibrium.

Some substances move more rapidly across a biological membrane than can be accounted for a process of diffusion due to concentration gradient. It is found that the transport of molecules is aided by a active carrier substance as in active transport. There is a greater permeability to the drug-carrier complex than to the drug alone so that the transport rate is increased. The accelerated movement is called facilitated diffusion. As carrier molecules are used for the transport, it requires energy. It is also found that facilitated diffusion will transport a molecule along its electrochemical gradient.

13.5 Ion pair transport

Drugs such as quarternary ammonium compounds and sulphonic acids which ionise under all pH values are absorbed through G-I membrane by ion-pair transport. Though they have low O/W partition coefficient values, they pass through the membrane by forming reversible neutral complexes with endogenous ions (like mucin) of the gastrointestinal tract. Such a phenomenon is called ion-pair transport. The mechanism is depicted below.

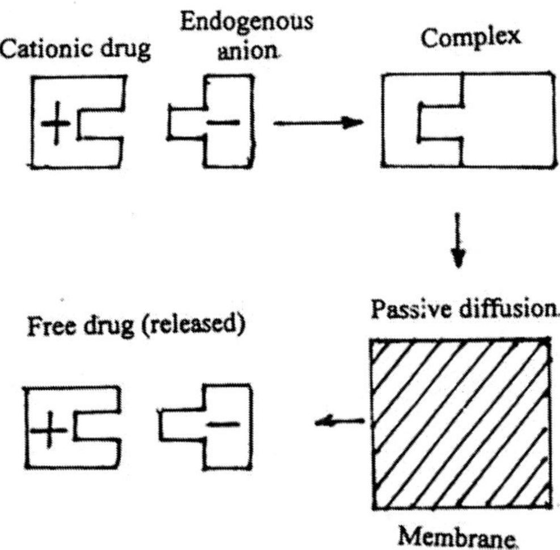

Fig. 148 Ion pair transport

Neutral complexes such as these have both the required lipophilicity as well as aqueous solubility for passive diffusion.

13.6. Pinocytosis

It is a process that resembles phagocytosis. The cell membrane has been observed to fold into a saccular structure. Extra cellular materials are getting collected into these sacs. The cell membrane closes at the top of the sac and subsequently the sac becomes a vesicle or vacuole within the interior of the cell. Pinocytosis shows some of the characteristics as that of active transport. The gastrointestinal absorption and pinocytosis play a vital role in absorbing macromolecules. It explains the oral efficacy of *Polio vaccine*.

14. CATALYSIS

Catalysis is a process of increasing the rate of a chemical reaction by an external agent termed catalyst. A catalyst is, therefore, defined as a substance that influences the rate of a chemical reaction (it may either increase or decrease the rate of chemical reaction) without itself altered in mass and chemical composition at the end of the reaction or at equilibrium. A catalyst is effective only when it comes in contact with reactant(s). A catalyst may be a positive or negative catalyst. A *positive catalyst* is one which accelerates the speed of a reaction. A *negative catalyst* or *an inhibitor* is one which retards the rate of a chemical reaction.

Catalysis may be of two types viz homogeneous catalysis and heterogeneous catalysis. A catalyst which is of biological interest is enzyme catalyst.

14.1. Homogeneous and Heterogeneous Catalysis

If the catalyst and the reactants are in the same phase (i.e. gaseous or liquid phase) then, the process of catalysis is termed *homogeneous catalysis* i.e. the catalyst mixes homogeneously with the reactant(s) and forms a single phase. The most important type of homogeneous catalysis is the acid-base catalysis.

If the catalyst and the reactants form separate phases in the mixture (i.e. a solid phase and a liquid or gaseous phase), then, the process of catalysis is termed *heterogeneous catalysis*. As this type of catalysis occurs at the surface of the solid catalyst, it is also called *surface catalysis*. The hydrogenation of unsaturated fatty acids by finely divided nickel (catalyst) is an example for heterogeneous catalysis because unsaturated fatty acid is the liquid phase and the catalyst nickel is the solid phase. Another example is the decomposition of hydrogen peroxide solution in water catalysed by solid magnesium oxide in colloidal state.

14.2. Characteristics of Catalysts

1. A catalyst remains unchanged in mass and in chemical component usually till the end of the reaction.
2. A very small quantity of catalyst is needed to bring about unlimited reaction.
3. The effect of catalytic action of a catalyst is increased by increasing the surface area. This may be achieved by reducing the catalyst to a fine powder or to a colloidal state.
4. Catalysts are *specific* in their action. That is, a catalyst may be effective for one reaction and ineffective for another reaction.
5. Generally catalysts *do not initiate a reaction*. They can speed up a reaction which has been already started.
6. Catalysts help in reaching the equilibrium state at a relatively shorter period of time. However, they do not affect equilibrium.
7. Change of temperature brings about an alteration in the catalytic reaction. However, the rate of reaction is at maximum at a particular temperature called the optimum temperature.

14.3. Theories of Catalysis

There are two main theories of catalysis

1. Intermediate compound formation theory
2. Adsorption theory.

Intermediate Compound Formation Theory Generally this theory applies to homogeneous catalytic reactions. According to this theory, the catalyst combines with the reactant specifically and forms an intermediate complex. This complex decomposes regenerating the catalyst and yielding the products. Simply the catalyst decreases the energy of activation by changing the pathway (mechanism) of the reaction. Consequently, the rate of reaction is increased. Alternatively a free radical may be formed and they may bring about fast chain reactions. Chain reactions include a series of steps involving free atoms or radicals that act as intermediates. A chain reaction may be stopped by a chain breaking or terminating step.

The intermediate compound formation theory may be illustrated as follows:

$$A + B \longrightarrow AB \qquad \text{... (1)}$$

If a catalyst '*C*' is added, the reaction proceeds through an intermediate compound formed

i.e. $A + C \longrightarrow AC$ (intermediate compound) ... (2)

$$AC + B \longrightarrow AB + C \qquad \text{... (3)}$$

The activation energies of the reactions (2) and (3) are lower than the reaction (1). In this way, the rate of reaction is increased. In many cases, the intermediate compounds which are as a rule unstable cannot be isolated. This theory is also called the '*chemical theory*'.

Adsorption Theory This theory applies to heterogeneous catalytic reactions. According to this theory, the reactant molecules are adsorbed on the surface of the catalyst presumably at adjacent sites. It involves most probably chemisorption (chemical adsorption). In chemisorption, the reactant is converted into an almost atomic state and in this state, it can form an activated complex which decomposes to form the product. The product is desorbed from the surface making room for the fresh reactant to get adsorbed and undergo reaction in the same way. This occurs at a fast but definite rate. For the same reactant a different product may be formed if the catalyst is changed.

When molecules of a gas get adsorbed on the surface of a catalyst, the molecules are brought very close together facilitating reaction between molecules whereas in the bulk of the gas, the molecules are far apart and hence the chances of reaction are rare.

Hydrogenation of ethylene molecule in the presence of nickel catalyst may be depicted as follows.

H – H

(Ni) (Ni)–(Ni) (Ni) (Ni)→

Adsorption of H_2 molecules

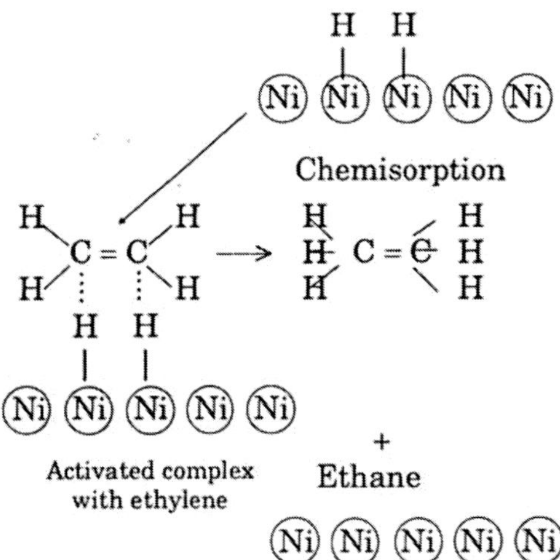

Regenerated Catalyst

Thus a heterogeneously catalysed reaction usually involves the following steps.

1. Chemisorption of reactants on the surface.
2. Diffusion and chemical reaction at the surface. In this chemical reaction, surface intermediates are often formed which then give rise to the ultimate products.
3. Desorption of products from the surface.

Adsorption theory is also regarded as *'Physical theory'*.

Active Centers It is believed that the entire surface of the catalyst is not uniformly active and that catalytic activity is concentrated only at specific points on the surface of the catalyst. Such specific points are called *active centers*. For greater activity, larger number of such active centers must be available. There fore, a catalyst with large surface area and hence maximum number of active centers is preferred.

Promotors A substance which itself is not a catalyst or a feeble catalyst can promote the activity of a catalyst. Such a substance is called a *promotor*. For example, cupric ions promote the catalytic action of ferric ions in the decomposition of hydrogen peroxide.

Catalytic poisoning Catalysts may be poisoned by extraneous substances. Such substances suppress the catalytic action of a catalyst and the process is called *catalytic poisoning*. For example, carbon monoxide poisons the catalytic action of copper in the hydrogenation of ethylene probably the carbon monoxide gets adsorbed on the copper surface in preference to the reactant. Thus it acts as a catalytic poison.

Autocatalysis

One of the products formed because of a chemical reaction between reactants may act as a catalyst for that reaction. Such a phenomenon is termed *autocatalysis*. For example, in the following reaction

$$CH_3COOC_2H_5 + H_2O \rightleftharpoons CH_3COOH + C_2H_5OH$$

The acetic acid formed as a product acts a catalyst (i.e. autocatalyst)

14.4. Enzyme Catalysis

Enzymes are complex protein molecules which are produced by living organisms. They are very effective catalyst. Enzyme catalysis occurs in most of the biological processes taking place in plants and animals. Each enzyme is produced in a particular living cell to catalyse the reactions occurring in that cell. The catalytic effect is produced by enzymes is so large and fast that the reaction may be completed within 10^{-4} or 10^{-6} seconds.

Each enzyme molecule is of rigid colloidal dimensions with cavities on their surface. These cavities are abound in active groups (such as ($-NH_2$, $-COOH$, $-SH$, and $-OH$). A molecule which has complimentary shape fit into these activities. As a result, the enzyme may form with the molecules (adsorbed) an activated complex which subsequently decompose to yield the products. It may be depicted as shown in Fig. 149.

Characteristics of enzyme catalysis

1. Enzyme catalysts are exceedingly efficient.
2. Enzyme catalyst is exceedingly selective in action.
3. Rate of enzyme catalysed reaction is maximum at optimum temperature i.e. it is active at relatively low temperature.
4. Catalytic activity of an enzyme may be initiated or destroyed by certain substances. The activity may also be enhanced by the presence of activators or coenzymes.

The physiological activity of drugs is due to the action of enzyme inhibitors in the body.

15. Applications of Catalysis

1. Number of chemical reactions are accelerated by using specific catalysts. For example, hydrogenation of unsaturated vegetable oils is catalysed by using finely divided nickel as catalyst.
2. Fermentation technology in the production of important organic chemicals and drugs, is fully based on the use of enzymes (organic catalyst) of micro-organisms. For example, production of alcohol, lactic acid, antibiotics etc are enzyme catalysed. Now-a-days enzymes are isolated and immobilised on solid inert material to

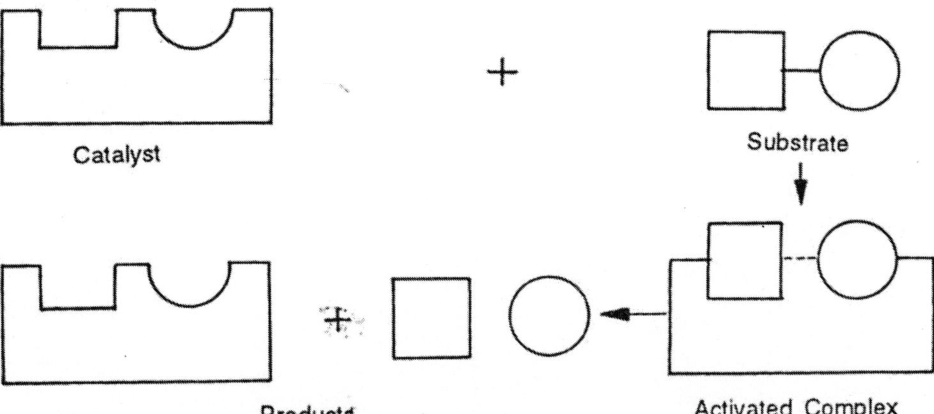

Fig.149. Representation of enzyme catalysis.

produce continuous bioconversions (solid state fermentation).

3. Microbial transformation is a technique of carrying out selective oxidation or reduction on a particular part of molecule by using enzymes of micro-organisms. Unlike chemical transformation, this technique gives more yield without much side products. Eg. Conversion of cortisone to hydrocortisone by using certain microbes having reductase enzyme.

4. Most of the biochemical reactions are carried out in our body by enzymes (organic catalysts) at body temperatures. A number of co-factors have been identified for the efficient action of enzymes. A number of digestive enzymes are isolated and are available in the market as dosage forms (either as tablets or capsules as a substitute for digestive enzymes for the patients).

5. Most of the chemical and polymeric reactions are effectively catalysed to produce the desired product in larger amounts.

6. In the preparation of Malt Extract, digestion of malt is aided by the enzyme diastase. The Malt Extract is an important ingredient in the marketed food products.

7. Sometimes catalyst may not be beneficial. For example, the antibiotic penicillin is destroyed by the enzyme penicillinase or by acid or base aided catalysts. The oxidation of many of the drugs is accelerated in the presence of heavy metals. Likewise a number of examples may be quoted. Hence proper steps should be taken to avoid catalysis in the above cases.

8. Bioconversion in the world is fully carried out by nature with the help of enzymes only. As example, degradation of all dead materials of animal and plant origin to simpler molecules may be cited. Conversion of simpler molecules to bioactive molecules are also carried out by the enzymes.

Thus the inorganic catalyst, organic catalyst, and the co-factors of the catalysts play a vital role in the various chemical biochemical and bioconversion processes.

SUGGESTIONS FOR PRACTICALS

1. Determination of specific rate constant, order of a chemical reaction and $t_{1/2}$ of the reaction

Principle

Determination depends on the estimation of the remaining concentration of a reactant at different time intervals during the decomposition of a reactant. The concentrations remaining at different times and the corresponding times are substituted in the appropriate equation to obtain the specific rate constant.

Procedure

Prepare 200 ml of 0.1 N hydrogen peroxide and place in a 500 ml container and close it. Withdraw 20 ml of the solution and keep aside. Add 2 ml of 5% ferric chloride solution to the solution in the flask. The decomposition will occur as follows:

$$H_2O_2 \xrightarrow{Fe^{3+}} H_2O + (O)$$

At an interval of 2 minutes, withdraw 20 ml of the hydrogen peroxide solution from the flask. To this add 10 ml of cold water and 15 ml of dilute sulphuric acid and also to the solution withdrawn and set aside initially. Titrate the solutions against $N/10$ potassium permanganate solution which has been standardised already with standard $N/10$ oxalic acid. Withdraw again after 4 minutes 20 ml of the solution, add 10 ml of water and 15 ml of dilute sulphuric acid and titrate immediately against $N/10$ potassium permanganate solution. The same is repeated for all the solutions withdrawn after 6 minutes, 8 minutes and 10 minutes. The results may be tabulated as follows:

	Time interval (t)	Volume of $N/10$ potassium permanganate consumed
(t_0)	0 (i.e. the solution withdrawn before the addition of 5% $FeCl_3$ solution)	$a = V_{t_0}$
(t_1)	120 seconds	$(a - x_1) = V_{t_1}$
(t_2)	240 seconds	$(a - x_2) = V_{t_2}$
(t_3)	360 seconds	$(a - x_3) = V_{t_3}$
(t_4)	480 seconds	$(a - x_4) = V_{t_4}$
(t_5)	600 seconds	$(a - x_5) = V_{t_5}$

Substitute the values in the following equation

(a) $kt = x$ (Zero order) or $k = \frac{x}{t}$

(b) $k = \frac{2.303}{t} \cdot \log \frac{a}{(a-x)}$ (First order)

(c) $k = \frac{1}{t} \frac{a}{(a-x)}$ (Second order)

(d) $k = \frac{1}{t} \cdot \frac{x(2a-x)}{2a^2(a-x)^2}$ (Third order)

The equation which gives constant values for k indicates the order of reaction and the k value is the specific rate constant.

For example if the reaction is first order, the substitution of the values is shown below:

$$\text{At time } t_1,\ k = \frac{2.303}{t_1} \log \frac{V_t}{V_{t_1}}$$

$$\text{At time } t_2,\ k = \frac{2.303}{t_2} \log \frac{V_t}{V_{t_2}}$$

$$\text{At time } t_3,\ k = \frac{2.303}{t_3} \log \frac{V_t}{V_{t_3}}$$

$$\text{At time } t_4,\ k = \frac{2.303}{t_4} \log \frac{V_t}{V_{t_4}}$$

$$\text{At time } t_5,\ k = \frac{2.303}{t_5} \log \frac{V_t}{V_{t_5}}$$

This reaction being first order $t_{1/2} = \frac{0.693}{k}$

Report: The specific rate constant and the order of the chemical reaction are to be reported.

2. Effect of temperature on specific rate constant and determination of energy of activation of a chemical reaction

Principle

This study involves the determination of specific rate constants (k values) of a reaction undergoing at different temperatures and finding out the influence of temperature on specific rate constant.

The energy activation is found from two different k values at two different temperatures.

Procedure

Mix 5 ml of ethyl acetate with 100 ml of 0.1 N hydrochloric acid taken in a conical flask and maintain at a temperature of 40°C. Withdraw 10 ml of aliquot of the reaction mixture at regular intervals say every 30 minutes. Transfer each reaction mixture into 30 ml of ice cold water and titrate against standardised 0.1 N sodium hydroxide using phenolphthalein as indicator. Titrate each reaction mixture immediately after transferring into the ice cold water and mixing with the indicator. A final titration is done after 24 hours which indicates the near completion of the reaction. Tabulate the results as shown.

	Time in minutes	**ml of alkali consumed**
(t_0)	0	V_{t_0}
(t_1)	30	V_{t_1}
(t_2)	60	V_{t_2}
(t_3)	90	V_{t_3}
(t_4)	120	V_{t_4}
(t_5)	150	V_{t_5}
(t_6)	180	V_{t_6}
(t_∞)	1440	V_{t_∞}

The reaction is a unimolecular reaction and hence it is first order reaction. Then,

$$k = \frac{2.303}{t} \cdot \log \frac{a}{(a-x)}$$

where $a = V_{t_\infty} - V_{t_0}$

$$x = V_{t_1} - V_{t_0}$$

$$(a - x) = V_{t_\infty} - V_{t_0} - (V_{t_1} - V_{t_0})$$

$$= V_{t_\infty} - V_{t_0} - V_{t_1} + V_{t_0}$$

$$= V_{t_\infty} - V_{t_1}$$

Substituting for a and $a - x$

$$k = \frac{2.303}{t} \cdot \log \frac{V_{t_\infty} - V_{t_0}}{V_{t_\infty} - V_{t_1}} \text{ after 30 minutes}$$

$$k = \frac{2.303}{t} \cdot \log \frac{V_{t_\infty} - V_{t_0}}{V_{t_\infty} - V_{t_2}} \text{ after 60 minutes}$$

In the same way calculate the k values for all the other reaction mixtures withdrawn and titrated at different time intervals

[**Note:** V_{t_∞} represents the volume of $N/10$ sodium hydroxide required in ml to neutralise the acid added and the acetic acid resulting from the complete hydrolysis of the ester. (This acetic acid concentration is equivalent to the initial concentration of the ester). V_{t_0} gives the volume of $N/10$ sodium hydroxide consumed to neutralise the acid added. Hence the difference ($V_{t_\infty} - V_{t_0}$) gives the initial concentration 'a'. ($V_{t_\infty} - V_{t_1}$) gives the volume of $N/10$ sodium hydroxide consumed at the time interval t_1 and ($V_{t_\infty} - V_{t_2}$) gives the volume of sodium hydroxide consumed at the time interval t_2 and so on].

Repeat the experiment in the same way but maintaining the temperature this time at 50°C. Again repeat at 60°C, 70°C and 80°C and calculate the k values from the data obtained at each of the above temperatures.

Repeat the observation

To obtain the ΔE value (Energy of Activation for the reaction), the following equation is used.

$$\log \frac{k_2}{k_1} = \frac{\Delta E_a}{2.303R}\left(\frac{T_2 - T_1}{T_2 T_1}\right)$$

Substitute the k values obtained at two different temperatures (say k_1 at 40°C and k_2 at 50°C or k_1 at 40°C and k_2 at 60°C) $R = 1.987$ calories/degree/mole and find out the ΔE_a value. T values indicate absolute temperature.

It is possible to find out k value at unknown temperature provided the k value at some other temperature and ΔE_a for the reaction are known.

Report the k values of the chemical reaction at different temperatures and ΔE_a of the chemical reaction.

XII MICROMERITICS

Mircromeritics is defined as the science and technology of small particles. This field has wider applications in pharmacy. They are:

1. The differentiation of solutions, colloids and suspensions depends upon the particle size of the dispersed phase only. In colloids, the particle size ranges from 1 nm to 0.5 nm and in suspensions, the particle size exceeds 0.5 nm.
2. The particle size in colloids and in suspensions decides their stability. The stability of the preparations decreases as the particle size increases and this leads to faster sedimentation.
3. The particle size of powder preparations is indirectly proportional to their surface area. The surface area of the given amount of powder gets increased as its particle size is decreased by size reduction. The relation between surface area and particle size is given by the expression.

$$S = \frac{6m}{d\,\rho} \quad \text{... (1)}$$

where S = surface area

m = mass of the powder

d diameter of the particles

ρ = density of the particles.

For a mass of 1 gram, assume that the diameter and the density have unit values, then the surface area is

$$S = \frac{6 \times 1}{1 \times 1 = 6}$$

If the diameter is reduced 10 times the original value, the surface area is

$$S = \frac{6 \times 1}{0.1 \times 1} = 60$$

That is, the surface area is increased ten times the original surface area. The increased surface area enhances the contact surface with the solvent. This leads to increased rate of dissolution of drug powder. This, in turn, increases the absorption of the drug from the gastrointestinal tract and hence the bioavailability of the drug. The increased rate of bioavailability of drugs from gastrointestinal tract is as follows.

Tablets and Capsules < Big particles < Micronized powder < suspensions < colloids < true solution

4. The particle size of the dispersed drug in ointment or suppositories affects its release characteristics from the dosage form to the skin or the mucous membrane.
5. The particle size decides the spreading ability and performance of some cosmetic preparations like dusting powder, face power, etc.

6. The size and shape of the particles in a powder decide its flow properties. The asymmetric particles have very poor flow properties. Hence granulation techniques are used to convert drug and the additive powders into symmetric spherical granules with good flow properties. This permits uniform supply of the drug powder from the hopper to the dies of the tablet machine. The tablets so produced will show uniform weights.
7. Particle size has a great effect on mixing of solids.
8. Process of separation of solids from fluids involves filtration and it is influenced by the particle size. Sedimentation also is influenced by particle size of powders.
9. Process factors such as loss as dust and explosion risk depend upon particle size of powders.
10. Extraction and drying are enhanced with smaller particle size of the material.
11. Adsorption capacity of a material will increase as the particle size decreases.

1. Particle size

For a symmetric particle like sphere, it is easy to describe the size by its diameter. But most of the drug powders do not show symmetry in their shapes. Hence the particle size of asymmetric particles are expressed in terms of '*equivalent spherical diameters*'. The various ways of expressing equivalent diameters are the following.

i)Surface diameter (d_s): It is the diameter of a sphere having same surface area as that of the asymmetric particle in question.

ii) volume diameter (d_v): It is the diameter of a sphere having same volume as that of the asymmetric particle in question.

iii) Projected diameter (d_p: It is the diameter of a sphere having same observed area as that of the asymmetric particle when viewed normal to its most stable plane by using a microscope.

iv) Stoke's diameter or sedimentation diameter (d_{st}): It is the diameter of a sphere which undergoes sedimentation at the same rate as that of the asymmetric particle.

2. Particle size distribution

Any powder (collection of particles) is polydisperse, i.e., a mixture of different sized particles. Hence it is necessary to know the size of particles and how many particles are present in each size range or what is the weight of particles present in each size range. Such a distribution of different sized particles in a powder is called particle size distribution. From the data of particle size distribution, average particle size of the powder can be calculated.

3. Average particle size

Suppose a powder is analysed microscopically. The number of particles in each size range is found out. A typical data may be presented as follows in table 1.

The average particle size is

$$\frac{\Sigma\, nd}{\Sigma\, n} = \frac{414}{204} = 2.028\ \mu m.$$

In the above method, only the total number and mean size of the particle have been considered to express the average particle size. The expression of average particle size can further be extended to take into account the surface and the volume of the particles. Edmundson has derived a general equation

Table 1. Particle Size Distribution Data

Size range in μm	Mean size range in $\mu m(d)$	No. of particles in each size range (n) obtained by microscopy	$d \times n$	Weight of powder in each size range by sedimentation technique
0.5 – 1.0	0.75	12	9.00	6 mg
1.00 – 1.5	1.25	24	30.00	11 mg
1.5 – 2.0	1.75	54	94.50	48 mg
2.0 – 2.5	2.25	84	189.00	64 mg
2.5 – 3.0	2.75	17	46.75	22 mg
3.0 – 3.5	3.25	8	26.00	12 mg
3.5 – 4.0	3.75	5	18.75	3 mg
		204	414.00	

to express the average particle size. It is given as

$$d_{mean} = \left(\frac{\Sigma nd^{p+f}}{\Sigma nd^{f}} \right)^{1/p}$$

where n = number of particles in each size range whose mid point is d which is one of the equivalent diameters.

p = it is an index related to size of an individual particle $p = 1, p = 2, or\ p = 3$ expresses particle length, surface or volume respectively

If the value of p is positive the mean is *arithmetic*, if p is zero, the mean is *geometric* and if p is negative, the mean is *harmonic*.

For a collection of particles, the frequency with which a particle in certain size range occurs is expressed by nd^f in which f is called frequency index which has values 0,1,2 or 3 thus the size frequency distribution is expressed in terms of total number or length or surface or volume of the particles respectively.

4. Scientific ways of expressing particle size distribution

Any given powder is polydisperse and it may be quantified by two ways.

1. Number of particles present in each size range (found out by microscopy)
2. Weight of particles present in each size range (found out by sedimentation or sieving techniques)

A plot of size range (or mid point of size range) against the number of particles in each size range frequency or weight of particles in each size range for the values found in table 1) is called *frequency distribution curve.*

The graph represents a plot of the number of particles against the size range. (histogram Fig.150). The mid points of the size ranges may also be

Some of the more significant arithmetic mean diameters (p is positive) are summarised as follows.

Statistical diameters

Size index (p)	Frequency index (f)	Edumundson equation $d_{mean}=\left(\frac{\Sigma nd^{p+f}}{\Sigma nd^{f}}\right)^{1/p}$	Type of mean	Mean diameter is based on
1	0	$\Sigma nd/\Sigma n$	Arithmetic	length number mean (d_{ln}
2	0	$\sqrt{\frac{\Sigma nd^2}{\Sigma n}}$	Arithmetic	Surface-number mean (d_{sn}
3	0	$\sqrt{\frac{\Sigma nd^3}{\Sigma n}}$	Arithmetic	volume number mean (d_{vn})
1	1	$\frac{\Sigma nd^2}{\Sigma nd}$	Arithmetic	Length weighted mean
1	2	$\frac{\Sigma nd^3}{\Sigma nd^2}$	Arithmetic	Surface weighted mean
1	3	$\frac{\Sigma nd^4}{\Sigma nd^3}$	Arithmetic	volume weighted mean

size index $p = 1$ means length is considered as a size parameter
size index $p = 2$ means surface is considered as a size parameter
size index $p = 3$ means volume is considered as a size parameter
Frequency index $f = 0$ means number is considered as a frequency parameter
Frequency index $f = 1$ means length is considered as a frequency parameter
Frequency index $f = 2$ means surface is considered as a frequency parameter

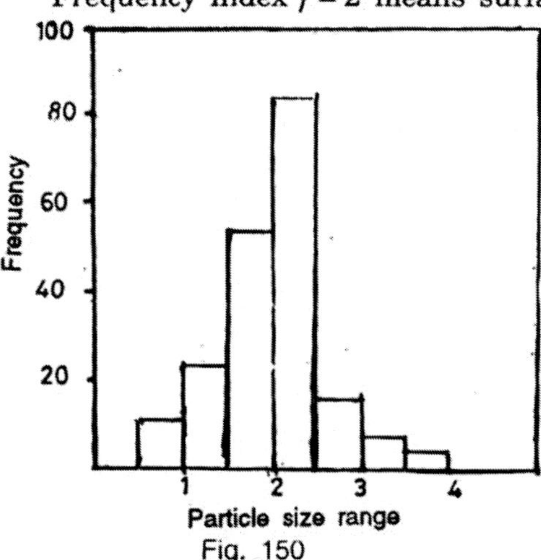

Fig. 150

plotted against the number of particles. It is called *number frequency distribution curve*. It is shown in the figure 151.

Graph (Fig. 152) indicates a plot of the weight of particles against the size range (histogram). The mid points of each size range may also be plotted against the weight of the particles. It is called *weight distribution frequency curve* and is also shown in Fig 152.

Both the figures provide a clear visible representation of the distribution of particles in a powder whereas the ex-

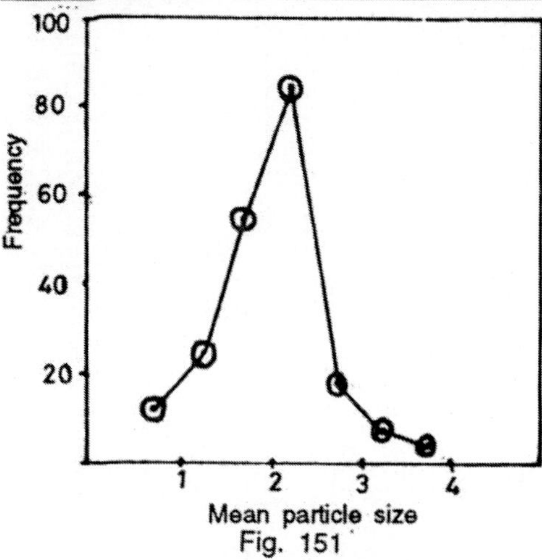

Fig. 151

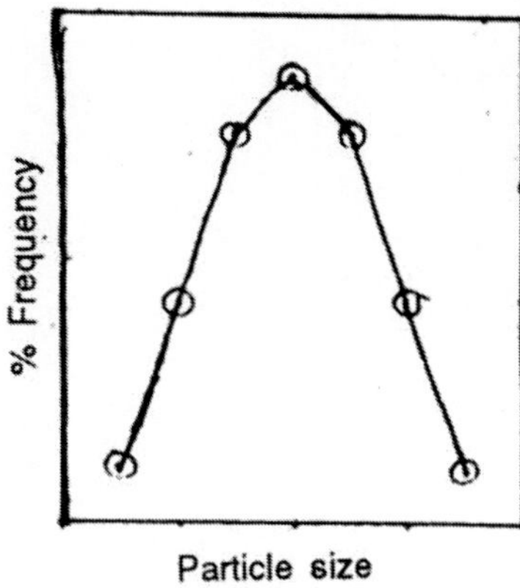

Fig. 153

pression of size in terms of average diameter does not give such a clear expression. Two powders having the same average diameter may not have the same frequency distribution. From the graph, we can make out the particle size which occurs more frequently and that size is called the *mode* of the sample.

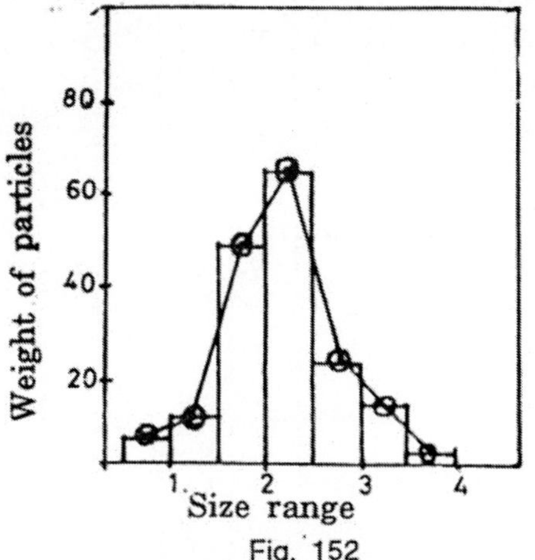

Fig. 152

A polydisperse powder is said to have normal distribution if the data plotted show a typical bell shaped curve (Fig. 153). In this one half of the curve is superimposable with another half, that is, the distribution of particles is symmetric around the mean. In this case *mode* and *average size* are same. The standard deviation (σ) is the indication of the distribution about the mean. In a normal distribution, 68% of the particles lie within ± 1σ from the mean, 95% of the particles lie within ± 1σ from the mean and 99.7% lie within ± 3σ from the mean. Most of the powders (i.e after size reduction) do not show this distribution.

The particle size distribution of most of the powders tends to be unsymmetric or skewed as shown in the Fig.154. However if the log of particle size is plotted against frequency (either number or weight) a typical bell shaped curve may be obtained. Frequently such a curve is called *log normal distribution curve* as shown in Fig: 155. For this, a semi-log, paper is used if arithmetic values are used.

We can represent the particle size distribution by preparing various

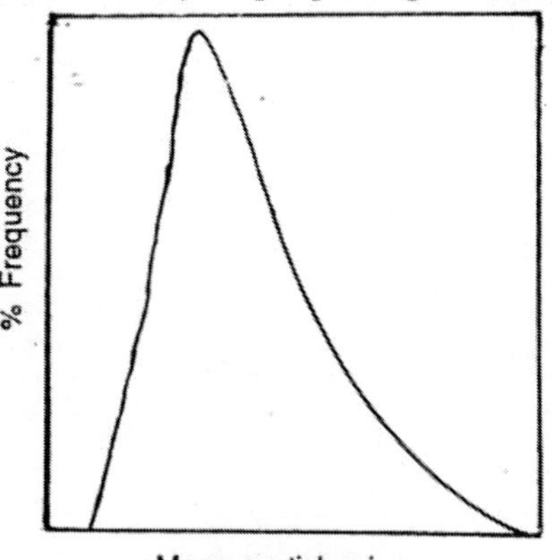

Fig. 154

The particle size data distribution of a given powder can be scientifically represented as follows in Table 2.

1	2	3	4	5	6	7	8	9	10	11	12	13	14	15	16
								Cumulative frequency Number distribution				Cumulative frequency weight distribution			
Size range µm)	Mean size (d)	No. of particles (n)	% Frequency	$n \times d$	$n \times d^2$	$n \times d^3$ (Weight)	percent $n \times d^3$ (weight)	under size	under size in %	over size	over size in %	under size	under size in %	over size	over size in %
0 – 2	1.0	3	1	3		3	0.0020	3	1	297	99		.002		99.99
2 – 4	3.0	45	15	135		1215	0.80	48	16	252	84		.802		99.20
4 – 6	5.0	96	32	480		14900	9.300	144	48	156	52		10.10		89.90
6 – 8	7.0	72	24	504		24696	15.40	216	72	139	28		25.50		74.50
8 – 10	9.0	42	14	378		30618	18.80	258	86	97	14		44.30		55.70
10 – 12	11.0	21	7	231		27951	17.30	279	93	76	7		61.60		38.40
12 – 14	13.0	12	4	156		26364	16.40	291	97	62	3		78.00		22.00
14 – 16	15.0	6	2	90		20250	12.60	297	99	58	1		90.60		9.40
16 – 18	17.0	3	1	51		14739	9.30	300	100	55	0		99.90		0.10
TOTAL		300	100			160736	99.90,								

Data for column no.3 is obtained by microscopy. Column No.3 become weight of particles if the estimation is done by sedimentation or sieving techniques. Number distribution may be converted to weight distribution by multiplying n and d^3 provided the general shape and density of the particles do not depend on the size range of the sample.

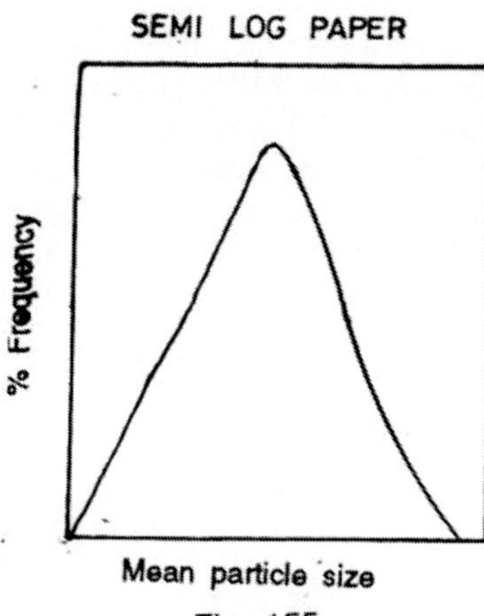

Fig. 155

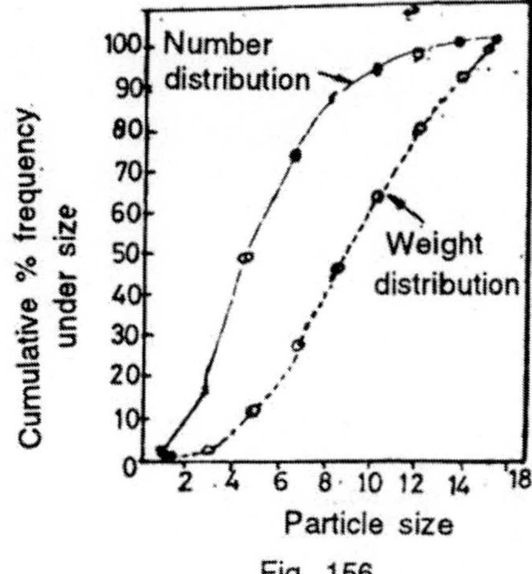

Fig. 156

graphs. That is parameters in column 2 in the table are taken on x-axis and plotted against the parameters appearing in column 3, 4, 9, 10, 11, 12, 13, 14, 15, or 16 on y-axis in an arithmetic graph paper (i.e. rectangular co-ordinate graph paper)

In order to obtain log-normal curve, parameters in column 2 in the table taken on x-axis (in log scale) can be plotted against the parameters appearing in column 3, 4, 9, 10, 11, 12, 13, 14, 15 or 16 on y-axis (arithmetic scale) of a semilog graph paper.

Thus the data obtained from the particle size analysis of a sample of powder can be represented scientifically to visualise the particle size distribution clearly.

Plotting either the cumulative percent oversize or undersize against the particle size gives a sigmoidal curve with the mode being at the greatest slope as shown in Fig. 156.

Determination of geometric mean diameter and geometric mean deviation of a powder.

Geometric mean diameter is based on

a) number distribution which is denoted as d_g and

Mean size range	Log of mean size	Cumulative % frequency under size (number)	Probit values for cumulative % frequency undersize (number)	Cumulative % frequency under size (weight)	Probit values for cumulative % frequency undersize (weight)
1	0.0000	1	2.674	0.002	–
3	0.4771	16	4.006	0.802	–
5	0.6990	48	4.950	10.10	3.718
7	0.8451	72	5.583	25.50	4.326
9	0.9542	86	6.080	44.30	4.849
11	1.0414	93	6.476	61.60	5.279
13	1.1139	97	6.881	78.00	5.772
15	1.1761	99	7.326	90.60	6.282
17	1.2304	100	10.00	99.00	7.326

Probit values for percentage values are given under practical section as empirical probits.

b) weight distribution which is denoted as d'_g and

geometric mean deviation based on

a) number distribution which is denoted as σ_g

b) weight distribution which is denoted as σ_g

The above parameters can be obtained as follows:

The data of log of particle size and probit *values** of cumulative per cent frequency undersize (number or weight) are obtained for the data given in table 2, and may be presented as follows:

By plotting the log mean size on x axis against empirical probit values for cumulative percentage frequency undersize (number) on y axis using an ordinary arithemtic graph paper as shown in Fig. 157 one obtains a straight line. The line so obtained may be characterized by two parameters that are the slope of the line and the reference point. The reference point is the logarithm of the particle size equivalent to 50% on the probit scale which is called geometric mean diameter. In this case, value of log particle size corresponding to 50%

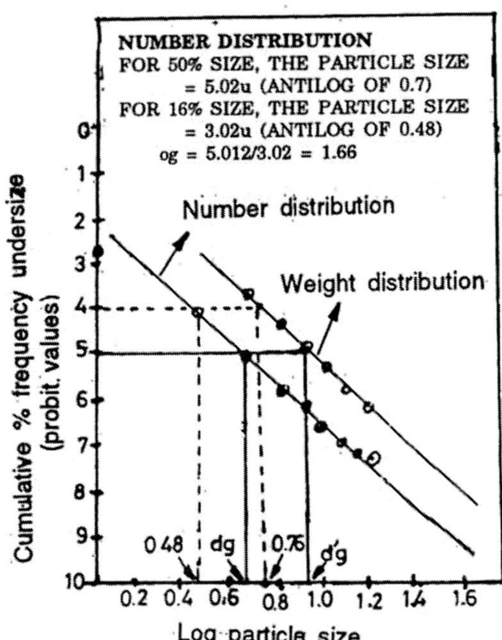

Fig. 157

probit value is 5.000) is 0.7. The antilog of 0.7 is 5.012 μm which is the geometric mean diameter (d_g) of the powder. If the geometric mean diameter is derived from the similar type of graph using weight distribution, the geometric mean diameter of the powder is designated as d_g. This value comes out to be 9.55 μm in the present example Fig. 157)

The geometric mean deviation

$$\sigma_g = \frac{84\% \text{ undersize or } 16\% \text{ oversize}}{50\% \text{ size}}$$

$$\text{or, } \frac{50\% \text{ size}}{16\% \text{ undersize or } 84\% \text{ oversize}}$$

From the data obtained,

$$\sigma_g = \frac{50\% \text{ size}}{16\% \text{ undersize}} = \frac{5.012}{3.02} = 1.66$$

Using the weight distribution data, the geometric mean deviation (σ_g) comes out to be 1.66 (as for number distribution) in the present example.

Equations developed by *Hatch-Choate* are available to convert weight distribution data into number distribution data and *vice versa*. It is also made possible to calculate statistical diameters such as mean surface diameter (d_s) mean volume diameter (d_v) and mean volume-surface diameter (d_{vs}) from the geometric mean diameter and the geometric mean deviation (either of number distribution or of weight distribution).

5. Particle Number (N)

It is defined as the number of particles per unit weight.

Assume the particles of a powder are spherical. Then, the volume of a single particle is $\pi d^3_{vn}/6$ where d_{vn} is the mean diameter based on volume and number. The mass of the particle is $\pi d^3_{vn}\, \rho/6$ (i.e. mass = volume × density) where ρ is density of the particle.

Number of particles per gram (N)

$$= \frac{1 \text{ gm of the powder}}{\text{Mass of one particle}}$$

$$= \frac{1}{\pi d^3_{vn}\, \rho/6}$$

$$N = \frac{6}{\pi d^3_{vn}\, \rho} \quad \text{... (6)}$$

Thus if mean volume number diameter of a powder and density of the powder are known, the number of particles per gram can be calculated.

6. Determination of average particle size and particle size distribution.

The various methods are

1. Microscopic technique
2. Sieving technique
3. Sedimentation technique
4. Coulter counter (electrical method) technique
5. Low angle light scattering technique

6.1. Microscopic Technique

An ordinary compound microscope is used for determination. First of all, an eye piece micrometer which may be square or linear type should be calibrated. For calibration a standard stage micrometer is used. In this 'one millimeter is divided into 100 equal divisions and hence each division is equal to 10 μ. The eye piece micrometer which is linear consists of 100 divisions. Calibration is undertaken to find out the measure of each division using the standard micrometer. After calibration, the eye piece micrometer is used for particle size determination.

A suspension (diluted) of the powder particles whose sizes are to be determined is prepared in a liquid vehicle in which it is insoluble. If it is slightly soluble, a saturated solution of the powder can be used for the preparation of the suspension. A drop of the suspension is mounted on a slide and observed under the microscope. About 300 particles are measured with the help of the eye piece micrometer. About 300 particles are measured with the help of the eye piece micrometer. All the particles in a field should be counted. The data may be presented as follows.

S.No.	Diameter of the particles
1	
2	
.	
.	
n	

The above data may be rearranged as follows:

Size range	mid point	No.of particles in each size range
...	...	...
...	...	...
...	...	...

The data can be scientifically represented as size-frequency distribution curve as described earlier. From the data, the average particle size as well as the size distribution can be found out. Particles in the size range of 0.2 μm to about 100 μm can be measured by this technique.

Disadvantages

1. The diameter of the particles represents two dimensions only i.e. length and breadth and not the depth.
2. At least 300 to 500 particle should be counted to get a reliable data and hence the method is tedious.

Advantages

The presence of agglomerates can easily be detected and avoided.

Improvements

1. The field viewed through the microscope can be projected for easy counting and measurement of the particles.
2. The field of the microscope can be photographed for measurement of the particles.
3. Particles may be counted with electronic scanners to avoid the strain of visual observation.
4. A double image microscope may be used. In this, the image of the particle is split until the two images are just separated using a calibrated image splitting device. The adjustment needed for this gives the particle diameter.
5. By using an electron microscope particles from 1 Å to 1 μm can also be measured.

6.2. Sieving Technique

A series of standard sieves are stacked one above the other so that sieves with larger pore size (less sieve numbers) occupy top portion followed by sieves of decreasing pore sizes (larger sieve numbers) towards the bottom. (The sieve number indicates the number of pores per linear inch Suppose the sieve number is 10, it indicates that it contains 10 pores (meshes) per linear inch or 100 pores per square inch)

Sieve apertures (which represent the actual or effective pore sizes) ranging from 90 μm down to as low as 5 μm are available. A definite mass of the sample is placed on the top sieve and the whole set-up is shaken mechanically for a definite period of time. The powder remaining on each sieve after the agitation is over, is collected separately and weighted. The data are summarized as follows.

S. No.	Sieve No.	Sieve aperture size μm)	Weight of powder detained in each sieve
...	...	...	...
...	...	...	...

For aperture size of standard sieve refer under practical. The geometric mean diameter (d'_g and standard deviation (σ'_g can be obtained by the method described earlier.

Disadvantage

Sieving errors may occur due to sieve loading and duration and intensity of agitation. Sieving may also cause attrition of granular pharmaceutical material (this produces size reduction). Hence enough care should be exercised to avoid errors introduced due to sieving conditions.

Depending upon the sieve number. powder particles may be classified as follows:

Sieve number (All the particles passes through)	Sieve Number Not more than 40% of powder pass through	Grade of the powder
10	44	Coarse powder
22	60	Moderately coarse powder
44	85	Moderately fine powder
85	–	Fine powder
120	–	Very fine powder

6.3. Sedimentation technique

This may be carried out by using an Andreason pipette (Fig. 158). It consists of a 550 ml vessel containing a

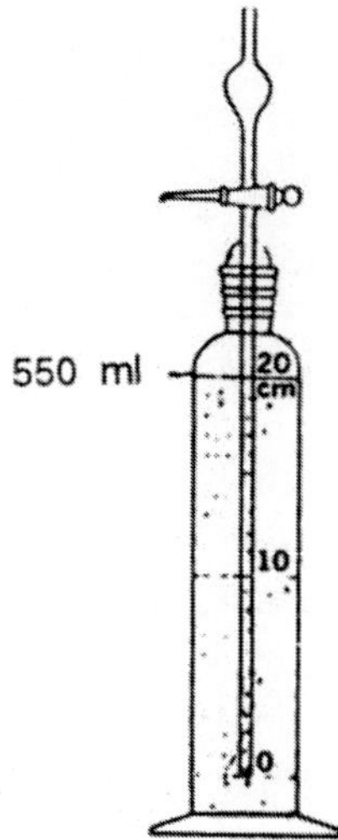

Fig. 158: Andreasean apparatus

10 ml pipette sealed into a ground glass stopper. When the pipette is in its place in the cylinder, the lower tip is 20 cm below the surface of the suspension.

For analysis, 1 to 2% suspension of the particles in a medium containing a suitable deflocculating agent (to separate any aggregate) is introduced into the vessel upto the mark 20 cm and that represents a total volume of 550 ml. The vessel is stoppered and shaken to distribute the particles uniformly within the medium. Having placed the pipette securely in its place, the vessel is clamped in a constant temperature bath. At various time intervals 10 ml samples are withdrawn into a previously weighed china dish everytime. Each sample is evaporated and weighed separately and necessary correction is made for the deflocculating agent.

The particle diameter corresponding to the various time period is calculated as follows by using Stoke's equation:

$$v = \frac{d^2_{st}(\rho - \rho_1 g}{18\eta_l} \quad \text{... (7)}$$

where v = rate of sedimentation

d_{st} = sedimentation diameter of the particle i.e. Stoke's diameter

ρ_s = density of the powder

ρ_l = density of the medium

g = acceleration due to gravity

η_l = viscosity of the medium

The rate of sedimentation is

$$v = \frac{h}{t} \quad \text{... (8)}$$

where $h$is the distance of the fall of particles in time t.

On rearrangement, the equation becomes:

$$d_{st} = \sqrt{\frac{18\,\eta_l\,h}{(\rho_s - \rho_l)gt}} \quad \text{... (9)}$$

Substituting appropriate values, d_{st} of particles at different time intervals can be calculated.

To apply Stoke's law, flow of dispersion medium around the particle as it sediments should be laminar or streamline. Whether the flow is laminar or turbulent is indicated by Reynold's number (R_e)

$$R_e = \frac{vd\rho_l}{\eta_l} \quad \text{... (10)}$$

$$\text{Now } v = \frac{R_e\,\eta_l}{d\,\rho_l}$$

$$\text{Thus } \frac{R_e\,\eta_l}{d\,\rho_l} = \frac{d^2(rho_s - \rho_l)g}{18\,\eta_l}$$

$$d^3 = \frac{18R_e\,\eta^2_l}{(rho_s - \rho_l)\,\rho_l\,g} \quad \text{... (18)}$$

This expression gives maximum diameter that could be calculated for a given density of liquid, set of density and viscosity conditions provided and the Reynold's number should not exceed 0.2.

The results are tabulated as follows

S. No.	Time period in minutes (t)	d_{st} at t	Weight of powder collected at different time intervals
...	...	...	...
...	...	...	...
...	...	...	...

From the data, various graphs needed may be obtained. Then the geometric mean diameter (d'_g)and standard deviation (σ'_g)for this weight distribution can also be calculated.

The improved technique of sedmimentation method is the centrifugal method. When the particles are very small, normal sedimentation is very slow. Hence centrifugal force is used to accelerate sedimentation instead of gravitational sedimentation. The particle size of the sediment at different time intervals is monitored by turbidoemetric method. In this, a beam of light is passed through the suspension. Some of the light is scattered and can be measured and from this the surface area of the particles can be calculated. Using appropriate equations, the particle size can be found. This method has a special advantage that suspension is not disturbed as in pipette sampling.

6.4. Coulter counter method (Electrical method to measure particle volume)

A Coulter consists of the following parts as shown in Fig. 159.

It consists of two electrodes of which one is dipped into a vessel containing the electrolyte and the particles and the other is dipped in the electrolyte solution in a tube which in turn is dipped into the vessel. The tube and the vessel are connected through an orifice. The terminals are connected to an amplifier. The tube is connected to the counter device via mercury in a tube.

A known volume of dilute suspension in an electrolyte solution is kept in

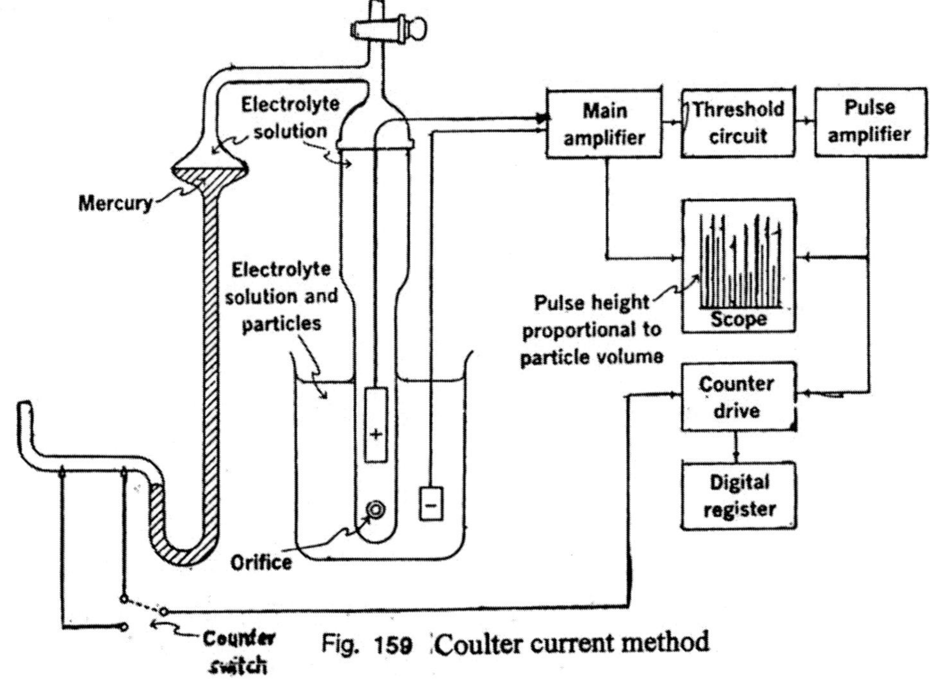

Fig. 159 Coulter current method

the vessel. The dispersion is pumped through the orifice into the tube. The suspension should be so dilute that at a time only one particle passes through the orifice. A constant voltage is applied across the electrodes. As the particle travels through the orifice, it displaces its own volume of the electrolyte and this results in an increased resistance between the two electrodes. The change in resistance which is related to particle volume causes a voltage pulse. The pulse is amplified and fed to an oscilloscope (pulse height analyser) calibrated in terms of particle size.

To avoid overcrowding, the electronic circuit is provided with a threshold selector which can be set for any particle size range. Suppose we get the instrument for the particle size range from 10 μm to 100 μm, the instrument will detect only those particles in that range. A typical print out will have the following data.

Number of particles counted	Pulse height	Particle size
...	...	...
...	...	...
...	...	...

Using this instrument, all the particles can be counted. The instrument is capable of counting at the rate of 4000 particles per second approximately. The instrument is also used to find out particulate contamination in parentral solution as per USP specifications.

From the pulse height, volume distribution can be obtained and this can be converted to weight distribution.

The choice of the method for particle size analysis is summarised as follows:

Method	Size range
Sieving	10 μm to 10,000 μm
Optical microscope	1 μm to 100 μm
Electron microscope	1Å to 1 μm
Sedimentation	1 μm to 660 μm
Ultracentrifuge	10 Å to 1 μm
coulter counter	0.5 μm to 1000 μm

6.5. Low angle Laser Light Scattering Technique

In this Laser diffraction principle (more correctly - low angle laser light scattering - LALLS) particle size is measured accurately and precisely. It is important because particle size influence stability, dissolution rates and material strength of drugs. Particles are irregular in shape and hence their size can vary greatly depending upon chosen dimension for measurement and the results vary depending upon different techniques of measurement. LALLS technique is speedy, easy and reproducible for particle size determination. Particles ranging from 0.5 μm to 3500 μm can be measured. A wide range of samples including dry powders, liquid suspension, aerosols, emulsions, particulate contaminant in injections can be anaylsed. Small amount of samples (10 mg) is enough. The technique is non - destructive.

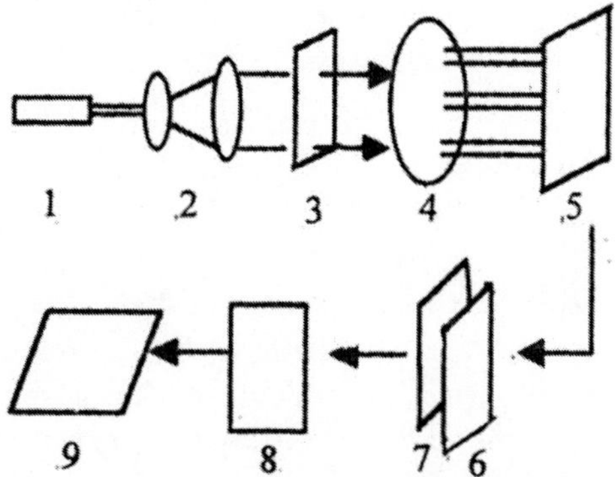

Fig. 160 Malveran Mastersizor

No calibration against a standard is necessary. The instrument used for this purpose is called Malveran Master sizer. (Fig.160) It comprises the following.

1. Laser source: He Ne laser providing light of wavelength 0.633 μm
2. Spartial filter.
3. Sample passing: samples are exposed to laser beam directly or through transparent cell. While exposing, no contamination from environment should occur.
4. Fourier lens
5. Detector: The light scattered from the sample is focussed by (4) to photo sensitizing silicon detector (5) comprising a number of discrete elements. The signal from each element is proportional to the amount of light falling on it. The light is received by scanning receiver (6) and subsequently amplified by an amplifier (7) Windows based software is used in a computer (8) for analysis and the data that come out are collected in a printer. The light falling on the detector is measured and integrated which is a statistical representation of the material.

USP prescribes the following standard to limit particulate contamination in parenterals. The injection meets the requirement of the quality control test if the average number of particles present in the units tested do not exceed the appropriate value in the given table as per light obscuration particle count test.

	Injection	>10 μm	>25 μm
a)	small volume parenterals (SVP)	6000	600 per container
b)	large volume parenterals (LVP)	25	3 per ml.

For the test, USP does not prescribe any instrument specifically. because of sophistication, Malveran Master sizer is extensively used in pharmaceutical industries. While measurement, test environment, glassware, closures or necessary equipment should not contribute any significant amount of particulate matter.

If the average number of particles exceeds the limit, they are to be tested by microscope particle count test as per USP requirement. In this method, the parenteral solution is filtered through membrane filter of minimum diameter of 21 mm and the porosity of 1.0 μm or finer. Necessary care is taken that no particulate contamination occurs from environment, container, closure or from the necessary equipments. The particle size and the count is made using microscope as per the procedure given in USP. The injection meets. the requirments if the average number of particles present in the unit does not exceed the given value.

Injection	>10 μm	>25μm
(LVP)	12	2 per ml

7. Particle shape

Particle shape affects the flow characteristics and packing properties of a powder.

A sphere has minimum surface area per unit volume. The more asymmetric the particle becomes, the greater is the surface area per unit volume. Hence it may be necessary to know the extent of asymmetry in a particle.

The surface area or volume of a **sphere is given by**

$$\text{Surface area} = \pi d^2 \quad \dots (12)$$

$$\text{volume} = \frac{\pi d^3}{6} \quad \dots (13)$$

To estimate the surface area or volume of an asymmetric particle, we must choose a diameter that relates this to the surface area or the volume of a sphere through a correction factor.

Suppose we obtain the size of a particle microscopically, then the size is given in terms of diameter as projected diameter d_p for the particle. Now the square and cube of this chosen diameter (*i.e.* d_p) are proportional to the surface area and volume respectively. Making use of proportionality constant, we can write.

$$\text{surface area} = \alpha_s\, d_p^2$$

where α_s is the surface area facter and d_s is the equivalent surface diameter (i.e spherical particle)

$$\text{Then, } \alpha_s = \frac{\pi d_s^2}{d_p^2} = 3.142$$

Thus, the shape factor α_s is the ratio of one diameter to another.

For volume , we can write

$$\text{volume} = \alpha_v\, d_p^3 = \frac{\pi d_v^3}{6}$$

where α_v is the volume factor and d_v is the equivalent volume diameter

$$\text{Then, } \alpha_v = \frac{\pi d_v^3}{d_p^3 .6} = 0.524 \quad \dots (14)$$

Each and every particle has its own volume and shape factors.

Taking the ratio of surface area factor and volume factor, we get

$$\frac{\alpha_s}{\alpha_v} = \frac{\pi d_s^2\, d_p^3\, 6}{d_p^2\, \pi d_v^3}$$

If the particle is spherical

$$\frac{\alpha_s}{\alpha_v} = 6$$

(since all the other terms get cancelled for a spherical particle)

If this ratio (α_s/α_v) exceeds 6, then the particle deviates from being a sphere and it can be said, the more this ratio exceeds this minimum value of 6, the more asymmetric the particle becomes.

8. Specific surface

Specific surface is defined as the surface area per unit volume (S_v) or per unit weight (S_w)

Taking into account, the surface area factor and volume factor for *n* number of asymmetric particles, specific surface per unit volume is

$$S_v = \frac{\text{Surface area of n particles}}{\text{volume of n particles}}$$

$$= \frac{n\, \alpha_s d^2}{n\, \alpha_v\, d^3} = \frac{\alpha_s}{\alpha_{vd}}$$

Specific surface area per unit weight is

$$S_w = \frac{\text{Surface area of n particles}}{\text{Volume of n particles} \times \text{density}}$$

$$S_w = \frac{n\, \alpha_s\, d^2}{n\, \alpha_x\, d^3\, \rho}$$

where ρ = true density of the particle

$$= \frac{\alpha_s}{\alpha_v\, d\rho}$$

$$\text{or } S_w = \frac{S_v}{\rho} \; (\text{where } S_v = \frac{\alpha_s}{\alpha_{vd}}) \quad \dots (15)$$

Defining the dimesions as d_{vs} which is volume surface diameter characteristics of specific surface, the above equation is written as

$$S_w = \frac{\alpha_s}{\alpha_v\, d_{vs}\, \rho} \qquad \text{... (16)}$$

For spherical particles

$S_w = \frac{6}{D_{vs}\, \rho}$ (since $\frac{\alpha_s}{\alpha_v} = 6$ for spherical particles)

8.1. Determination of surface area of powders.

The surface area of a powder can be derived indirectly from the size and size distribution obtained by the methods (such as microscopy, sieving, sedimentation and volume determined by Coulter counter) already described. Direct calculation of surface area may be done using two methods. They are the adsportion and air permeability methods.

8.1.1. Adsorption method

In this method, the amount of liquid solute or a gas that is adsorbed onto a sample of powder to form a monolayer is found out and from this data, surface area of the powder may be determined.

a) By using a solute which forms a monolayer: This involves the adsorption of a solute from its solution onto the surface of a powder (i.e. adsorbent)

Methanolic solution of stearic acid is first prepared. Stearic acid being a linear molecule, the molecules get adsorbed on solid surface (i.e. on powder surface) as a monolayer. The method is applicable to powders insoluble in methanol.

A known amount of the powder is treated with excess amount of methanolic solution of stearic acid. The contents are stirred. After one hour or after ensuring so, that adsorption has attained equilibrium it is filtered. The filtrate contains unadsorbed stearic acid. It is estimated by titrating with a standard solution of sodium hydroxide. A blank tritration is performed to find out the amount of stearic acid originally present in the solution. The difference between these values gives the amount of stearic acid adsorbed by the quantity of the powder added. From this value, the amount of stearic acid adsorbed per gram of the material can be calculated. Assume this to be 'x' grams. The number of molecules present in 1 gram mole of stearic acid (i.e. 284 gm) is given by Avogadro's number, 6.0223×10^{23}. From these data it is quite simple to find out what will be the number of molecules present in x grams of stearic acid. Let the number of molecules present in x grams be n and since one molecule of stearic acid occupies an area of 20.46×10^{-16} sq. cm., the total surface area of stearic acid molecules in x grams is $n \times 20.46 \times 10^{-16}$ sq. cm. This gives the specific surface. The specific surface may also be expressed in square meters per gram.

b) By using adsorption of gas on powder For this an instrument called *Quantasorb* may be used. The powder whose surface area is to be determined is introduced into a cell in the instrument and nitrogen which is the adsorbate gas and helium which is an inert gas and not adsorbed are passed through the powder in the cell. A thermal conductivity detector measures the amount of nitrogen adsorpbed at every equilibrium pressure and a bell shaped curve is obtained on a strip-chart recorder. The signal height gives the rate of adsorption of nitrogen gas and the area under the curve provides the amount of gas adsorbed on the powder sample.

The volume of nitrogen gas V_m in cm^3 adsorbed by 1 gram of the powder when the monolayer is complete is given by BET equation as.

$$\frac{p}{V(p_o - p)} = \frac{1}{V_m b} + \frac{(b-1)p}{V_m b p_o} \quad \ldots (17)$$

where v = volume of gas in cm^3 adsorbed per gram of powder at pressure p

p_o = saturated vapour pressure of liquified nitrogen at the temperature of the experiment.

b = a constant and it gives the difference between the heat of adsorption and the heat of liquefaction of the nitrogen gas.

A plot of $p/V(p_o - p)$ against p/p_o ordinarily yields straight line. The intercept on the ordinate gives the value of V_m. (Fig.161)

The specific surface of the powder is then obtained by applying the equation given below.

$$S_w = \frac{A_m N}{m/\rho} \times V_m$$

where m/ρ = molar volume of the gas at N.T.P.

N = Avogadro's number 6.02×10^{23}

A_m = area of a single close packed gas molecule adsorbed as a monolayer on the surface of the powder particles. For nitrogen the value is 1.62×10^{-16} cm^2.

Quantasorb may be used to determine the true density of powders and to obtain pore size and pore volume distributions for porous materials.

8.1.2. Air permeability method

Surface area determination by air permeability method can be carried out with an instrument called *Fisher sub-sieve sizer*. The instrument is shown in Fig. 162.

A plug of powder is considered to have a series of capillaries whose diameter is related to average particle size. According to Poiseuille's equation.

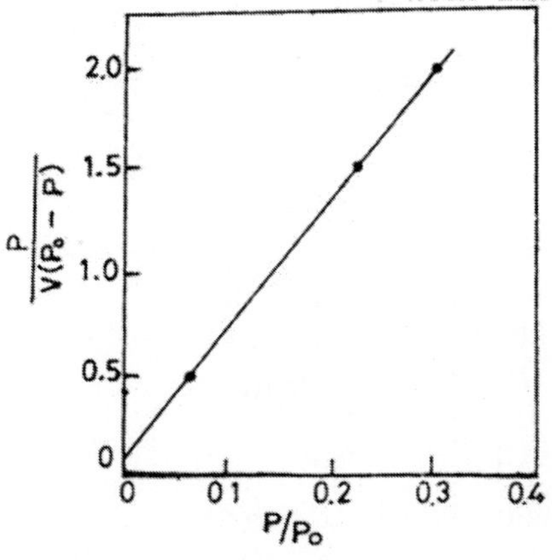

Fig. 161

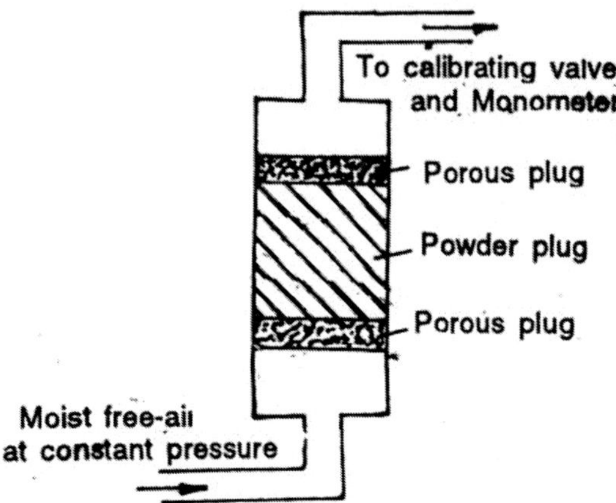

Fig. 162. Fisher Subsieve Sizer

$$v = \frac{\pi d^4 \Delta pt}{8l\eta}$$

where v is the volume of air flowing through a capillary of internal diameter d and length l in t seconds under a pressure difference of Δp. The viscosity of the fluid (air) is η poise.

When the air is allowed to pass through the plug of a compacted powder, resistance to the flow of air occurs. This resistance is related to the surface area of the powder. As per Kozency-Carman equation derived from Poiseuille's equation.

$$v = \frac{A}{\eta S_w^2} \cdot \frac{\Delta pt}{kl} \frac{\varepsilon^3}{(1-\varepsilon)^2}$$

where A = cross sectional area of the plug.

k = a constant (usually 5.0 ± 0.5)

ε = porosity

From the values of A, k, ε (See under porosity of powders), ΔP (which is obtained from the manometer) η (the visocity of the fluid air), and v (the volume of the air that flowed in time t), the specific surface (S) can be calculated.

This method is widely used to control batch to batch variations in specific surface of powders. As the porosity of powder decreases, surface area of the powder is also decreased.

9. Derived properties of powders

The size *distribution* and the *surface area* are the two fundamental properties of the powders.Based upon these two properties, there are a number of derived properties. They are as follows.

9.1. Dissolution and dissolution rate

Dissolution and dissolution rate are a direct property of surface area increase due to size reduction. The student is directed to refer under dissolution and it needs no further discussion here.

9.2. Densities of powders

a) **Bulk density**: It is the ratio between a given mass of a powder and its bulk volume.

$$\text{Bulk density} = \frac{\text{Mass of a powder}}{\text{Bulk volume of the powder}}$$

A given quantity of the powder is transferred to a measuring cylinder and is tapped mechanically either manually or using some tapping device till a constant volume is obtained. This volume is the bulk volume (v) and it includes the true volume of the powder and the void space among the powder particles.

A given pack of powder has air spaces between the particles. This air space is called void space or void volume (Fig. 163). Thus the bulk volume is true

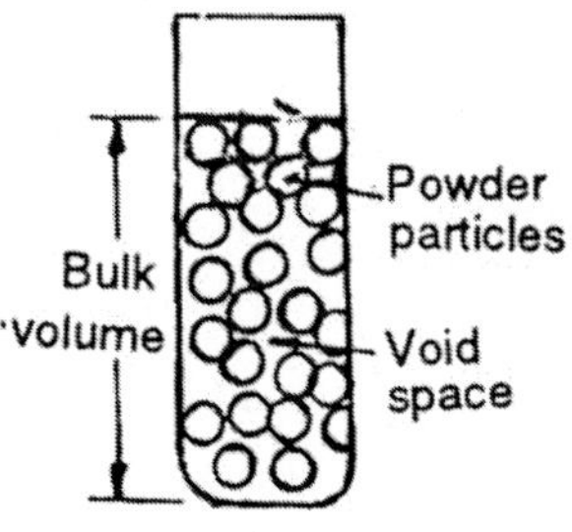

Fig. 163

volume of the powder plus the void volume.

b) **True density**: The ratio between a given mass of a powder and its true volume (v) is called true density.

True volume = bulk volume-void volume

The true density of a powder can be determined as follows:

i) Liquid displacement method: A 25cc standard flask may be used for the determination of true volume. Some amount of powder whose true density is to be found out, is added into the flask and the weight is found out. Now a liquid in which the powder is insoluble is added to occupy the void spaces within the powder until the powder and liquid together occupy the volume i.e 25cc. Again it is weighted.Empty the contents of the flask and add only the liquid upto the 25cc mark and weigh it. The calculation may be carried out as given below.

Weight of the empty bottle = a grams

Weight of the bottle + liquid = b grams

Weight of the bottle + powder = c grams

Weight of the bottle + liquid + powder = d grams

The weight of the powder = $c - a$ grams

$$\text{Density of the liquid } (\rho) = \frac{b-a}{25}$$

$$\text{True density} = \frac{\text{weight of the powder}}{\text{true volume}}$$

$$= \frac{c-a}{25 - \left(\frac{d-c}{\rho}\right)}$$

$$\text{or } \frac{c-a}{\left(\frac{(b-a)}{\rho}\right) - \left(\frac{d-c}{\rho}\right)}$$

A pycnometer can be used for better results.

The liquid displacement method by using water or alcohol gives a density slightly less than true density of the powder since these liquids cannot enter into the smallest void space. This results in possible change in the true density values.

ii) Gas displacement method: A weighted amount of the powder is introduced into the sample tube and already adsorbed gases are removed by degassing procedure. Helium gas which is not adsorbed by the powder is introduced. The pressure difference before and after the introduction of helium gas is obtained from a manometer. By applying gas laws, volume of helium surrounding the particles and penetrating into the small cracks and pores is calculated. The difference between the volume of helium filling the empty apparatus and the volume of helium filling in the presence of the powder gives the true volume of the powder. The true density can then be calculated. This method gives the closest value to true density as the helium can enter into all void spaces including pores and cracks.

9.3. Granular density (ρ_g)

It is determined by the method similar to liquid displacement method but mercury is employed as displacement liquid. The liquid mercury will not enter into the internal pores of the particles. Thus the granule volume represents the volume of the particles and intraparticle spaces.

Granular density

$$= \frac{\text{mass of the granular powder}}{\text{granule volume}}$$

9.4 High compression density

In this method, the powder is highly compressed under a pressure of 100,000 lb/sq. inch into tablets. The ratio of the weight and its volume (obtained from tablet dimensions) gives the high compression density. These values are closer to true density.

9.5. Porosity of powders (ε)

Porosity is defined as the ratio of the void volume to the bulk volume of a powder packing

$$\varepsilon = \frac{\text{bulk volume} - \text{true volume}}{\text{bulk volume}}$$

$$= \frac{V_b - V_t}{V_b} = 1 - \frac{V_t}{V_b}$$

Porosity is also given as

$$\varepsilon = 1 - \frac{\text{weight/true density}}{\text{weight/bulk density}}$$

$$= 1 - \frac{\text{bulk density}}{\text{true density}}$$

$$\text{or } \frac{\text{true density} - \text{bulk density}}{\text{true density}}$$

The porosity calculated by using the true density value obtained from the gas adsorption method gives total porosity (ε_{total}) since the void space determined takes into account the intraparticle space and pores and cracks within the particles. (Fig. 164)

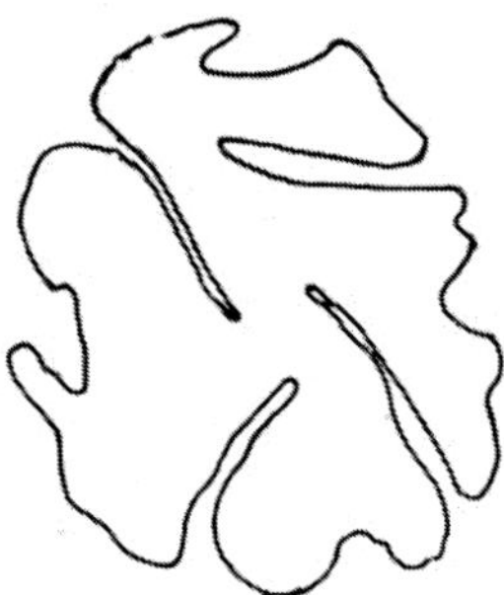

Fig. 164. Pores and Crevices in a Granule particle

$$\varepsilon_{total} = 1 - \frac{\text{bulk density}}{\text{true density}}$$

similarly

$$\varepsilon_{interspace} = 1 - \frac{\text{bulk density}}{\text{granule density}}$$

$$\text{and } \varepsilon_{intraparticle} = 1 - \frac{\text{granule density}}{\text{true density}}$$

Porosity is usually expressed as percent i.e $\varepsilon \times 100$

9.6. Bulkiness

The reciprocal of bulk density is called bulk or bulkiness. It increases with a decrease in particle size. In a mixture of different sized particles, the bulkiness gets reduced since the smaller particles sift between the bigger particles. It is an important factor to be considered in the selection of suitable capsule size for a given dose of drug powder. It also serves as a guideline in choosing the containers for packaging.

9.7. Packing arrangements of powder beds and heaps

A bed or a heap of powder contains a number of particles each in contact with its neighbours. Theoretically two types of packaging is possible. They are close packing or *rhombohedral packing* and open packing or *cubical packing* (Fig. 165).

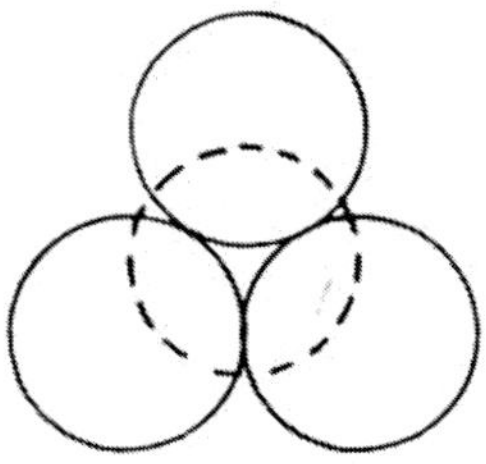

Rhombohedral packing

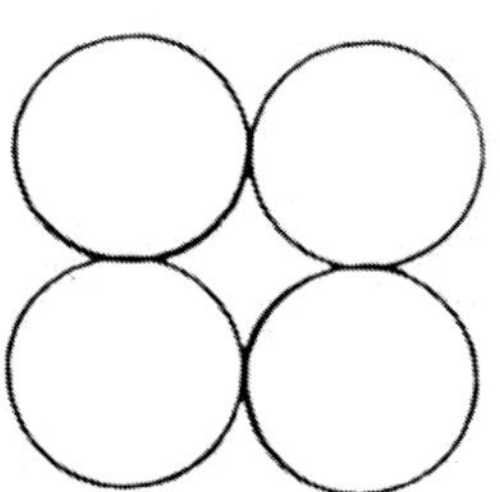

Cubical packing

Fig. 165. Powder Packing

The fraction of powder bed occupied by free space is called porosity. If the powder consists of isodiametric particles (spherical particles) and if the packing is open type the theoretical porosity is 48% and for close packing, it is 26%. But in practical situation, only a mixture of these two types of packing is possible and the porosity is around 30% or above. However if the powder consists of different sized particles, the porosity may go below the theoretical minimum of 26%. This is because the smaller particles fill up the void spaces between the larger particles. On the other hand, if powder contains floccules or aggregates which lead to formation of bridges and arches in the packing, the porosity may go above the theoretical maximum of 48%.

Crystalline materials compressed into a hard core under a force of 100,000 lb/sq. inch can have porosities less than 1%.

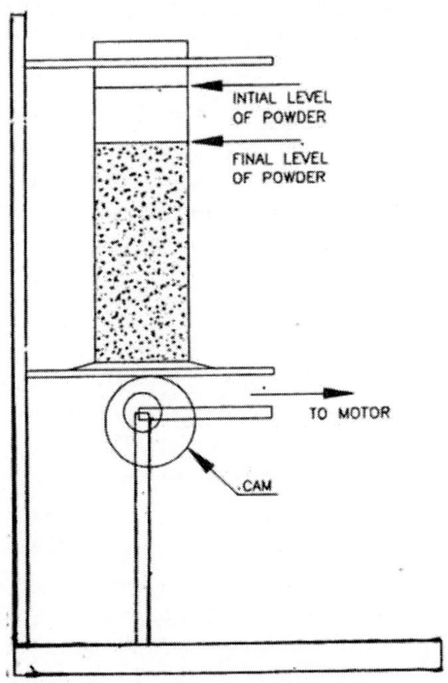

Fig. 166. Mechanical Tapping Device

If a powder is placed in a mechanical tapping device (Fig. 166) and tapped with the help of a rotating cam operated by a motor at a desired constant speed, there occurs a change in volume due to reduction in void space as more and more packing of particles occurs (i.e packing down). If the particles are spherical and monosize, it will take less time for packing down to a constant volume under the given condition. Powders composed of non-isodiametric particles take much longer time to pack down to a constant volume.

It is obvious that tablet granules (i.e granules for tableting) which are mostly both monosize and spherical will pack down rapidly. It helps to ensure uniform filling of the die to get constant weight tablets. That is why granulation is undertaken before compression of the drug powder into tablets.

9.8. Flow properties of powders and granules

A bulk powder is somewhat analogous to a non-Newtonian liquid as it exhibits plastic flow and sometimes dilatancy. In a powder, the flow of particles are influenced by attractive forces to varying degrees. Accordingly, the particles may be free flowing or sticky (cohesive). The various factors which decide the flow properties are particle size, shape, porosity, density and surface texture. The factors affecting flow properties may be called collectively as cohesive which is due to

1. surface force. between particles like *van der Waals* forces, surface tension, and electrostatic forces. These forces may cause the particles to adhere to the container.
2. inter particulate friction if the surface are rough and pitted.
3. interlocking of powder particles causing 'bridging" and 'arching'.

For many powders these factors are difficult to be overcome by gravitational forces. Such powders are called sticky or cohesive.

The cohesion may be quantified as follows by using *Jenike cell* (Fig. 167)

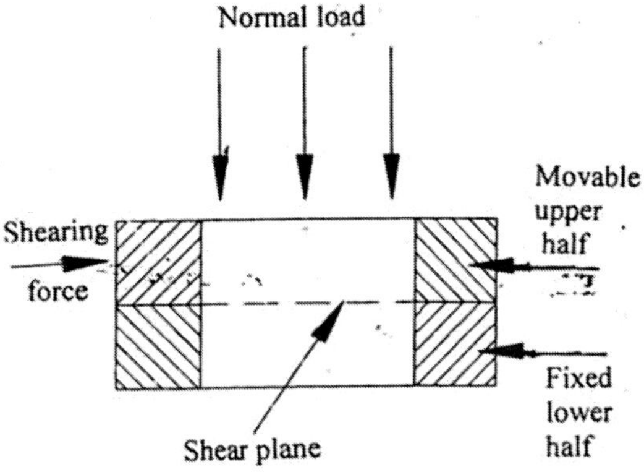

Fig. 167. Jenike Cell

The powder is packed carefully into the two equal segments of a cell and a lid is placed on the top segment. A load is placed on the lid. The force required to just shear (that is the force just required to make the upper half to move) is found out by using a gauge. The experiment is repeated under different weights. The results are summarized as follows.

S.No.	Weight	Force required to shear
1	W_1	-
2	W_2	-
3	W_3	-
n	W_n	-

The values are plotted as follows shown in Fig. 168.

The straight line obtained is extrapolated to meet the y-axis. The intercept point c which is the stress required to shear the bed under zero load is the actual cohesion force that exists between the particles of the powder. A highly cohesive powder tends to pack on

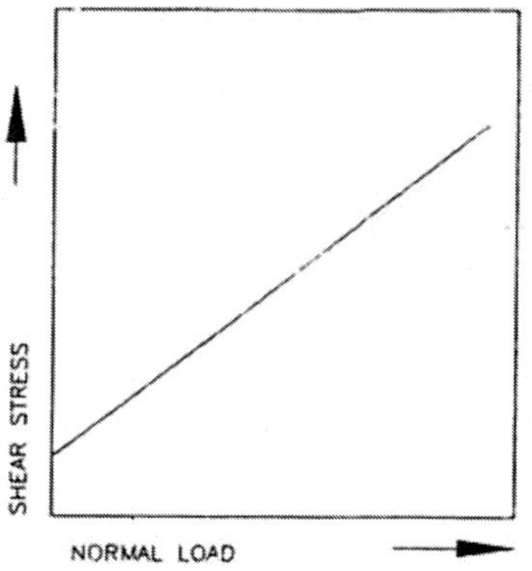

Fig. 168

storage and flow with difficulty and hence causes blocking of pipes and orifices. The cohesion is influenced by the following factors.

a) **Average particle size**: Cohesion is a surface effect. Hence fine powders are more cohesive than coarse ones. Below 10 microns in size, the particles of most powders are extremely cohesive.

b) **Particle density**: Dense substances are less cohesive than lighter ones.

c) **Nature of the surface**: The surface of any particle is associated with surface free energy which is reduced by adsorption of gases and water vapour. In the absence of adsorption, there will be enormous cohesion. However. A continuous film of moisture also increases cohesion to a great extent.

10. Assessment of flow properties of powders

Flow property of a powder is usually assessed by determining angle of repose of the powders. For this, the powder is allowed to fall through an orifice from certain height, to form a conical heap of powder on a horizontal surface. The particle will slip and roll over each other when the heap is formed until the gravitational forces just balance the interparticular forces. The slanting side of the heap forms an angle with the horizontal surface which is known as

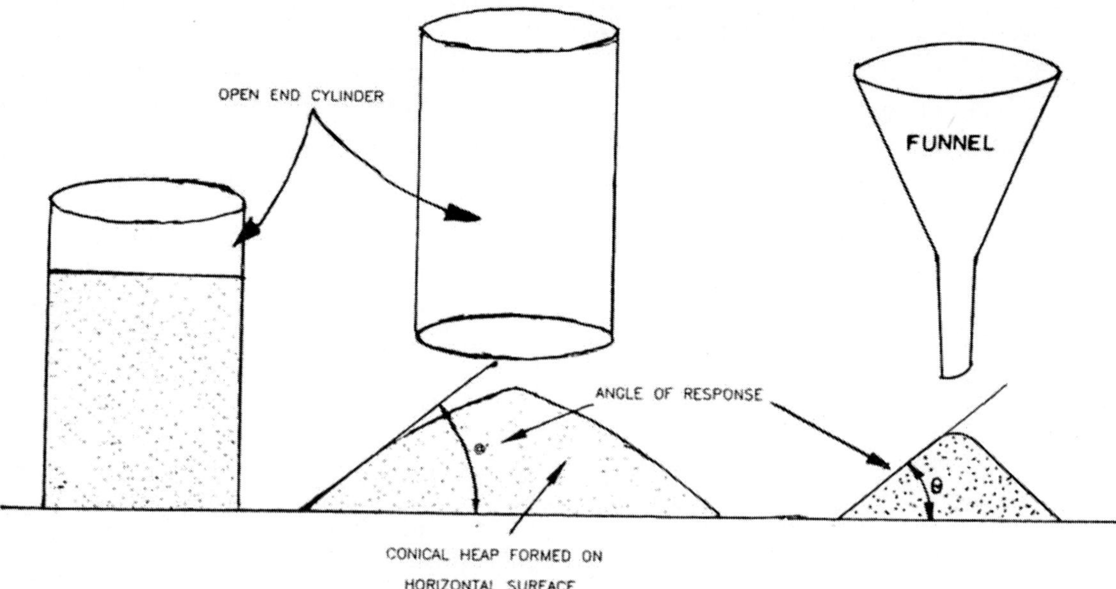

Fig. 169. Measurement of Anale of Repose

Fig. 170

angle of repose. The angle of repose is high if the cohesive and other forces are high. The angle of repose between 35° and 45° indicates the powder does not have satisfactory flow property. When the angle of repose is around 25°, it indicates very good flow property. Flow property of powders play an important role during tablet manufacture and during capsule filling.

The angle of repose is measured as follows:

i) The powder is allowed to fall over a paper placed on a horizontal surface through a funnel or an orifice kept at a certain convenient height (Fig. 169) or

ii) a cylindrical tube open at both the ends is placed on a paper on a horizontal surface so that one of the two open ends is closed. The powder is then, poured into the cylinder and the tube is gradually withdrawn without any shaking movements allowing the powder to form a heap on the horizontal surface. (Fig. 170)

The height of the heap formed is measured by a suitable method and then the circumference of the base of the heap is drawn on the paper with the help of a pencil. The radius of the circle obtained is measured. The angle of repose is then given as

$$\tan \theta = \frac{h}{r}$$

where θ = angle of repose

h = height of the heap

r = radius of the base of the heap (cone shaped heap)

The disadvantage of the funnel method is that it is suitable for free flowing powder only and it does not give reproducible results. The height through which the funnel should be raised to form heap is also critical and the force of fall of the powder through the funnel tube may compress the powder reducing the height of the powder. These difficulties may be overcome in the open ended cylindrical tube method.

In a dynamic method, a cylinder containing half filled powder is rotated slowly on a plane about its horizontal axis till the powder begins to cascade. The angle between horizontal plane and slanting plane of the powder heap is the angle of repose. In yet an another dynamic method, the powder is taken fully in a rectangular box and the box is slowly lifted till the powder slides down. The angle between the horizontal surface and slanting plane of the powder heap is the angle of repose.

Flow rates Granular powders (have little cohesiveness because of symmetry of particles) show better flow rate than fine powders. As the proportion of fines increases, the flow rate of granules are decreased (above 40% fine, flow rate is suddenly decreased to low values)

Flow rate can be assessed by finding out compressibility index *(I)*.

$$I = \left(1 - \frac{V}{V_o}\right) \times 100$$

where V = volume occupied by a sample of the powder after being tapped by a standardized tapping procedure.

V_o = volume before tapping.

For a powder with good flow property and flow rate, the value is below 15% and the values above 25% indicate poor flow property and the values between 15% and 25% indicate moderate flow property.

10.1. Improving the flow properties of powders

a) If the powders contain a large proportion of fines, they may be removed by sieving or adsorbed over larger particles.

b) If the cohesion is due to moisture present, the powder may be dried.

c) By increasing the average size of the particle, the flow may be improved. Finer powders show cohesion. Granulation may be undertaken to increase the size and thus the flow property. In tablet technology, fine powder of the drugs and additives are converted to granules by dry granulation or by wet granulation techniques. Such a technique of conversion into granules is used even for nutritional foods and detergents.

d) Presence of a small proportion of fine powder may improve the flow property due to the filling up of small crevices and pits present in coarse powders. In the absence of fine powder, a little amount of fine powder may be added.

e) By producing isodiametric and symmetric particles like monosized spheres, the flow property can be increased. Such a requirement is met with spray dried products.

f) Required particle size powders may be produced by suitable crystallisation or precipitation.

g) By using additives like lubricants and glidants, the flow property may be increased. This is adopted to improve the flow property of granules in tablet technology.

Powders with improved flow properties are very essential in tablet technology wherein granules have to flow uniformly from the hopper to the die to produce tablets having uniform weights. In capsule technology also, uniform filling of capsules is assured only with free flowing powders. In cos-

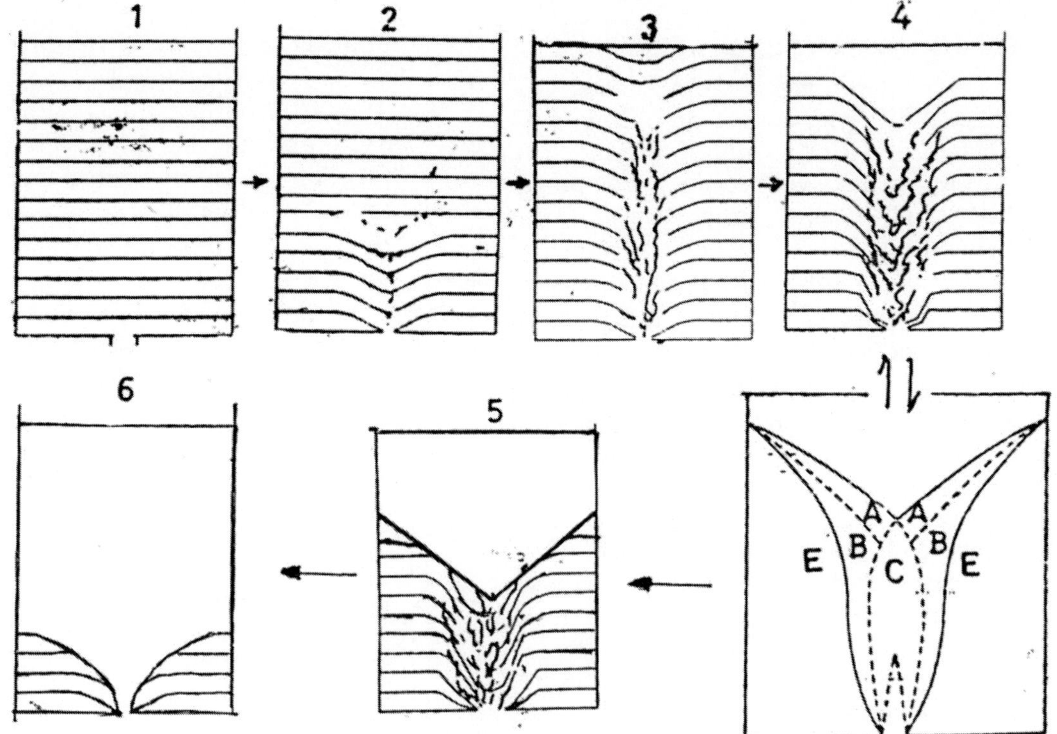

Fig. 171. Gradual Development of flow through an orifice

metic technology flow of powders such as face powders, tooth powders, dusting powders out of sifter top containers should be smooth enough.

The free flowing powders are characterized by dustability. The dustibility of Lycopodium (Pollen grains) is arbitrarily taken as 100% . Talcum powder has a value of 57% and potato starch 27%.

11. Nature of flow of powders through orifice

The powder or granules have to flow uniformly through hopper into the die or into the capsules. The nature of the flow can be scientifically explained as follows. (Fig. 171)

1. On opening the orifice, there is no instantaneous movement at the surface but the particles just above the orifice fall freely through (fig 1 and 2).
2. A depression forms at the surface and spreads outwards to the sides of the container.
3. If the container is tall and not too narrow, the flow pattern follows as described and shown in Fig.171.
4. The particles in zone A falls rapidly over the slower moving particles in zone B while the particles in E are at rest. Particles from zone A is fed into zone C from which the particles flow down quickly. The particles from the slower zone B do not enter this zone. Both streams B and C converge to a *'tongue'* just above the orifice. If the container is repeatedly refilled and partially emptied, the particles in zone E remains static.
5. The flow pattern comes down towards the orifice and the particles are emptied as in fig 5 and 6.

12. Compaction of powders.

Powders are heterogeneous because of differing shapes and sizes of individual particles randomly interspersed with air spaces (void spaces). For an industrial pharmacist, properties of an individual particle and of bulk powder are of very important in handling powders.

Compaction includes compression and consolidation.

Compression means applying mechanical force on powders with subsequent reduction in bulk volume of the powder as a result of displacement of gaseous phase (i.e reduction in void space) Thus compacts are formed. Consolidation means increase in mechanical strength of the compact resulting from particle - particle interactions due to compression. For better understanding of these processes, the following inherent properties of the powder are to be understood.

Solid - air interface

Atoms or ions at the surface of the powder are having unsatisfied attractive molecular forces extending beyond solid surface to small distances whereas atoms or ions at the bulk of the powders experience intermolecular and intramolecular bonding. Fig. 172 The unsatisfied attractive molecular force is called free surface energy of the solid,

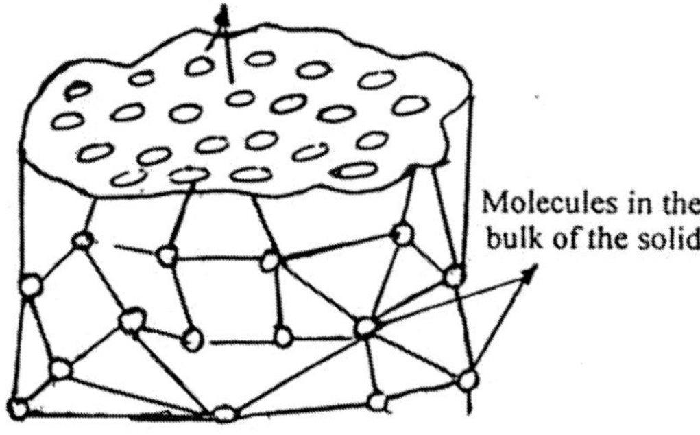

Fig. 172

which plays sizeable role in the interaction between particles and a particle with its environment. Various phenomena due to this manifestations are adsorption, cohesion, adhesion, rate of solution, crystallisation etc.

Because of unsatisfied bonding forces at the surface of particles, particles of the same powder are inherently attracted and tend to stick to one another. This attraction between like particles are cohesion. If the attraction occurs with particles of other type or solid surfaces, it is called adhesion. These attractive properties result in an intrinsic property of all bulk powdered solids that they resist any external force when they are agitated. Because of this, they influence several operations such as flow of powder from hopper to die or from feed frame to die in a tablet machine, relative motion of powders in a mixer and compression to produce tablets.

Two other factors also play a major role in affecting overall resistance.

1. Due to friction between particles, particles develop electrostatic force. The force depends on nature of material and type of motion. The forces although small, they act over greater distance than molecular forces.
2. The development of adsorbed layer of water on the particles reduces the effect of electrostatic forces by forming conductive path for charge dissipation. Nonetheless, particles are held together by moisture film by surface tension effect.

Neumann found that when the powders were compressed under a pressure of 5 kg/cm^2, the porosities of the powder composed of rigid particles (sodium carbonate for example) were

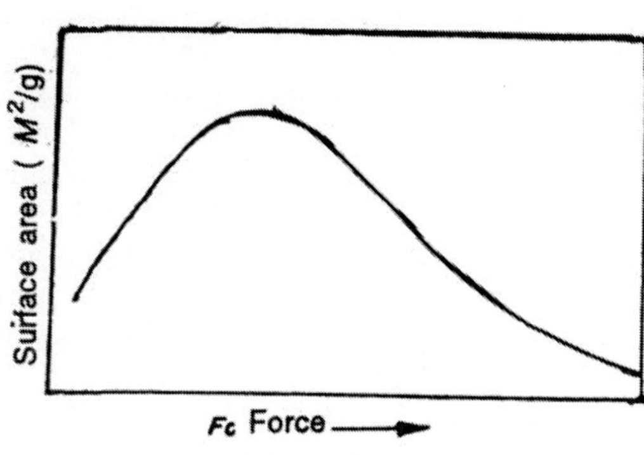

Fig. 173. Influence of compressional force on specific surface of granules

higher than the powders in close packing. Thus, the powders show dilatancy due to expansion by stress. However, the powders having soft and spongy particles (example kaolin) are deformed on compression and their porosities are decreased on compression.

Influence of compression force on specific surface area, granule density, tablet hardness and disintegration time in pharmaceutical tablets has been studied.

On compressing *sulphathiazcle* granules, the surface area increases to a maximum initially (due to the formation of new surface area as a result of fragmentation) followed by decrease in surface area beyond a compressional force of 2500 pounds (resulting from cold bonding between particles). It was also observed that porosity decreased and density increased as a linear function of logarithm of compression force. Hardness, fracture resistance, and disintegration have been found to increase as the compression is increased. The strength of the compressed tablet depends upon compression force and particle size. An ideal lubricant distributes the compression force uniformly throughout the tablet.

Suggestions for Practicals

1. Study of particle size distribution of a given powder by sieving method:

For methodology refer the text. The experiment may be done with 100 grams of the powder. The powders on all the sieves are collected separately and weighed individually. From the data, prepare a chart consisting the particle size range, mean size and cumulative frequency weight distribution (under size and under size in percentage or over size and over size in percentage):

Then, prepare various plots. a) particle size (arithmetic mean size of openings of two successive sieves on x axis versus weight of particles on y axis b) particle size versus % frequency c) log of particle size versus % frequency d) particle size versus cumulative % frequency undersize (or oversize) on probability scale to find out σ_g (geometric mean deviation and d'_g geometric mean weight diameter)

Alternatively the particle sizes are converted to log of particle sizes and the cumulative % frequency undersize (or oversize) to empirical probits using the table shown below:

The d_{st} of the particles and weight of the fractions collected (to be corrected for defloccnlating agent added) at different time levels intervals are tabulated. The weight of each sample residue is called the weight undersize and the sum of the successive weight is known as cumulative weight undersize. Proceed on similar line as given under the sieving method to represent the particle size distribution graphically to find out d_g and σ_g and to find out various statistical diameters.

(The density of calamine $\rho_s = 1.855\, g/cc$. The density of water $\rho_o = 1\, g/cc$, the viscosity of water is taken as (η_o) 1 centipoise, $g = 980\, cm/sec^2$ and height of the sample from pipette, i.e., $h = 20cm$. if Andreason apparatus is used).

Normal dimensions of standard sieves:

Sieve No.	Sieve openings (apertures)	
	in mm	in μm
2	9.52	9520
4	4.76	4760
8	2.38	2380
10	2.00	2000
20	0.84	840
30	0.59	590
40	0.42	420
50	0.297	297
60	0.250	250
70	0.210	210
80	0.177	177
100	0.149	149
120	0.125	125
200	0.074	74

2. Study of particle size distribution of a given powder by sedimentation method

Empirical Probits

%	0	1	2	3	4	5	6	7	8	9
0	...	2.674	2.946	3.119	3.249	3.355	3.445	3.524	3.595	3.659
10	3.718	3.773	3.825	3.874	3.920	3.964	4.006	4,046	4.085	4.122
20	4.158	4.194	4.228	4.261	4.294	4.326	4.357	4.387	4.417	4.447
30	4.476	4.504	4.532	4.560	4.587	4.615	4.642	4.668	4.695	4.721
40	4.747	4.773	4.798	4.824	4.849	4.874	4.900	4.925	4.950	4.975
50	5.000	5.025	5.050	5.075	5.100	5.126	5.151	5.176	5.202	5.227
60	5.253	5.279	5.305	5.332	5.358	5.385	5.413	5.440	5.468	5.496
70	5.524	5.553	5.583	5.613	5.643	5.674	5.706	5.739	5.772	5.806
80	5.842	5.878	5.915	5.954	5.994	6.036	6.80	6.126	6.175	6.227
90	6.282	6.341	6.405	6.476	6.555	6.645	6.751	6.881	7.054	7.326

5.5 gram of calamine (or zinc oxide) is dispersed in 50 ml of a solution in water containing 2.75 g of sodium citrate (deflocculating agent). Add more water with trituration to obtain 550 ml of the dispersion. for methodology refer the text. The results are tabulated as follows:

S.No.	Time	Height of the suspension	h (incm)/t(insec)
1	5	20	-
2	10	20	-
.	.	.	.
.	.	.	.
.	.	.	.
n	t	20	-

The d_{st} of particles collected at different time intervals will be

$$d_{st} = \sqrt{\frac{18\,\eta_o}{(\rho_s\,\rho_o\,g} \times \frac{h}{t}}$$

where η_o = viscosity of the medium

ρ_o = density of the medium

ρ_s = density of the particles

g = acceleration due to gravity

$\frac{h}{t}$ = rate of settling of particles

Both the parameters are plotted. The logarithm of the particles size equivalent to 50% on the probit scale is called geometric mean weight distribution (d_g). The slope of the line is called geometric mean deviation (σ_g) and is given by

$$\sigma_g = \frac{50\%\text{ size}}{16\%\text{ undersize}} \text{ or } \frac{84\%\text{ undersize}}{50\%\text{ size}}$$

Hatch-Choate equations for computing statistical diameters from number and weight distribution. Using the equations number distribution can be converted into weight distribution and vice-versa.

(*Note:* The value of geometric deviation derived from weight distribution and number distribution is same. Hence it is designated by σ_g).

3. Study of particle size distribution of a given powder by microscopy

For methodology, refer the text. Represent the particle size range and the number of particles in each size range graphically as given in the text. Also find out the geometric mean diameter (d_g), geometric mean deviation (σ_g) and various statistical diameters using d_g and σ_g.

For measuring particle size diameter, use eye piece micrometer (either square type or linear type) which has been calibrated by using a standard (stage) micrometer in which 1mm is divided into 100 divisions and therefore 1 division equals 10 µ. For calibration of eye piece micrometer, find out the number of divisions of eye piece micrometer that is equal to the number of divisions of standard micrometer. (For this adjust the zero division of eye piece micrometer that exactly coincides with the standard stage micrometer). From the values obtained, the measure of each division of eye piece micrometer is obtained as given below:

Each division of eyepiece micrometer

Hatch-Choate Equations for Computing Statistical Diameters from Number and Weight Distributions

Diameter	Number Distribution	Weight Distribution
Length-number mean	$\log d_{ln} = \log d_g + 1.151 \log^2 \sigma_g$	$\log d_{ln} = \log d'_g - 5.757 \log^2 \sigma_g$
Surface-number mean	$\log d_{sn} = \log d_g + 2.303 \log^2 \sigma_g$	$\log d_{sn} = \log d'_g - 4.606 \log^2 \sigma_g$
volume-number mean	$\log d_{vn} + 3.454 \log^2 \sigma_g$	$\log d_{vn} = \log d'_g - 3.454 \log^2 \sigma_g$
Volume-surface mean	$\log d_{vs} = \log d_g + 5.757 \log^2 \sigma_g$	$\log d_{vs} = \log d'_g - 1.151 \log^2 \sigma_g$
Weight-moment mean	$\log d_{wm} = \log d_g + 8.059 \log^2 \sigma_g$	$\log d_{wm} = \log d'_g + 1.151 \log^2 \sigma_g$

$$= \frac{\text{number of divisions of standard micrometer} \times 10\ \mu}{\text{number of divisions of eyepiece micrometer that coincides}}$$

4. Determination of angle of repose of a given powder

Find out the angle of repose as described in the text using calcium carbonate, potassium dichromate, tannic acid (dry), sodium bicarbonate, powdered potassium bicarbonate or oxalic acid. Report whether the powder is free flowing.

Choose a powder having poor flow property, mix with a suitable lubricant with such as talk or boric acid in the ratios of 1%, 2%, 3%, etc. with the powder and find out whether the flow property is improved or not. Report the result.

Again choose a powder such as sodium bicarbonate with poor flow property, granulate with suitable granulating agent and find out whether the flow property is improved because of granulation.

5. Determination of Bulk density, True density and porosity of a given powder

Refer the text for methodology. Find out the bulk density, true density (by liquid displacement method) and porosity of the powder. Report the results.

6. Determination of specific surface area of a given powder by adsorption method

For methodology, refer the text. For the experiment, prepare 0.5% stearic acid in neutralised methanol. For 5 gram of the powder, use 50 ml of the stearic acid solution. Titrate against $N/50$ sodium hydroxide using pheolphtalein as indicator.

The amount of stearic acid adsorbed is given by

$$= \frac{\text{(blank titre value} - \text{titre value)} \times \text{real normality}}{\text{actual normality}(0.02) \times 0.0056\ \text{g}}$$

Calculate the specific surface area of the powder as described in the text.

XIII PHOTOCHEMISTRY

For a chemical reaction to occur, it is necessary that reacting molecules should possess the required energy of activation. This energy may be obtained by the molecules through heat or light. The chemical reactions produced directly or indirectly by means of light are called photochemical reactions and the study of those reactions is called photochemistry. In this, the molecules are activated by photons of high energy radiations like visible rays, ultraviolet rays, X-rays, *γ–rays* or any other part of the electromagnetic spectrum. Reaction between hydrogen and chlorine in the presence of light to form hydrogen chloride is a classical example of photochemical reaction. The energy of a photon is given by

$$E = hu = hc/\lambda$$

where $h =$ the Plank's constant (6.62×10^{-27})

$c =$ the velocity of radiation in vacuum $3 \times 10^{10}\ cmsec^{-1}$

$\lambda =$ wavelength of the radiant energy

$v =$ frequency of radiant energy

If v is expressed in cycles sec^{-1} and λ in cm, the energy is given in ergs. The energy of an *Avogadro's number* ($6.026 \times 10\ 23$) of photons is called an Einstein (Ei) which is equal to $\frac{2.859}{\lambda} \times 10\ ^5$k.cal $mole^{-1}$. From this, it is found that one Einstein of a visible light of wavelength 6000$\mathring{A}$ has energy equal to 45 k.calories $mole^{-1}$. Hence absorption of radiations in the visible or ultraviolet region can induce a chemical reaction by breaking a chemical bond or producing a high energy reactive complex. The infra red radiation has practically no effect on chemical reaction. The X-rays and γ rays are associated with so much energy that they can induce ionisation reactions. The energy of an electromagnetic spectrum is shown below.

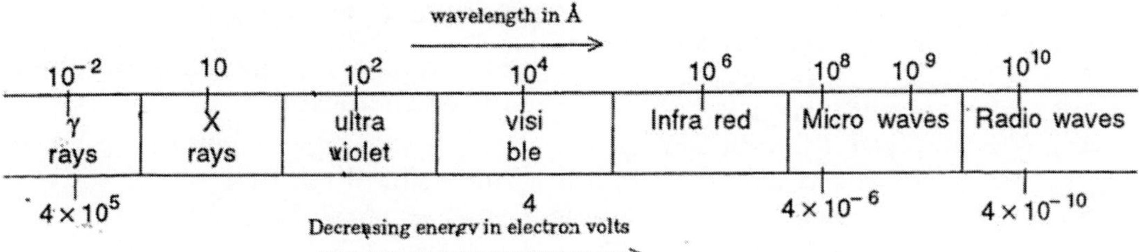

The energy of various radiations are

Radiation region	Wave length in Å	Energy per mole in	
		kcal	ev
Infra red	1×10^5	2.86	0.12
Red	8000	35.7	1.55
Blue	5000	56.9	2.48
Violet	4000	71.6	3.10
Ultraviolet	1000	286.0	12.4
X-ray	1.0	2.86×10^5	12.4×10^3
γ-ray	0.01	2.86×10^7	12.4×10^5

1. Sources of photochemical radiations

1.1. Sunlight

It is rich in ultraviolet radiation. The intensity of the radiation varies with place, season and time. Hence it is not useful for quantitative study of photochemical reactions.

1.2. Arc Light

An arc can be produced between electrodes of iron and carbon. This is a good source of ultraviolet radiation.

1.3. Mercury Vapour Lamp

When mercury is evaporated in an electric arc, a brilliant light is emitted and it is also a good source of ultraviolet radiation.

2. Measurement of intensity of radiation (Radiometry)

2.1. By Radiomicrometer

It consists of a couple of unlike metals say bismuth and silver connected in a circuit that is suspended between poles of an electro magnet. When the couple is exposed to radiation at the junction, a current is produced in the circuit. In the presence of the magnetic field, the coil of the circuit is deflected which is measured by a lamp and scale arrangement. The deflection is directly proportional to the intensity of light.

The other techniques are by using photoelectric cell, chemical Actionmeters or a Thermopile. A Thermopile consists of a series of junctions of unlike metals (bismuth and silver) connected to a galvanometer. Alternate junctions of the thermopile are heated by exposure to light when the galvanometer deflection corresponds to the intensity of light.

3. Laws of photochemistry

There are two basic laws:

First Law (Grotthus Draper Law)

It states that only those radiations which are absorbed by the reactants can produce a chemical reaction. The consequences of light absorption are summarized as follows:

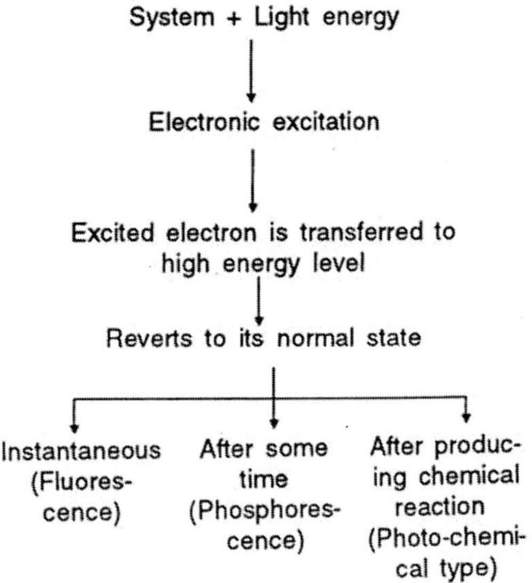

Second Law

Einstein Stark law of photochemical equivalence.

It is the quantum mechanical statement of the first law. It states that when a substance undergoes a photochemical reaction, each photon or quantum of radiation absorbed results in the decomposition of only one molecule That is,

$$AB + hv = A + B$$

In a primary process, each reacting molecule absorbs one photon and **gives one product** molecule. It is called **Quantum yield** (ϕ) or Quantum efficiency.

$$\phi = \frac{\text{Number of molecules decomposed}}{\text{Number of photons absorbed}}$$

Deviations

1. Theoretically the quantum yield should be only one. But in many reactions, the value of ϕ is more than one indicating that one photon can induce decomposition in more molecules which is due to secondary process or secondary reaction.

eg: Photochemical decomposition of hydrogen iodide

$HI + hv = H^\circ + 1^\circ$ (primary process)

$H^\circ + HI = H_2 + I^\circ$

$I^\circ + I^\circ = I_2$ Secondary process

$2HI + hv = H_2 + I_2$

where H° and I° are free radicals.

In this reaction, one photon has decomposed two molecules. It is due to the secondary reaction. The reaction showed high quantum yield of two.

2. There are photochemical reactions in which low quantum yield occur - i.e number of molecules decomposed are less than number of photons participated in the reaction. The reasons are

a) deactivation of excited molecules before they react by some process.

b) some of the excited molecules may not receive energy sufficient enough to react.

c) some of the dissociated fragments from the excitation recombine and so the yield is less.

4. Photochemical reaction

a typical photochemical reaction involves a primary process followed by a secondary process. eg: combination of hydrogen and chlorine.

1. $Cl_2 + hv = Cl^\circ + Cl^\circ$ (primary process)

2. $Cl^\circ + H_2 = HCl + H^\circ$ (Secondary process)

3. $H^\circ + Cl_2 = HCl + Cl^\circ$

The reactions 2 and 3 repeat many times till combination of millions of molecules takes place (chain reaction). The cycle continues till one of the reactants is fully consumed.

Such a photochemical reaction in which series of reactions are set up and millions of molecules react for each quantum of light absorbed is called chain reaction in which a high quantum yield is obtained.

However presence of traces of foreign materials (inhibitors) can retard the chain reaction. For example, explosion of petrol in a combustion engine is a chain reaction and presence of traces of lead tetra ethyl $Pb(C_2H_5)_4$ can inhibit the chain reaction.

5. Photosensitisation

Certain reactants which are not sensitive to light are made sensitive in the presence of a small quantity of a foreign substance. This foreign substance absorb light and stimulate the reaction without taking part in the chemical reaction.

eg:1. Hydrogen molecule cannot be decomposed by light. But in the presence of mercury, hydrogen molecule can be decomposed as follows:

$$Hg + hv \rightarrow Hg^* \text{ (Activated mercury)}$$

$$Hg^* + H_2 \rightarrow 2H + Hg$$

In this reaction, mercury acts as a photosensitizer.

2. Similarly, decomposition of ozone into oxygen is photo sensitized by chlorine.

The substance which induces such a chemical reaction is called photosensitizer and the phenomenon is called photosensitisation.

6. Photochemical equilibrium

If a reversible reaction is sensitive to light, then under constant illumination, a chemical equilibrium is set up. For example, decomposition of sulphur dioxide occurs very slowly in the dark. In the presence of light, both forward and backward reactions are induced by the light and a chemical equilibrium is set up under constant illumination.

$$2SO_3 \rightleftharpoons 2SO_2 + O_2$$

7. Significance of photochemistry in pharmacy.

The study of photochemistry indicates that organic molecules absorb light and undergo decomposition. Even on exposure to light, some chemical molecules will undergo chain reaction with one photon of light. Some of the chemical reactions can be made photo sensitive in the presence of a photosensitizer.

The Pharmacopoeia lists out a number of drugs which are photosensitive and affected by light. eg: Number of organic molecules, enzymes, vaccines, fixed oil, etc. Hence necessary care should be taken to protect the drugs from photodegradation. Some measures may be preserving the drugs in dark places, shady places, hermetically sealed metal containers, in amber coloured glass containers or vials or ampoules, by using ultra violet stabilisers (as the part of the glass container composition) which absorb ultraviolet radiation and dispose of energy without forming free radical. eg:Phenyl salicylate and 2-hydroxy benzophenone and strip packing of tablets.

8. Applications of photochemistry.

a) **Photography**: A photographic plate coated with gelatin-silver bromide is sensitive only to blue violet part of the spectrum. If the same plate is dyed with eosin, it is made photosensitive to green, yellow and orange part of the spectrum as well (orthochromic plates) cyanin, erysthrosin, pinaschrome and orthochrome T are also used for this purpose. Pinacyanol sensitises the plate even to red part of the spectrum (Panchromatic plates)

b) **Photosynthesis in plants**: The photochemical reaction between carbondioxide and water occurring in plants is photosensitised by chlorophyll

$$CO_2 + H_2O + h\nu\text{(light)} \xrightarrow{\text{Chlorophyll}} \underset{\text{Formaldehyde}}{CH_2O} + O_2$$

The formaldehyde is converted to cellulose and other carbohydrates. c) Irradiation of ergocalciferol by ultraviolet light in our body produces calciferol (vitamin D) which is essential for bone development. Hence children should be encouraged to play in the evening sunlight.

d) **Luminescence**: (Cold light) Electrons of atoms or molecules can be excited by heat, electricity, light, or any other forms of energy. The excited electrons while returning to ground state will emit light (luminescence) in the following ways:

i) **Resonance radiation**: The absorbed radiation is emitted instanteously (10^{-8}) with the same frequency.

ii) **Fluorescence**: The excited atom or molecules by the incident light emit radiations of different frequency which are less energetic than incident light. A soon as incident radiation is cut off, fluorescence ceases. eg: organic dyestuffs, quinine sulfate, fluorescein, eosin, chlorophyll etc. Fluorescence of substances on exposure to ultra violet light is used as tools for analysis of chemical molecules. Fluorescence produced by X-rays falling on a film of barium platinocyanide is employed for diagnosis by X-rays.

iii) **Phosphorescence**: Many substances continue to emit after the incident light is cut off. This is known as phosphorescence. eg: Zinc sulphide, Strontium sulphide, etc.

iv) **Chemiluminescence**: It refers to emission of light as a result of chemical reactions at ordinary temperatures. eg: Yellow phosphorous on exposure to air gets oxidised and produces light. Fireflies glow in darkness which is due to oxidation of luciferin (a protein) in the presence of an enzyme.

v) **Laser technique**: In this, the excited molecules are made to interact with impinging photons. Thus, the intensity of light radiations are amplified. Lasers are very much useful in communications, printing, surgery etc.

XIV. COMPLEXATION AND PROTEIN BINDING

Complexation

A complex may simply be defined as a species formed by the association of two or more interactant molecules or ions. Such an association takes place because one of the interactants called the ***substrate*** accepts a pair of electrons donated by the other interactant called the ***ligand***. As a result a bond is formed between the two interactants (substrate and ligand) and the compound thus formed is called the complex. Thus, the complex may be considered as a species of definite substrate to ligand stoichiometry which can be formed in an equilibrium process in solution, and also may exist in solid state. The complex formation may be represented by the following chemical equation.

$$mS + nL \rightleftharpoons S_mL_n$$

where m = number of substrate molecules

n = number of ligands

S = substrate

L = ligand

$S_m L_n$ = complex

Some of the properties of the complex thus formed are different from those of its constituents. The properties that may be altered are solubility, light absorption, conductance, partitioning behaviour and chemical reactivity.

1. Types of complexes

Two main types or groups of complexes are recognised based on chemical bonding involved. They are the metal-ion co-ordination complexes and molecular complexes.

1.1 Metal-ion coordination complexes

In metal-ion coordination complexes, one interactant is the metal ion (substrate) and the other interactant is the inorganic or organic molecule or ion (ligand). They are formed by transfer of a pair of electrons, in some degree from one interactant (ligand) to the other interactant (metal-ion). The bond formed as a result of such transfer of a pair of electrons is called coordinate bond. Therefore, the complexes may be considered as products of Lewis acid-base reactions.

The metal-ion coordination complexes consist of a central metal ion (the substrate) bonded to an electron pair donor (the ligand). The ligand may be a base such as NH_3, an ion such as Cl^- or an aromatic compound such as benzene, toluene etc. The metal ion coordination complexes may be neutral or charged.

The number of bonds between the metal ion and the ligand is called coordination number of the complex. Thus the coordination number of $Cu(NH_3)_2^{2+}$ and $Cu(NH_3)_4^{2+}$ are 2 and 4 respectively. Most complexes with coordination number 4 have the square planar structure but some are tetrahedral. Nearly all complexes of coordination number 6 are octahedral.

Ammonia has a single basic group capable of bonding to a metal ion and hence it is a unidentate ligand whereas ethylene diamine has two accessible basic binding sites and it is a bidentate ligand. Thus ligands having more than one binding site are called multidentate ligand. Ethylene diamine tetraacetate (EDTA) is a multidentate (i.e. hexadentate) ligand and it can also have a coordination number of 4 or 5. If a metal ion binds with a multidentate ligand (i.e. with two or more binding sites) it usually forms with the ligand a cyclic complex called chelate.

If the ligand forms a stable, water soluble metal chelate, it is called a sequestering agent.

1.2 Organic Molecular complexes

In molecular complexes, both the interactants are organic molecules. They may result from noncovalent interactions between the substrate and ligand.

The noncovalent forces are due to

(a) electrostatic forces among ions and molecules with permanent dipole moments, (i.e. ion-ion, ion-dipole and dipole-dipole).

(b) induction forces or polarization forces between an ion or polar molecule and a non-polar molecule, (i.e. ion-induced dipole and dipole-induced dipole) and

(c) dispersion (London) forces operating between all molecules (i.e. induced dipole-induced dipole).

Most molecular complexes probably involve a combination of noncovalent interactions.

A molecular complex may be a charge transfer complex of donor-acceptor complex. In charge transfer complex, there is transfer of electron from a donor to an acceptor molecule. The bond resulting from charge transfer may have some covalent character in addition to non covalent forces. In these complexes resonance between the charged species and uncharged species contributes greatly to the stability of the complex.

In donor acceptor complex the resonance between the charged and the uncharged moieties of the complex is fairly weak and the stability is mainly due to *van-der-waals* forces, dipole-dipole interactions and hydrogen bonding and it lacks charge transfer.

In both charge transfer and donor acceptor complexes new absorption band occurs in u.v. spectra.

2. Classification of complexes

In general, complexes can further be classified as follows.

I. Metal ion coordination complexes

(a) Inorganic type

(b) Chelate

(c) Olefin type

(d) Aromatic type

II. Organic molecular complexes

1. *Based on bonding or interaction*

(a) Charge transfer

(b) Hydrogen bonding

(c) Hydrophobic interaction

(d) Stacking interaction

2. *Based on structure of interactants*
   (a) Small molecule - small molecule complex
   (b) Small molecule - macromolecule complex
   (c) Drug - protein complex
   (d) Drug - receptor complex
   (e) Antigen - antibody complex
3. *Based on structure of complex*
   (a) Self associated aggregates
   (b) Micelle
   (c) Inclusion compounds
   (d) Clathrate

2.1 Metal - ion coordination complexes

Inorganic type: They include the simple inorganic complexes first described by Werner. When ammonia is treated with cobalt chloride, a complex called hexamine cobalt III chloride, $[CO(NH_3)_6]^{3+} Cl_3^-$ is formed. In this each ammonia molecule donates a pair of electrons and forms a coordinate bond with cobalt ion. Some other examples in this group are $[Ag(NH_3)_2]^+ Cl^-$, and $[Cr(H_2O)_6]^{3+}$

Chelates: A substance containing two or more donor groups (chelating agent) may combine with a metal to form a chelate. For example ethylene diamine forms a chelate (a cyclic complex) with Cu (II)

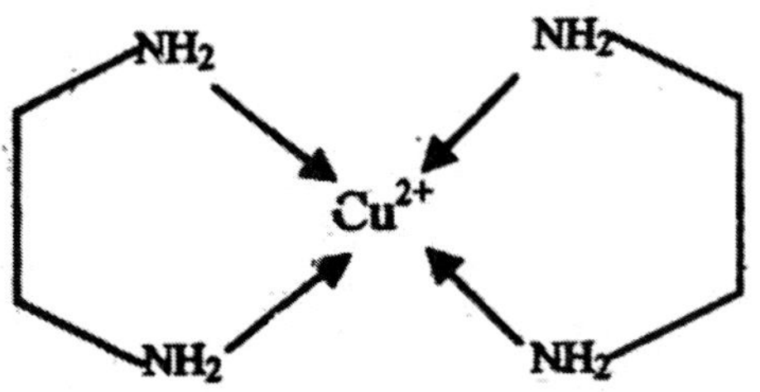

ETHYLENE DIAMINE COMPLEX WITH Cu (II)

Some other chelating agents are 1,10-phenanthroline, 8-hydroxy quinoline, dimethyl glyoxime and ethylene diamine-tetra acetic acid. Chelation places stringent steric requirements on both metal and ligands. Chelates can exhibit geometrical isomerism and hence only the cis-coordinated ligands adjacent on a molecule are readily replaced when reacted with a chelating agent.

For example in Vitamin B_{12}, only the trans coordination positions of the metal ion (cobalt ion) are available and hence they are not able to react with chelating agents.

Chlorophyll and hemoglobin are two naturally occurring chelates in plants and animals respectively.

EDTA can sequester iron and copper ions. It is also used to sequester calcium ions.

Olefin complexes: They are formed by reacting olefin with metal ions. Aqueous solutions of platinum or silver absorb olefins forming a water soluble complex. These complexes are used as catalysts.

Aromatic type complexes: They are formed with aromatic bases and metal ions by Lewis acid-base reactions. They may be pi-bond complex, sigma bond complex or sandwich complexes. Aromatic bases such as benzene and toluene form pi-bond complexes with silver ions. A carbon of aromatic ring forms a sigma (σ) bond complex with a metal ion such as aluminium. Such a σ bond complex occurs in Friedel-Crafts reaction. An example of sandwich complex is ferrocene. It is dicyclopentadienyl iron II. It is referred to as sandwich complex because two molecules of cyclo pentadienyl sandwiches iron II

2.2 Organic molecular complexes

These complexes are formed by the union of two organic molecules. Of these two molecules, one acts as the substrate and the other as the ligand.

Charge transfer complexes They are formed as a consequence of the transfer of an electron from a molecular orbital on an electron-donor molecule to an orbital on an electron-acceptor molecule. Hence charge transfer complexes are also called as electron-donor-acceptor complexes. In the case of charge transfer complexes, a change in electron configuration occurs producing a change in electronic energy levels. This leads to change in UV absorption spectra resulting in the appearance of new absorption bands. As the bond formed may have some covalent character in addition to non covalent forces, the bonding in the complex is somewhat stronger. A good example of charge transfer complex is solution of iodine in organic solvent. In this complex solvent is the electron-donor and the iodine is the electron-acceptor. eg: Solutions of iodine in benzene and in ether. Iodine also forms 1:1 charge transfer complexes with drugs such as disulfiram, chlomethizole, and tolnaftate.

Benzene is an electron-donor. But substitution of benzene by alkyl groups enhances its donor properties. For example hexamethyl benzene is a good electron donor. Lewis acids are electron acceptors. They may be unsaturated and aromatic compounds substituted with electron-withdrawing groups eg: tetracyanoethylene and picric acid. Picric acid forms a charge transfer complex, butesin picrate, with butesin.

The stability of charge transfer complexes seems to be due to the number of electron withdrawing groups (such as nitro group) on the first compound and the presence of electron releasing groups (such as methyl and amino groups) on the second compound and the formation of complex also depends on steric factors.

Hydrogen bonded complexes: In non-covalent interactions, an additional type of bonding called hydrogen bonding is often involved. It occurs between a proton donor and a proton acceptor part of molecules. The hydrogen bonds are relatively weak bonds with about 10% of the strength of an ordinary covalent bond. Its strength is controlled in part by the acid strength of proton donor and the base strength of the proton acceptor. The solvent has also a role to play. The following structures show hydrogen bonding

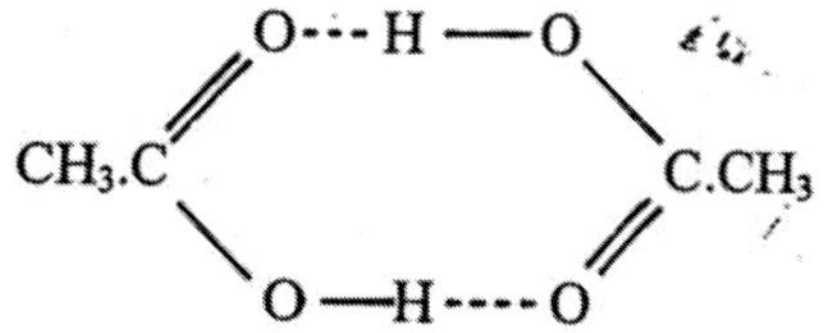

O---H—O
$CH_3.C$ C.CH_3
O—H----O

Dimer of acetic acid
(Intermolecular hydrogen bond)

O —O
C H
O

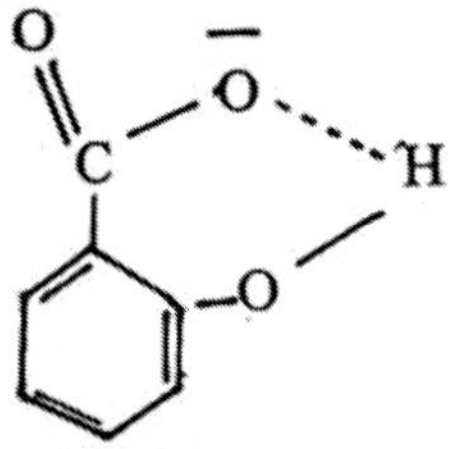

Salicyclic acid
(Intramolecular hydrogen bond)

Some other examples of hydrogen bonded complexes are phenol-pyridine complex in inert solvents, adenine-thymine and guamine-cytosine complexes in the double helix structure of DNA molecule.

Hydrophobic interaction

In this there is no bond formation but there is a tendency for hydrophobic molecules or hydrophobic parts of a molecule to remain together in an aqueous environment. This is because of the tendency of hydrophobic parts of the molecule to avoid water. This tendency resulting out of unwelcome reception in water makes the molecules come closer and remain together usually in a spherical form (micelle) is what is called as hydrophobic interaction. It involves *van der Waals* forces, hydrogen bonding between molecules of water in a three dimensional structure and other reactions.

Proteins are largely hydrophobic and they associate into miscelle - like structure and they acquire spherical shape in water. In this spherical shape, polar ends occupy the surface and make contact with water and the non-polar ends constitute the central portion of micelle in an aqueous environment. This type of hydrophobic attraction as explained earlier is 'called hydrophobic bonding' or 'hydrophobic interaction'. Globular proteins are thought to maintain their ball-like structure in water because of hydrophobic effect.

The interactions of drugs with proteins in the body may involve hydrophobic bond at least in part. Insulin shows concentration dependent self association due to hydrophobic interaction which may affect solubility, diffusion, transport through membrane and therapeutic action. Addition of urea at non-toxic concentrations (1.0 to 3.0 mg /ml) has been shown to inhibit self association of insulin. Urea breaks up "icebergs" in liquid water and associates with structured water by hydrogen

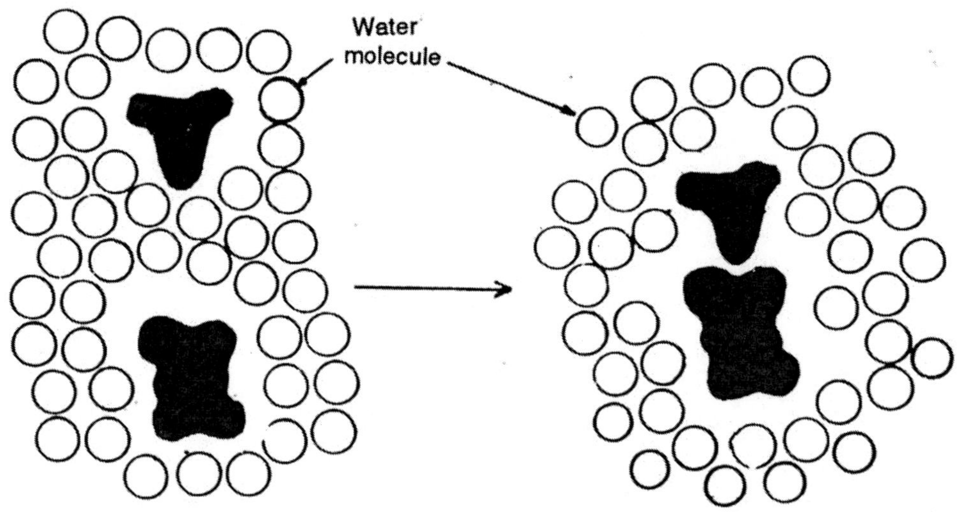

Ordered water molecules surrounding two large non-polar molecules

Hydrophobic interaction with squeezing out of water molecules.

Fig. 174. Hydrophobic Interaction

bonding, taking an active part in the formation of a more open "lattice" structure. Similarly inhibition of aggregation of procaine insulin by sodium salicylate results in about 7800 fold increase in solubility.

Ligand (drug) hydrophobicity (logarithm of ligand partition coefficient between octanol and water is a measure of hydrophobicity) is the main contribution to the formation of water soluble complexes. For example, hydrophobic chlorobiocin analogs show highest percent of drug bound to hydrophobic portion of human serum albumin and hence formation of more soluble water complexes. Significant correlation has been established between stability constant of the complex and hydrophobicity of the ligand.

Solvents other than water also can lead to complex formation. However they are less effective than water because of their low surface tensions. When solvents other than water are involved, the interaction is termed as solvophobic interaction or effect.

As there is increase in entropy (disorder) during the hydrophobic interaction, it is thermodynamically favoured. Fledman and Gibaldi attributed the enhancement in the solubility of benzoic and salicylic acids by urea and its derivatives such as 1, 3 dimethyl urea to hydrophobic interaction rather than complexation. The driving force for the solubilisation was the increase in entropy due to the breaking up of hydrogen-bonded water clusters. There is a possibility of ureas forming channel complexes with these aromatic acids.

Hydrophobic interaction may be illustrated as in Fig 174.

Stacking interactions: Two planar molecules may undergo plane-to-plane contact as a result of hydrophobic association in an attempt to reduce total surface area exposed to water. Such a plane-to-plane orientation is called stacking interaction. The purine-pyrimidine hydrogen bonded base pairs in DNA molecule undergo stacking interactions with adjacent pairs.

Small molecule - small molecule complex: When the two interactants involved in the formation of complex are of small sizes, the complex is termed as small molecule - small molecule complex. There are many examples of this type. Butesin picrate is a small molecule small molecule complex. Many drug complexes such as benzocaine - caffeine, salicylamide - caffeine are also of this type.

Small molecule macromolecule complex: Polymer-drug complexes constitute this type of complex. Polymers such as sodium carboxy methyl cellulose and povidone being macromolecules form complexes with various drugs. Crosspovidone, a cross linked insoluble povidone interact with drugs such as acetaminophen, benzocaine, benzoic acid etc. Polymer-drug complexes are used to modify biopharmaceutical parameters of drugs and hence are used in sustained action dosage forms. Complexation may provide slow sustained release of drugs from membrane encapsulated devices. The forces involved in the formation may be mainly the dipole-dipole and hydrogen bonding.

Drug - serum protein complexes: They are discussed under protein binding. Some examples may be cited here and may be protein warfarin, protein-phenytoin, protein-tetracyline complexes.

Drug - receptor complex: Many drugs act by combining with some key substance called receptor in the biological system to elicit pharmacological effect. The drug-receptor interaction is mainly due to complex formation. The receptor is considered mostly to be a cellular constituent. In few instances it may be extra-cellular.

Antigen antibody complex: Antigens are a group of proteins which are toxic to biological system. Antibodies are also a group of proteins used to nullify the effects of antigen. Antigen-antibody reaction is specific-that is, antibody with a specific chemical affinity and stearic requirements only can react with antigen. Antigen-antibody reaction is a typical complex formation.

Self associated aggregates: Self associated aggregates are formed because of self association of molecules of same species. This type of complex is exemplified by a hydrogen bonded dimer of acetic acid which can exist in the vapour phase and in inert solvents. Benzene also forms dimers in aqueous solutions; Benzene-benzene complex (a dimer) may undergo hydrophobic stacking interactions in water. A Micelle is an aggregated complex. In this surfactant is the interactant. A surfactant molecule has both a polar and a non-polar portions. In water above a concentration called critical micellar concentration, the surfactant molecules form micelles which may be considered as a complex. (Refer under colloids for more details.)

2.3 Inclusion complexes (No bond complexes)

Inclusion complexes comprise mono-molecular inclusion compound, macromolecular inclusion compound, clathrates, channel lattice complexes and layer type complexes.

2.3.1 Monomolecular complexes: These are formed when a macrocyclic compound with an intermolecular cavity of molecule dimension interacts with a small molecule that can have access into the cavity i.e. this complexation involves the entrapment of a guest molecule into the cage like structure of a simple host molecule. These complexes or compounds are characterised by lack of adhesive forces between the components of the complex.

Cyclodextins are macrocyclic hosts which can take in guest molecules such as benzocaine, mitomycin-c etc within their cavities. It should be pointed at this juncture that some drugs may be too large to be taken totally into the cavity. For example mitomycin-C (in γ-cyclodextrin) and indomethacin (in β-cyclodextrin) are only partly accommodated in the cavities.

Cyclodextrins consist of α-D glucose joined with glycosidic linkages. The three commercially available cyclodextrins are α-, β- and γ-cyclodextrins (cyclohexa-amylose, cycloheptaamylose and cyclo-octa-amylose respectively). β-cyclodextrin can take up a single molecule of tamotidine or tolbutamide to form inclusion complex.

Cyclodextrin may improve the organoleptic characteristics of oral liquid formulations by entrapping the drug (the guest molecule) which is bitter in taste within the cavity of the cyclodextrin and then formulating the complex thus formed into oral liquid formulation. For example, the bitter taste of femoxetine is greatly suppressed by formulating the β-cyclodextrin femoxetine inclusion complex as a suspension.

2.3.2 Macromolecular complexes They are also called as molecular sieves. In this the atoms of a macromolecule are arranged in three dimensions to provide cages and channels and the guest molecules can be entrapped within. Synthetic zeolites, dextrins and silica gels are examples of macromolecular inclusion compounds.

Clathrates This is a special type of inclusion complex wherein the host molecules form a crystal lattice containing cavities into which guest molecules can fit. The crystal lattice is a cage like structure and is formed by the combination of several molecules of the host compound. The entrapped guest molecule may be a solid, liquid or gas. In this complex, the stoichiometry is not integral.

Clathrates are usually prepared by crystallisation of the host compound from a solution of guest compound. The host compound crystallises in a cage like structure entrapping within the guest molecule. For example hydroquinone crystallises in a cage like hydrogen bonded structure with holes of diameter 4.2 Å. This permits the entrapment of small molecules such as HCl, CH_3OH and CO_2.

Warfarin sodium USP is a clathrate of water, isopropyl alcohol, and sodium warfarin. It occurs as white crystalline powder.

"Gas" hydrates are also examples of clathrates. In this structure, a hydrogen-bonded network of water molecules encloses gaseous small molecules such as argon, methane and nitrogen (eg: $4CH_3 \cdot 23H_2O$).

The entrapped compound may be released by dissolving, heating or grinding the clathrates.

The stability of clathrates is due to the strength of the structure.

Channel lattice complexes These are inclusion complexes in which the host component crystallises in a channel like structure into which the guest molecule can fit. The guest molecule should be of a shape that fits into the channel

Deoxycholeic acid can take up paraffins, organic acids, esters, ketones and aromatic compounds into its channel like structure. Urea ($NH_2 \cdot CO \cdot NH_2$) forms channel clathrates and can take up long chain molecules. Starch-iodine solution is also a channel type complex.

Layer type complexes These are complexes in which the incalant or guest molecule is trapped between the layers of host lattices. For example, montmorillonite (a principle constituent of bentonite) can take up or intercalate the guest molecules between their layers. Montmorillonite can trap hydrocarbons, alcohols and glycols.

2.4. Applications of inclusion compounds

Hydroquinone can clathrate inert gases such as krypton 85 (a radioactive) making it possible to handle gases easily. Synthetic metal alumino-silicates (molecular sieves) can be used to store gaseous, volatile and toxic materials. The molecular sieves can also be used to dry gases and to separate gaseous mixtures. It is possible to load the molecular sieves with substances such as volatile oils, germicidal agents, detergents, and pesticides providing for a convenient dry material. Synthetic zeolites may be made to a desired pore size so as to separate molecules of different dimensions.

Channel lattice complexes provide a means of separation of petroleum products. The starch-iodine colour has been shown due to a channel type complex consisting of iodine molecules within the spirals of starch molecule. Monsostearin, an interfering substance in the assay of *dienestrol* can be removed easily from dermatologic creams by channel-type inclusion in urea.

Inclusion complexes can be used to prevent oxidation (vitamin A can be protected from oxygen by including in cyclodextin). Cyclodextrins have been used to entrap, stabilize and solubilize sulfonamides, tetracyclines, testosterone.

Cyclodextrins are of recent interest in forming inclusion compounds. They are cyclic oligosacchardies containing a minimum of six D-(+)-glucopyranose units attached by $\alpha - 1,4$ linkages produced by the action of *Bacillus macerans* amylase on starch.

The natural α, β, γ cyclodextrins consists of 6, 7 and 8 units of glucose respectively. They show a structure of torus or doughnut ring (truncated cone) as shown in Fig 175.

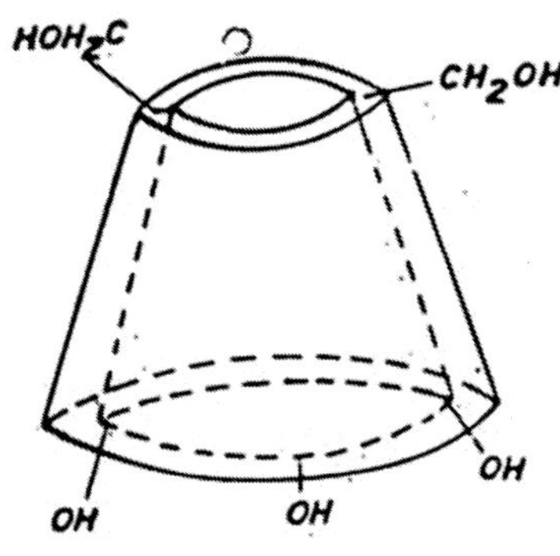

Fig. 175

The interior of the cavity is relatively hydrophobic because of the CH_2 groups whereas the entrances are hydrophilic owing to the presence of hydroxyl groups. The internal diameters are 5Å, 6Å, and 8Å for α, β, and γ forms of cyclodextrins respectively and of which β and γ are more useful because of larger diameters. Molecules of appropriate size and steriochemistry will get included in the cyclodextrin cavity by hydrophobic interaction by squeezing out water from the cavity. a) This type of trapping is found to stabilize and solubilize sulfonamides, tetracyclines, morphine, aspirin, benzocaine, ephedrine, reserpine, testosterone and retinoic acid b) The dissolution rate of famotidine (an antigastric ulceration drug) and tolbutamide (oral antidiabetic drug) are increased when complexed with β-cyclodextrins c) Cyclodextrin may increase or decrease the reactivity of guest molecules depending upon the orientation within the molecule d) β-cyclodextrins show poor water solubility (due to intramolecular hydrogen bonding) and nephro-toxicity when given parenterally. Hence derivates of natural cyclodextrins have been developed to improve aqueous solubility and to avoid nephrotoxicity. Partial methylation of some of the -OH groups is used to achieve this. Amorphous derivatives are more effective solubilising agents than parent cyclodextrins for sex hormones e) Complex forms of drugs (testosterone) are absorbed more when given sublingually f) Hydrophobic forms of β-cyclodextrins such as ethylated derivative form of complexes with drugs act as sustained action products. (eg. a calcium antagonist diltiazem and a vasodilator isosorbide dinitrate) f) Complexation with cyclodextrin mask the bitter taste of oral formulations (eg. an antidepressant femoxetine).

Prostoglandins yield insoluble inclusion compounds which may be dried and used in suspension, tablets and suppositories. Clathrates have been used to separate optical isomers. For example, *dl*-terpineol has been resolved by the use of digitonin.

2.5 Applications of Complexes

In general, the application of complexes may be summarised as below

1. Pharmaceutical properties affected by complexation.

Complex	Increased property
Aspirin - caffeine	solubility
Phenobarbital-cyclodextrin	dissolution rate
Benzoic acid - caffeine	partition coefficient
Prednisolone - dialkylamides	permeatribity
Salicytates - caffeine	Absorption rate
Digoxin - cyclodextrin	bioavailability
Indomethacin - cyclodextin	biological activity
vitamin A - cyclodextrin	(solid state) stability
Benzocaine - caffeine	chemical stability
Iodine - PVP	volatility reduction
Nitroglycerin - cyclodextrin	physical state
Resin-drug complex and polymer drug complex	Sustained action dosage torm.

2. In liquid dosage forms, heavy metals catalyse oxidation of drugs. These metals are complexed with EDTA to make them catalytically inactive.

3. In shampoos, EDTA is used to complex divalent metals in hard water so that shampoos will give more lather (or foam) during bathing. It is also used to remove kidney stones (calcium salt stones) in which EDTA sequesters calcium ions and dissolves the stones.

4. To the pharmaceutical investigator, the main concern is how the complex affects the safety, stability and therapeutic efficacy of a product. Sometimes drugs may have adverse effects due to complexation. To cite an example, the parabens (used as preservatives) may be inactivated due to complexation with non-ionic surfactant such as polysorbate 80.

5. For the determination of metals. Complexometric or chelatometric titrations are useful. Titration of a divalent or trivalent metal ions with a solution of EDTA gives an end point which is the result of 1:1 stoichiometry between metal ion and multidentate EDTA tetra anion. The end point is detected potentiometrically using ion selective membrane electrodes or with metallo-chromic indicators (solochrome T, or erythrochrome T)

   Very low concentrations of metals can be determined colorimetrically by complexation with a ligand. For example, determination of ferric ions by complexation with 1,10-phenanthroline and the complex has absorption in the visible range of light and determination of mercuric ions by complexation with diphenylthiocarbazone (i.e dithizone)

   Certain metals are analysed gravimetrically after precipitation with a ligand. (Nickel forms an insoluble complex with 8 - hydroxyquionline.

6. In ion-pair chromatographic technique: An amine sample in its cation form is complexed with a hydrophobic anion (Ex: Alkyl sulfonate, RSO_3^-) and reverse phase

liquid chromatography is performed.

In reverse phase liquid chromatography, mobile phase is aqueous (i.e polar) and the stationary phase is non-polar. The amine complex (ion-pair) with its hydrophobic counter ion can now partition between the two phases.

7. Affinity chromatography: There is a specific interaction between migrating solutes and a ligand which is chemically bonded to the stationary phase. For example, in the isolation of enzymes, a column is prepared with an inhibitor of the enzyme (ligand) and when the sample mixture is passed through the column, the enzyme inhibitor complexes the enzyme from the mixture. which is then subsequently eluted

8. Chiral chromatography: It is used to separate optical isomers based on interaction between isomers and a stationary phase that possesses chiral binding sites. For example, covalently bound cyclodextrins, a stationary phase, is used in chiral separations.

9. Complexes with metals occur in biological systems. Ex: haemoglobin (iron), cytochrome (iron), carbooxypetidase.A (zinc), carbonic anhydrase (zinc), vitamin B_{12} (cobalt) chlorophyll (magnesium) etc.

   DNA base pairing is also a complex. Charge transfer interactions play a role in physiological processes. Numerous antimicrobial and anti-neoplastic agents (planar in nature) exerts their action by complexing with DNA base pairs that is by intercalation between planar base pair assemblies in DNA double complex. Drugs such as quinicine, proflavin, adiamycin and actinomycin D can be intercalated.

10. Many metal ion poisoning can be treated by agents that form strong co-ordination complexes. i.e chelates. These complexes are easily excreted and thus it aids in the excretion of the metal ion (chelation therapy) This chelation therapy is applied in ion, copper, lead, cobalt, nickel, mercury and zinc poisoning. The chelating agents used for the purpose are EDTA, dimercaprol (BAL) and D. penicillamine.

11. Polymerisation: Metal olefin complexes (platinum olefin complex, silver olefin complex) are considered to enter into the polymerisation of ethylene and propylene to form poly .ethylene and polypropylene

3. Methods of Analysis

Complexes are analysed for

i) stoichiometric ratio of ligand to metal (or donor to acceptor ratio) and

ii) stability constant of the complex

The various methods are

3.1. Job's method of continuous variation.

Additive properties such as spectrophotometric extinction coefficient., dielectric constant or square of the refractive index are used in this method.

By using dielectric constant: Solutions of two species A and B are prepared such that each solution has equal molar concentration with the other solution. It means that the first solution contains only A and for which the mole fraction of B is zero. The

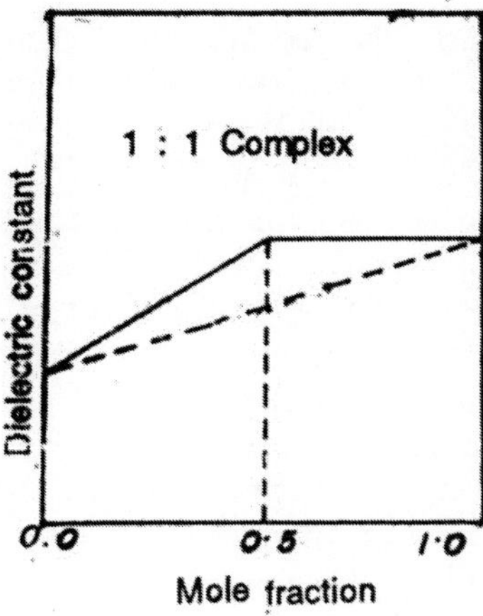

Fig. 176. Ligand-acceptor ratio

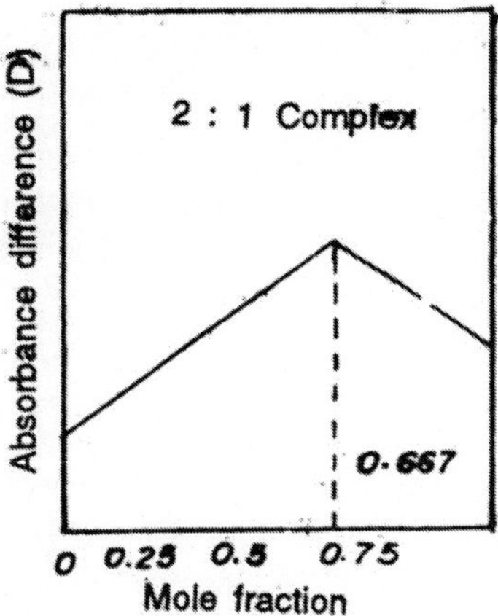

Fig. 177. Ligand-acceptor ratio

second solution contains A and B in the mole fractions of 0.9 and 0.1 (total 1) respectively and the remaining solutions of A and B are in the mole fractions of 0.8 and 0.2; 0.7 and 0.3; 0.6 and 0.4; 0.5 and 0.5; 0.4 and 0.6; 0.3 and 0.7; 0.2 and 0.8; 0.1 and 0.9 and 0.0 and 1.0 respectively. The dielectric constants of these solutions are found out. (Refer under introduction) Then the values of these dielectric constants are plotted against the mole fractions of 0 to 1 for one of the components in the mixture (Fig. 176). If it produces a straight line as indicated by the dotted line, it indicates no complexation has resulted. On the other hand, if the curve shows a maximum (or minimum) as shown in the figure by the continuous line, it indicates complexation between A and B has occurred. The complex is at its greatest concentration at a point where the species A and B are combined in the ratio in which they occur in the complex. As the change in slope occurs at a mole fraction of 0.5, it indicates that ligand metal ratio is 1:1.

By using absorbance: Solutions of two species A and B are prepared as described above under dielectric constant method so that each resulting solution has equal molar concentration. The absorbance of each solution is found out in a spectrophotometer. The observed values are subtracted from the corresponding values that would have been expected had no complex resulted (theoretical value). A zero difference indicates no complexation. If there is a difference, plot the difference in absorbance obtained from each corresponding solution against mole fractions of one of the components either A or B. (fig 177) From the maximum of the curve, the molar ratio of the complex can be read. In this case as shown in the figure the ratio is 2:1

The equation for complexation between a metal (M) and a ligand (L) may be written as

$$M + nL = ML_n \qquad \text{... (1)}$$

The stability constant is

$$K = \frac{[ML_n]}{[M]\,[L]^n} \qquad \text{... (2)}$$

Taking logarithm,

$$\log[ML_n] = \log K + \log [M] + n \log[L]$$

where $[ML_n]$ = concentration of the complex

$[M]$ = concentration of uncomplex metal

[L] = concentration of uncomplexed ligand

n = number of moles of ligand combined with one mole of metal

K = equilibrium constant or stability constant

Keeping the concentration of metal ion constant, the concentration of the ligand is varied and the corresponding concentration $[ML_n]$ of the complex formed is obtained by spectroscopic analysis. When the log $[ML_n]$ is plotted against log [L], the slope of the line yields the stoichiometric ratio (number 'n' of ligand molecules co-ordinated with one metal ion) and the intercept on the ordinate the stability constant since [M] is a known quantity.

3.2. pH titration Method

This method is applicable when there is a change in pH during complexation. For example, the formation of copper-glycine is attended by a change in pH.

In this method, a solution of glycine is titrated against standard sodium hydroxide solution potentiometrically. A titration curve is obtained by plotting the pH against the equivalents of the base in ml added. Fig 178 Then, a solution of glycine and copper salt is separately titrated against standard sodium hydroxide (In this, the complexation is attended by a decrease in pH). Again a titration curve is obtained by plotting the pH against the equivalents of the base (NaOH) in ml added to the copper-glycine mixture on the same graph paper.

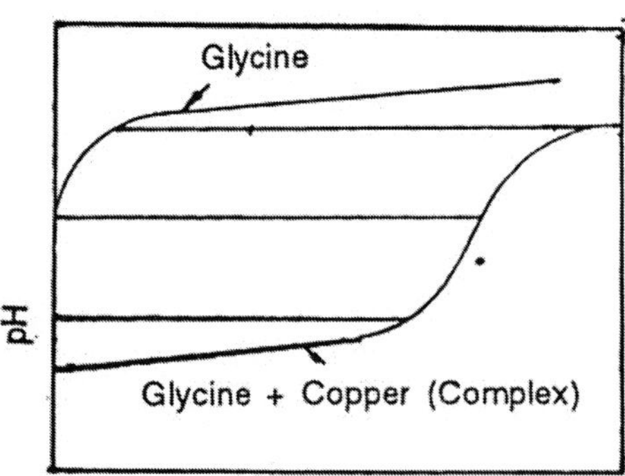

Fig. 178: pH Titration method

The complexation may be represented as

$$Cu^2 + 2NH^+{}_3\,CH_2\,COO^-$$

$$= Cu\,(NH_2\,CH_2\,COO)_2 + 2H^\cdot$$

The step wise equilibria between the metal M and glycine (i.e ligand) L may be given as

$$M + L = ML$$

$$K_1 = \frac{[ML]}{[M]\,[L]} \quad \text{... (3)}$$

$$ML + L = ML_2$$

$$K_2 = \frac{[ML_2]}{[ML]\,[L]} \quad \text{... (4)}$$

The overall reaction is

$$M + 2L = ML_2$$

$$\beta = K_1\,K_2 = \frac{[ML_2]}{[M]\,[L]^2} \quad \text{... (5)}$$

where K_1 and K_2 are called as *formation constants* for the first and subsequent steps whereas the equilibrium constant β for the overall reaction ($K_1 \times K_2$) is known as the *stability constant*

The average number of ligand groups (glycine) bound per metal ion is designated as $\overline{n}$ and is given by

$$\overline{n} = \frac{\text{total concentration of ligand bound}}{\text{total concentration of metal ion (both bound and unbound)}}$$

$$\text{or } \bar{n} = \frac{[ML] + 2[ML_2]}{[M] + [ML] + [ML_2]} \quad \ldots (6)$$

The term $[ML_2]$ in the numerator is multiplied by 2 to indicate that each **molecule of ML_2** contains 2 molecules of **the ligand. The** total concentration of **the metal ion** refers to both and bound **and unbound** metal ion concentrations.

If $\bar{n} = 1$, the equation is

$$\frac{[ML] + 2[ML_2]}{[M] + [ML] + [ML_2]} = 1$$

$$\text{or } [ML] + 2[ML_2] = [M] + [ML] + [ML_2]$$

$$[ML] + 2[ML_2] - [ML] - [ML_2] = [M]$$

$$[ML_2] = [M]$$

$$\text{Then } \beta = K_1 K_2 = \frac{[ML_2]}{[M]\,[L]^2}$$

$$= \frac{[M]}{[M]\,[L]^2}$$

$$(\text{since } [ML_2] = [M])$$

$$= \frac{1}{[L]^2} \quad \ldots (7)$$

$$\log \beta = -2\log[L] \quad \ldots (8)$$

$$\text{or } \frac{1}{2}\log \beta = P^{[L]} \text{ at } \bar{n} = 1$$

where $p[L] = -\log[L]$

It has been shown that

$$p[L] = \log K_1 \text{ at } \bar{n} = \frac{1}{2} \quad \ldots (9)$$

$$p[L] = \log K_2 \text{ at } \bar{n} = \frac{3}{2} \quad \ldots (10)$$

Therefore, the individual complex formation constants K_1 and K_2 and the overall stability constant β can be obtained if $\bar{n}$ and p[L] are known.

In order to obtain the value of $\bar{n}$, the concentration of ligand bound and the total concentration of metal ion should be known. The total concentration of metal ion is a known quantity since a known quantity is used. The total concentration of ligand bound is the quantity of alkali which is obtained from the horizontal distance represented by the line between the titration curve for glycine alone and for glycine - copper mixture at any pH. From these two values $\bar{n}$ can be obtained.

The other value needed is the concentration of free glycine i.e [L] at any pH. This may be obtained from the dissociation expression for glycine.

$$\text{i.e. } NH^+{}_3\,CH_2\,COO^- + H_2O = H_3O^+ + NH_2\,CH_2\,COO^-$$

$$Ka = \frac{[H_3O^+]\,[NH_2\,CH_2\,COO^-]}{[NH^{+}{}_3\,CH_2\,COO^-]}$$

$$\text{or } [NH_2\,CH_2\,COO^-] = [L]$$

$$= \frac{Ka[NH^{+}{}_3\,CH_2\,COO^-]}{[H_3O^+]}$$

$[NH^+{}_3\,CH_2\,COO^-]$ at any pH is taken as the difference between the initial concentration of glycine (i.e. $NH^+{}_3\,CH_2\,COO^-$ initial) and the concentration of alkali [NaOH] added.

$$[L] = Ka\frac{([NH^+{}_3\,CH_2\,COO^-]_{initial} - [NaOH])}{[H_3O^+]}$$

or,

$$\log[L] = \text{loga } Ka - \log [H_3O^+]$$

$$+ \log\left(NH^+{}_3\,CH_2\,COO^-]_{initial} - [NaOH] \right)$$

Reversing the sign

$$-\log[L] = -\log Ka + \log [H_3O^+]$$

$$- \log\left([NH^{+}{}_3\,CH_2\,COO^-]_{initial} - [NaOH] \right)$$

where [L] is the concentration of the free ligand, glycine.

The value of $\bar{n}$ against p[L] at various pH values are then plotted Fig 179. The curve that is obtained is the formation curve for glycine copper complex, it is seen to reach a limit at

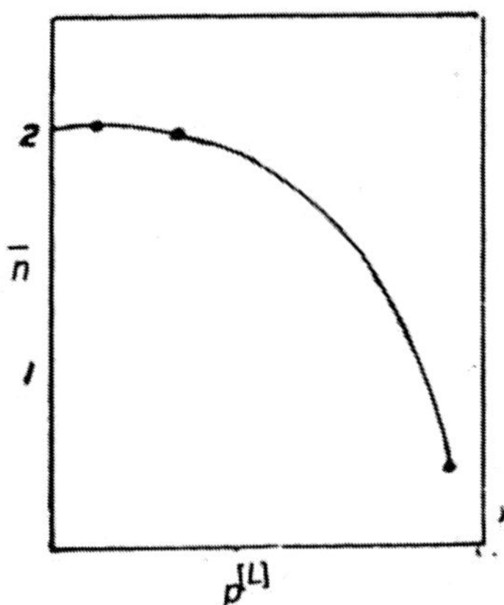

Fig. 179

$\bar{n} = 2$. This 2 indicates **the maximum** number of glycine molecules that can combine with one atom of copper.

From this curve at $\bar{n} = \frac{1}{2}$, at $\bar{n} = \frac{3}{2}$ and at $\bar{n} = 1.0$, the approximate values for $\log K_i$, $\log K_2$ and $\log \beta$ respectively are obtained.

3.3. Distribution Method

The stability constant for the complex formed as a result of interaction between iodine and potassium iodide can be determined by distribution method.

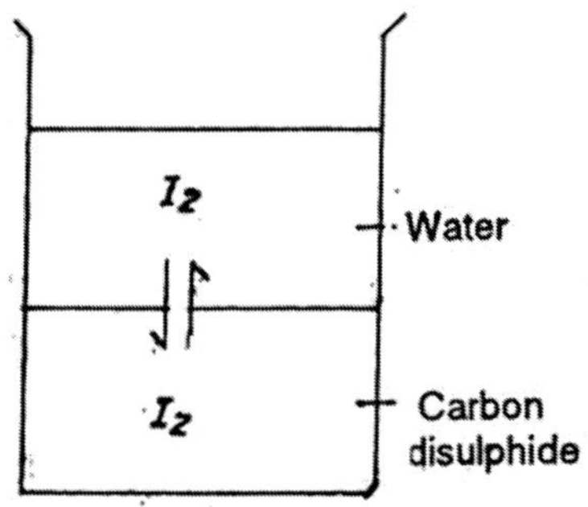

Fig. 180. Distribution Method

First, the iodine is added to an immiscible system containing carbon tetrachloride and water. Fig 180. The distribution coefficient is given by

$$K = \frac{[I]_o}{[I]_w} \quad \text{... (11)}$$

where K = distribution coefficient

$[I]_0$ = concentration of iodine in organic phase i.e. carbon tetrachloride.

$[I]_w$ = concentration of iodine in aqueous phase.

Iodine is, then, added to an immiscible system containing carbon-tetra chloride and an aqueous solution of potassium iodide so that iodine gets distributed between these two phases. After the equilibrium has been achieved and assuming a simple complex formation at lower concentration.

$$I_2 + I^-{}_3 \text{ (i.e. } I_2 + KL = KI_3)$$

the concentration of the free and total iodine (i.e. complexed and uncomplexed) and also that of potassium iodide in the aqueous phase (KI is insoluble in carbon tetra chloride) are determined. The species common to both phases is the free iodine and this is obtained from the distribution law. A chemical analysis yields the concentration of free and complexed iodine in the aqueous phase.

The concentration of the complexed iodine in the aqueous phase is given by

$$[I_2]_{\text{complexed}} = [I_2]_{\text{aq.total}} - [I_2]_{\text{aq.free}}$$

According to the equation $I_2 + I^- = I_3$ iodine and potassium iodide combine in equimolar concentrations to form the simple complex. Therefore,

$$[KI]_{\text{complexed}} = [I_2]_{\text{complexed}}$$

The concentration of free KI is

$$[KI]_{\text{free}} = [KI]_{\text{total}} - [KI]_{\text{complexed}}$$

The stability constant is now given by

$$K = \frac{[\text{complex}]}{[I_2]_{\text{free}}\,[KI]_{\text{free}}}$$

Stability constants for the complexes formed between a number of acidic drugs such as benzoic acid, salicylic acid and acetyl salicylic acid with caffeine, polyvinylpyrrolidone, and polyethylenegylcols have been investigated using the distribution method.

3.4. Solubility metnod

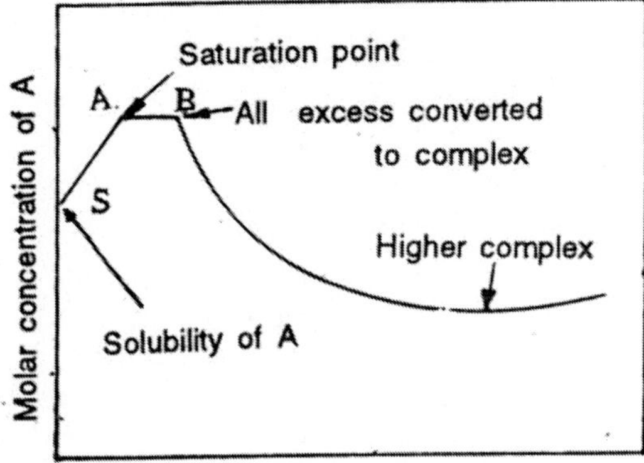

Fig. 181: Solubility Method

In this method, various concentrations of a complexing agent in aqueous vehicle is taken in well stoppered containers. To each of the containers, an excess quantity of drug is added. The containers are placed in a constant temperature bath and are agitated then and there until the equilibrium is attained. After the equilibrium has been achieved, aliquot portion of the supernatant liquid is removed and analysed.

The results are plotted as shown in Fig. 181.

S on the ordinate indicates the solubility of the drug. The solubility increases for the drug as the complexing agent is added due to complexation. The curve raises from S to A. At the point A, the solution is saturated with respect to both the drug and the complex. As the addition of the compexing agent is continued, the complex continues to form and the precipitate from the already saturated solution. The point B indicates that all the excess drug has been used up for complexation. On further addition of complexing agent, one or more secondary complexes are formed and that is indicated in the graph.

The stoichiometry of the interaction can be determined from the curve. The amount of drug entering into the complex from the point A to B is given by the difference between the total amount of drug added and the amount of drug in solution at point A. The amount of complexing agent can be read directly from the abscissa and is equal to

$$\frac{\text{moles of drug in complex}}{\text{moles of complexing agent in complex}}$$

If the ratio is 1, the complexing reaction may be written as

$$D + C = DC$$

and the stability constant is

$$K = \frac{[DC]}{[D]\,[C]} \quad \text{... (12)}$$

where [DC] = total drug in solution at point A less solubility of the uncomplexed drug (S).

[D] = solubility of the uncomplexed drug.

[C] = the concentration of complexing agent added to the system at point A less the amount of complexing agent in the drug complex [DC].

The stability constants for a number of caffeine complexes have been obtained by the solubility method and are available in literature.

3.5. Spectroscopy

The study of donor acceptor or charge transfer complexes can be undertaken with absorption spectroscopy in the visible and ultraviolet regions of the spectrum.

The stability constant k, may be obtained from the reaction between donor D and acceptor A

$$D + A \underset{k_2}{\overset{k_1}{\rightleftharpoons}} DA \quad \text{... (13)}$$

where $k = \frac{k_1}{k_2}$ is the equilibrium constant or stability constant of complex.

k_1 and $k_2 =$ interaction rate constants.

When two molecules (i.e. one molecule of donor and one molecule of accepter) associate to form a charge transfer complex and if the absorbance 'a' is measured at a definite wavelength, the stability constant of complex k is obtained from the Benesi - Hilderbrand equation

$$\frac{A_0}{a} = \frac{1}{\varepsilon} + \frac{1}{k, \varepsilon} \cdot \frac{1}{D_0} \quad \text{... (13)}$$

Where $A_0 =$ initial concentration of acceptor

$D_0 =$ initial concentration of donor

$\varepsilon =$ molar absorptivity at a particular wavelength

$k =$ stability constant of complex

$a =$ absorbance of the complex

Stability constant can be obtained from the slope of the line obtained by plotting $\frac{A_0}{a}$ versus $1/D_0$

Spectroscopy method has been used for investigating the interaction of nucleic acid bases (electron acceptors) with catechol, epinephrine and isoproterenol (electron donors)

The other methods used for studying the complexation include NMR and IR spectroscopy, polarography, circular dichroism, kinetics, X-ray diffraction and electron diffraction.

4. Protein binding

Protein binding refers to complex formation between small molecules (drug molecules) and blood proteins such as albumins and globulins.

Of all the constituents of blood that might take part in the formation of complexes with drugs, the most important and most studied is the protein serum albumin. The concentration of this normal human serum albumin (HSA) is remarkably high in the blood. The concentration may vary from 3.5 to 4.5 g/100 ml. This variance is due to age, exercise, stress, and disease. It consists of 5875 amino acid resudes. This albumin molecule appears to be flexible and is able to adapt its shape to fit the molecular shape of the ligand (drug ligand) binding to it. The principal binding force for complexation is hydrophobic interaction *which is explained latter in this chapter.* Hydrophobic compounds such as long chain fatty acids are found to be avidly bound to HSA. The extent of order of binding of drugs to various plasma proteins is albumin, α_1 acid glycoprotein, lipoprotein, globulins.

The study of protein binding is aimed at knowing the maximum number of small molecules which could be bound per protein molecule, the magnitude of association constant or constants, the chemical and conformational nature of this binding sites on the proteins and the nature and intermolecular forces involved in the complex formation. The other studies relate to action and uses of specific drugs due to protein binding. Thus, the binding of drugs to proteins in the body influences their actions and may

1. decrease the distribution of drugs by reducing concentration of free form of the drug.
2. inactivate a drug by reducing the concentration of free form of the drug needed for action.
3. retard the excretion of a drug since only the free form of the drug is excreted.
4. alter the duration of action of a drug by slowly releasing the free form of drug.

A protein molecule is a macromolecule composed of many hundreds of aminoacids linked together. The functional groups present in the side chains of the aminoacids provide sites for binding small molecules (i.e drug molecules). A macromolecule (protein) may have many and varied binding sites. These sites can be divided into different classes with different binding abilities. However sites within a class possess the same binding ability.

Binding is a function of the affinity of the protein molecule for the drug molecules and also the concentration of drugs and proteins. The interaction between protein (P) and drug (D) for a simple case of 1:1 protein drug complex can be represented as follows:

$$P + D \rightleftharpoons PD$$

Applying the law of mass action, the expression is

$$K = \frac{[PD]}{[P]\,[D]} \qquad \text{... (14)}$$

or, $[PD] = K[P]\,[D]$

where K = association constant

$[P]$ = concentration of unbound protein

$[C]$ = concentration of unbound drug

$[PD]$ = concentration of protein drug complex

Expressing the total protein concentration as $[P_t]$, we can write,

$$[P_t] = [P] + [PD]$$

or $[P] = [P_t] - [PD]$

substituting for [P],

$$[PD] = K[D]\left([P_t] - [PD]\right)$$

$$[PD] = [K[D][P_t]] - K\,[D]\,[PD]$$

or $[PD] + K[D][PD] = K[D][P_t]$

$$[PD](1 + K\,[D] = K[D]\,[P_t]$$

$$\text{or } \frac{[PD]}{P_t} = \frac{K\,[D]}{1 + K[D]} \qquad \text{... (15)}$$

$\frac{[PD]}{[P_t]}$ represent the average number of drug molecules bound per mole of protein $[p_t]$. Replacing $[PD]/[P_t]$ by r, we can write,

$$r = \frac{K[D]}{1 + K[D]} \qquad \text{... (16)}$$

If two independent and equivalent sites belonging to some particular class are considered, the approximate equation is

$$r = \frac{2K[D]}{1 + K\,[D]} \qquad \text{... (17)}$$

and for 'v' equivalent and independent sites, the equation is given as

$$r = \frac{v\,K[D]}{1 + K\,[D]} \qquad \text{... (18)}$$

where v = number of sites in a class of proteins

K = intrinsic association constant.

The above equation can be inverted for convenient plotting, Thus, inverting the equation, we get

$$\frac{1}{r} = \frac{1 + K[D]}{\upsilon K[D]}$$

$$\frac{1}{r} = \frac{1}{\upsilon K[D]} + \frac{1}{\upsilon}$$

$$\frac{1}{r} = \frac{1}{\upsilon K}\frac{1}{[D]} + \frac{1}{\upsilon} \quad \text{... (19)}$$

This equation is similar to Langmuir equation for adsorption.

The equation (18) can be modified to obtain a plot and is called *Scatchard plot*

$$\text{ie. } r = \frac{\upsilon K[D]}{1 + K[D]}$$

$$r(1 + K[D]) = \upsilon K[D]$$

$$r + rK[D] = \upsilon K[D]$$

$$r = \upsilon K[D] - rK[D]$$

$$= [D](\upsilon K - rK)$$

$$\text{or } \frac{r}{[D]} = \upsilon K - rK \quad \text{... (20)}$$

Graphical representation of data using the equation (19) is useful at low concentrations of free drug D, and at higher concentrations of free drug D, it misrepresents the protein binding behaviour. However equation (20) does not have this disadvantage and is used for plotting the data. The plot obtained using the data in equation (20) is called a *scatchard plot.*

Both these equations (19) and (20) cannot be used, if the nature and the amount of protein in the experimental system is unknown. Under these circumstances, a slightly modified form of the equation (20) is used.

$$\text{ie. } \frac{[D_b]}{[D]} = -[D_b]K + \upsilon K[P_t] \quad \text{... (21)}$$

where D_b is the concentration of the bound drug. The ratio $[D_b/[D]$ is plotted against $[D_b]$ and K is determined from the slope and $vK[P_t]$ is obtained from the intercept.

The *Scatchard plot* yields a straight line when only one class of binding sites is present. For n classes of binding sites, a plot of r/[D] against r (i.e $[PD]/[P_t]$ shows a curvature suggesting more than one class of binding sites. For example, *Scatchard plot* is shown for the binding of bishydroxycoumarin to human serum albumin at 20 ° and 40 ° C in Fig 182.

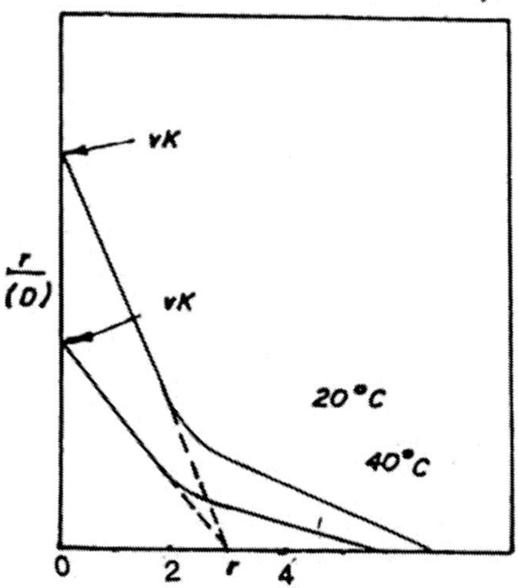

Fig. 182. A Scatchard Plot

The curvatures in both the plots at 20 ° and 40 °C indicate the presence of more than one type of binding sites. Extraploting the straight line portions of the plots at 20 ° and 40 ° C to abscissa, assuming a single class of binding sites without any electrostatic attraction, one can obtain the approximate value for υ number of sites in the single class. In this case, the value of υ is 3 i.e. three independent sites in the single class of binding sites.

A general expression for 'n' classes of sites can be given, designating each class as i and the number of sites as v, as

$$r = \sum_{i=1}^{n-1} \frac{v_i K_i [D]}{1 + K_i [D]} + V_n K_n [D] \quad \text{... (24)}$$

4.1. Experimental methods of determining protein binding.

A number of methods such as equilibrium dialysis, ultrafiltration and electrophoresis are available. The other methods include gel filtration, and nuclear magnetic resonance. The most commonly used technique is the equilibrium dialysis.

In this method, a protein solution is enclosed within a membrane (semi-permeable membrane such as cellophane) which is permeable to small drug molecules and not to macro-molecule, the protein molecules. The protein solution within the membrane is contacted with a solution of drug. The solution is agitated slightly until equilibrium has been achieved. Samples from both sides of the membrane are withdrawn and analysed. If the concentration of the drug within the membrane and outside the membrane (i.e. in the solution with which the membrane is contacted) are same, it indicates no protein binding has occurred. If the concentrations differs, that is, if the concentration within the membrane is more, it indicates protein binding has occurred. (The concentration is increased because both bound and unbound drug are present)

This may be depicted as follows in Fig. 180.

A kinetic method for equilibrium dialysis is called *dynamic dialysis*. This method is based on the rate of disappearance of drug from a dialysis cell.

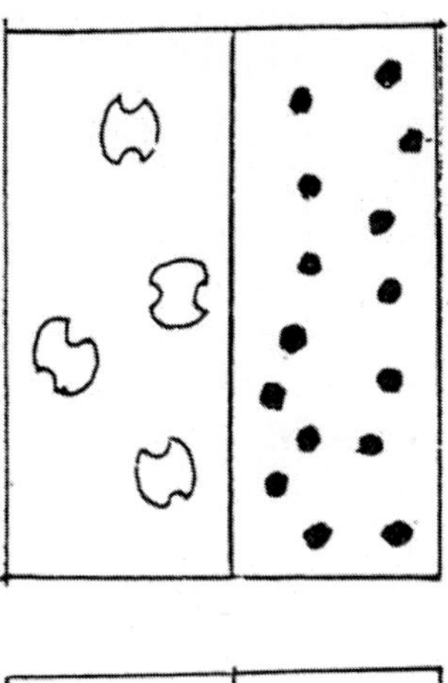

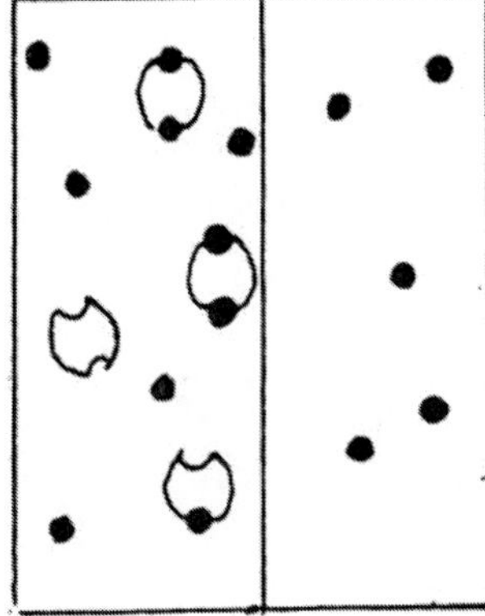

Fig. 183. Equilibrium Dialysis Experiment

This rate of disappearance is proportional to the concentration of unbound drug.

These experimental methods can be used

(a) to know the solubility behaviour of a drug in the presence and absence of protein. This may be used to assess the degree of interaction between various species, solvent, drug and protein.

(b) to study the influence of protein on the partitioning behaviour of drug molecules between an aqueous and an organic solvent that are immiscible.

(c) to study changes in spectral characteristics of drug molecules for assessing the degree of binding.

4.2. Competitive binding

In general, protein bound drug is not pharmacologically active. However this (inactivation) may be reversed by the addition of a competitive inhibitor to the binding system.

Consider the binding of drug (D) with protein (P)

$$P + D \rightleftharpoons PD$$

and also a competitor (C) which competes for the same binding site

$$P + C \rightleftharpoons PC$$

Applying Law of mass action, the equilibrium constant or association constant for the drug and protein is

$$K_D = \frac{[PD]}{[P]\,[D]}$$

and for the competitor and protein,

$$K_C = \frac{[PC]}{[P]\,[C]}$$

Rearranging the equation for [PD] and [PC]

$$[PD] = K_D\,[P]\,[D]$$

$$[PC] = K_C\,[P]\,[C]$$

The average number of drug molecules bound per mole of protein is given as

$$\frac{[PD]}{[P_t]}$$

where [PD] = concentration of protein drug complex

$[P_t]$ = the total protein concentration.

The total protein is actually the sum of [P], the concentration of free protein; [PD] the concentration of protein bound with the drug; and [PC], the concentration of protein bound with the competitor C:

Therefore

$$\frac{[PD]}{[P_t]} = \frac{[PD]}{[P] + [PD] + [PC]}$$

Substituting the values for [PD] and [PC] appearing in the denominators of the equation.

$$\frac{[PD]}{[P_t]} = \frac{[PD]}{[P] + K_D\,[P]\,[D] + K_C\,[P]\,[C]}$$

$$= \frac{[PD]}{[P]\,(1 + K_D\,[D] + K_C\,[C]}$$

$$\frac{[PD]}{[P_t]} = \frac{[K_D\,[D]}{1 + K_D\,[D] + K_C\,[C]}$$

$$\text{since}\ \frac{[PD]}{[P]\,[D]} = K_D \text{ and } \frac{[PD]}{[P]} = K_D\,[D]$$

Replacing $\frac{[PD]}{[P_t]}$ by r_D

$$r_D = \frac{K_D\,[D]}{1 + K_D\,[D] + K_C\,[C]}$$

where r_D = average number of drug molecules per mole of protein

K_D = association constant for the drug protein complex

K_C = association constant for the competitor-protein complex

[D] = concentration of unbound drug

[C] = concentration of unbound competitor.

It has been demonstrated that the antibacterial activity of sulfonamide in the presence of albumin (a protein) is increased markedly by the presence of a displacing agent (i.e competitor) such as phenylbutazone, ethyl biscoumacetate etc. This is because of replacement of sulfonamide from protein sulfonamide complex by the competitor. In the same way protein bound warfarin is displaced by phenyl butazone increasing the prothrombin time markedly. Thus a competitor can compete for the available protein binding sites and it results in an increase in plasma concentration of the displaced drugs. Such an effect may influence the dosage regimen. Normally the competitor show structural resemblance with drug molecules.

4.3. Significance of protein Binding

1. Plasma protein bound drugs are unable to penetrate biological membranes. Hence they cannot be excreted or biotransformed. Only free form of the drug is pharmacologically active.

2. Binding between plasma protein and drug is a reversible interaction. The bound drug acts as a reservoir which releases the drug in the free form to replace the drug which is removed from the body by excretion or biotransformation. This effect prolongs the duration of action of the drug. For example, drugs which are bound in larger proportions strongly to proteins (eq. sulphamethoxydiazine and hydroxocobalamine) get released slowly for the complex with longer $t_{1/2}$ (i.e biological half life) and hence are long acting. Whereas drugs which are bound in smaller proportions less strongly (eg. sulphathiazole and cyanocobalamine) show less duration of action since larger amount of drug in the free form are quickly excreted and metabolished.

3. Protein binding may lead to increase in solubility of certain drugs eg. discoumarol.

4. The pharmacological response to a drug is due the attainment of particular concentration of the drug at the site of action and to its interaction with the receptor site (a typical complexation phenomenon occurs). Such interactions are very specific.

5. Drugs may exhibit competitive binding due to differences in the affinities of the drugs for the binding sites in the protein molecule. Such competitive binding may be advantageous or disadvantageous. For example, displacement of antibiotics by other drugs provides better effect due to the release of free antibiotic for action. But displacement of protein bound anticoagulants may cause excessive bleeding.

   Thus, if any potent drug, which is bound to the extent of 85% to 90%, is displaced by another drug from protein, there will be observable clinical toxicity. The reaction is due to the amount of drug displaced which is more than 10% of the free form of the drug (concentration is more than doubled.)

6. Drugs may interact with other tissues also similar to drug protein binding. For example, very lipid soluble drugs like thiopentone accumulate in the body fat, and tetracyclines in teeth.

7. The concentration of a drug in the plasma is often a measure of drug distribution in the body since the drug distributed in various organs of the body show a dynamic equilibrium. There are exceptions. Chlorpromazine binds to lipoproteins of brain tissue fifty times more than the binding with blood proteins.

8. If a drug protein binding is very high, the concentration of free form of the drug may not be sufficient to elicit pharmacological activity. This can be remedied by giving sufficiently more amount of

drug to provide the required concentration for activity.

9. There are several pharmacological and pharmacokinetics consequences because of drug protein binding. Drugs not only bind to plasma proteins in the blood but also to the constituents of the tissues perfused by the blood supply. If drug binding is more to plasma proteins than to tissues, more drug will be retained in the blood. This affects distribution of the drug and therefore the apparent volume of distribution will be low. If drug binding is more to the tissues than to the plasma proteins, retention of drug in the tissues is more and this affects the distribution of drug. In this case the apparent volume of distribution will be high.

   Protein binding affects drug clearance also. If the excretion ratio for a tissue is high, protein binding has little effect on the clearance. On the other hand, if the excretion ratio for the tissue is small, the clearance depends upon protein binding. In the latter case, only the free drug is cleared. Volume of distribution and elimination rate constant become dose dependent if protein is saturated by the drug. In such a situation, a high loading dose is recommended to saturate the proteins followed by lower maintenance doses.

Recognised prefixes for SI units

Prefix	Symbol	Multiple
Pico	P	10^{-12}
nana	n	10^{-9}
micro	μ	10^{-6}
centi	c	10^{-2}
deci	d	10^{-1}
kilo	k	10^{3}
mega	M	10^{6}
giga	G	10^{9}
tera	T	10^{12}

For example, 1 nanometer = 10^{-9} meter or 10^{-3} milli meter

PHYSICAL CONSTANTS

	cgs units	SI units
Acceleration of gravity, *g*	$980.665 \text{cmsec}^{-2}$	9.80665ms^{-2}
Avagadro's number, *N*	$6.0221 \times 10^{23} \text{mole}^{-1}$	$6.0221 \times 10^{23} \text{mole}^{-1}$
Boltzman constant, *K=R/N*	$1.38066 \times 10^{-16} \text{ergdeg}^{-1} \text{molecule}^{-1}$	$1.38066 \times 10^{-23} \text{JK}^{-1}$
1 calorie (gram calorie)	$4.1840 \times 10^{7} \text{erg}$	4.1840 J
Electronic charge, *e* (electron volt)	$4.8030 \times 10^{-10} \text{esu}$ 1.16022×10^{-20} emu 1.6022×10^{-19} coulombs(C)	$1.6022 \times 10^{-19} \text{C}$
Faraday, *F*	96,485 coulomb Eq^{-1} 23,000 cal $\text{volt}^{-1} \text{Eq}^{-1}$	96,485 C mole^{-1}
Gas constant, *R*	$8.3143 \times 10^{7} \text{erg deg}^{-1} \text{mole}^{-1}$ 1.9872 cal $\text{deg}^{-1} \text{mole}^{-1}$ 0.821 litre atm deg $\text{sec}^{-1} \text{mole}^{-1}$	8.3143 $\text{JK}^{-1} \text{mole}^{-1}$
1 litre atmosphere	24.22 cal	
1 atmosphere	$1.01325 \times 10^{6} \text{dyne cm}^{-2}$ 760 mm Hg = 760 torr	101.325 Nm^{-2}
1 bar	0.987 atm = $10^{6} \text{dyne cm}^{-2}$	100,000 Nm^{-2}
1 kilobar (kbar)	987 atm	10^{8}Nm^{-2}
Planck's constant, *l*	6.6262×10^{-27} erg sec	$6.6262 \times 10^{-34} \text{Js}$
Velocity of light in a vaccum, *c*	$2.99792 \times 10^{10} \text{cm sec}^{-1}$	$2.99792 \times 10^{8} \text{ms}^{-1}$
Volume, ideal gas at STP	22.44 litre mole^{-1}	$22.414 \times 10^{-3} \text{m}^{3} \text{mole}^{-1}$

ln ($\log_e$) = $\log_{10} \times 2.303$

Ice point, 0°C = 273.15°K

Temperature conversion: $°C = \frac{5}{9} - (°F - 32)$

Circle: circumference, $C = 2\pi r = \pi D$

area, $A = \pi r^2 = \left(\frac{1}{4}\pi D^2\right)$

Sphere: area, $A = 4\pi r^2 = \pi D^2$

Volume, $V = \left(\frac{4}{3}\right)\pi r^3 = \left(\frac{1}{6}\right)\pi D^3$

Greek Alphabet

A	α	Alpha	N	ν	Nu
B	β	Beta	Ξ	Ξ	XI
Γ	Γ	Gamma	Γ	ο	Omicron
Δ	Δ	Delta	Π	Π	Pi
E	E	Epsilon	P	ρ	Rho
Z	ζ	Zeta	Σ	Σ	Sigma
H	η	Eta	T	τ	Tau
θ	θ	Theta	Υ	Y	Upsilon
I	ι	Iota	Φ	φ	Phi
K	κ	Kappa	X	χ	Chi
Λ	λ	Lambda	Ψ	Ψ	Psi
M	μ	Mu	Ω	Ω	Omega

Surface tension of some liquids at 20°C in dyne/cm		
Water	...	72.8
Glycerin	...	63.4
Oleic acid	...	32.5
Benzene	...	28.8
Chlorofom	...	27.1
1-Octanol	...	26.5
Carbontetra-chloride	...	26.8

Interfacial tension of some liquids agaisnt water at 20°Cin dynes/cm		
Chloroform	...	32.8
Benzene	...	35.0
Oleic acid	...	15.6
1- Octanol	...	8.51
Carbon tetrachloride	...	45.0

INDEX

REFERENCE MATERIALS

1. Physical Pharmacy by Alfred Martin etal.
2. Cooper and Gunn's Tutorial Pharmacy.
3. Remington's Pharmaceutical sciences.
4. Bentley's Text book of Pharmaceutics.
5. The theory and practice of Industrial Pharmacy by Leon Lachman etal.
6. Text book of Pharmaceutical formulation by B.M. Mithal.
7. Teaching materials developed by authors of this book during their teaching career.

9 789352 300785

Printed at Repro India Ltd.